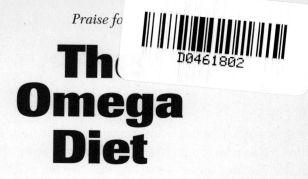

*Praise fo*

# The
# Omega
# Diet

"This is the most solidly based nutritional program currently available. The information is easily understandable, not obscured by technical jargon. And the recipes produce dishes that actually taste good! *The Omega Diet* is a major step forward for readers concerned with their own health."
—S. BOYD EATON, M.D., author of *The Paleolithic Prescription* and clinical associate professor of radiology, Emory University School of Medicine

"I'm not a betting woman, but if I were, I'd put my money on Dr. Artemis Simopoulos as most likely to be remembered as the great nutritional/geneticist breakthrough genius of our age. For those of us 'at sea' between the high-carb diets that may point us toward overweight and diabetes and the high protein/high fat diets that may be anathema to our hearts, here, at last, is good sense and great eating, based on serious science."
—BARBARA SEAMAN, author of *The Doctor's Case Against the Pill*, cofounder National Women's Health Network, and contributing editor *Ms.* magazine

"As a practicing internist and cardiologist, I have found *The Omega Diet* to be a great aid in my daily struggle to improve the health of my patients through nutrition and exercise. This should be required reading for all Primary Care Physicians."
—RICHARD M. DELANY, M.D., F.A.C.C. Medical Specialty Group

# The Omega Diet

The Lifesaving Nutritional
Program Based on the
Diet of the Island of Crete

*Previously published as* The Omega Plan

## Artemis P. Simopoulos, M.D.,
## and Jo Robinson

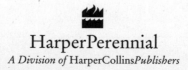

HarperPerennial
*A Division of* HarperCollins*Publishers*

First HarperPerennial edition published 1999.

*Designed by Laura Lindgren*

Library of Congress Cataloging-in-Publication Data

Simopoulos, Artemis P., 1933–
    The omega diet : the lifesaving nutritional program based on the diet of the
Island of Crete / by Artemis P. Simopoulos and Jo Robinson.
       p.    cm.
    Originally published by HarperCollins under the title: The Omega plan.
    Includes bibliographical references and index.
    ISBN 0-06-093023-3
    1. Omega-3 fatty acids—Health aspects. 2. Essential fatty acids in human
nutrition. 3. Nutrition. I. Robinson, Jo, 1947–    . II. Title.
QP752044S56   1999
613.2'84—dc21                98-33990

99 00 01 02 03 ❖/RRD 10 9 8 7 6 5 4 3

To my husband, Alan Lee Pinkerson, M.D., and my daughters, Daphne, Lee, and Alexandra Pinkerson, M.D., whose enthusiasm and support encouraged me to translate the latest nutrition knowledge and concepts into a book for the benefit of the general public

A.P.S.

# Contents

# Acknowledgments

I would like to thank my assistant, Peggy Roberts, whose knowledge, dedication, and discipline contributed enormously in pulling the information together.

My most sincere appreciation and thanks go to the scientists in the field of fatty acids and lipids, particularly those doing research on omega-3 fatty acids in health and disease and in growth and development, and on the ratio of omega-6 to omega-3 fatty acids. My special thanks to the scientists interviewed for the book.

—A.P.S.

My thanks, as always, to Frances Robinson, my unofficial editor, for her support, time, and invaluable insights. Sarah Scott, Michel Ottmar, and Elise Campbell, my research and editorial assistants, helped to assure accuracy, thoroughness, and timely delivery of the manuscript.

Thanks to Joelle Delbourgo, editor-in-chief at HarperCollins, who helped make the book more accessible to the general public without compromising its depth or scientific accuracy. I also wish to thank Richard Pine, our agent, for helping to shape the project at its inception.

Finally, Dr. Simopoulos and I want to acknowledge the many researchers who generously agreed to be interviewed for the book, including Marvin L. Bierenbaum, William E. Connor, Robert T. Dauchy, Joseph R. Hibbeln, S. Roy MacKintosh, Ronald S. Pardini, David P. Rose, Norman Salem Jr., Leonard A. Sauer, Laura J. Stevens, and Lilian U. Thompson. A special thanks to David E. Blask for inviting me into his laboratory and sharing the joy and tribulation of being a research scientist—plus giving me the original insight on fatty acids and cancer that stimulated my interest in this fascinating area of medical research.

—J.R.

# Introduction

In this book, I have the privilege of presenting some lifesaving new discoveries about diet and health. Careful research conducted over the past fifteen years has shown that fat is more than fuel—it is an essential nutrient that influences every aspect of your being from your ability to learn to the beating of your heart. Whether fat enhances or undermines your health depends on its unique blend of "fatty acids," the molecular building blocks of fats and oils. Eating a healthy balance of fatty acids will reduce your risk of a host of diseases, including cardiovascular disease, cancer, diabetes, obesity, arthritis, and asthma. It might even save your life.

In an ideal world, we should not have to know anything about fatty acids in order to eat a healthy diet; we should be able to shop at the local store, buy products that are readily available, and be confident that we are bringing home nutritionally balanced food. But we do not have this luxury. Unwittingly, we have allowed the food industry to make technological changes to our food supply without understanding the biological consequences. The net result is that our diet is so different from the natural human diet, the diet on which our species evolved, that it is at odds with our genetic makeup, increasing our risk of heart disease, cancer, diabetes, obesity, and immune disorders. **The Omega Diet**, the landmark medically proven program featured in this book, restores a healthy balance of essential nutrients to your diet. This simple and delicious program will help every cell and every system in your body function as nature intended.

As fortune would have it, I grew up eating a diet very similar to **The Omega Diet.** I was born in Greece, a country with a 5,000-

year tradition of good nutrition. My mother made a great effort to give us fresh, wholesome food, a task made easier by the fact that we had a large estate that had been in her family for generations. Within the stone walls of the estate were chickens, goats, sheep, and hundreds of trees that gave us olives, pears, figs, plums, and pomegranates. The mild climate allowed fruits and vegetables to grow year round. Given this bounty, everything we ate was impeccably fresh. The eggs that went into the spinach pie had been laid by our hens that very morning. The milk was from the day's first milking. The whole-wheat bread was freshly made, and the olive oil that anointed the bread had been pressed from our own olives. For lunch, we had charcoal-broiled fish that had been swimming in the Mediterranean Sea only the day before. One of my childhood delights was waking up in the morning and hurrying down to breakfast, knowing that I would be greeted by a bowl of ripe fruit. The fruit would be chilled—not because it had come from the refrigerator but because it had been picked before dawn.

Although the food was delicious and bountiful, it was eaten with restraint. As is true in most Greek households, a period of fasting preceded our holidays and feast days. During Lent, for example, we would go for several weeks without eating meat or dairy products. During Easter week, we would even forgo olive oil. It wasn't unusual for adults to lose ten pounds before Easter, a reversal of the American tradition of feasting during the holidays and *then* going on a punishing diet. Exercise was an integral part of our lives. We would walk to market, to school, and to church. In church, everyone would stand except the old people. In school, we had a full hour of physical activity every day. People from the wealthiest families even had personal exercise trainers—decades before the practice became fashionable in the United States.

I was in for a rude shock when I came to the United States in 1949 to study chemistry at Barnard College. To put it bluntly, I found much of the food inedible. I can still remember the first breakfast I ate in the dorm. The only bread available was white bread, which, to me, tasted like cotton. There was one kind of cheese, an intensely orange, bland, and rubbery cheese. The fruit *looked* appetizing, but it had so little flavor that it was hard to believe it was the same kind of fruit that grew in Greece. There were three other Greek students at Barnard, and they viewed the American diet with equal dismay. Eventually, we discovered that white bread tastes better when it's toasted, and that rye crackers are a reasonable stand-in for whole-grain bread.

The stark contrast between the American diet of the 1950s and the traditional Greek diet made such an impression on me that it helped shape my entire medical career. When I went to medical school, I specialized in pediatrics and focused much of my attention on infant and maternal nutrition. I began to realize that many of the children with serious diseases had been malnourished in the womb. This unfortunate start was made worse by the types of food eaten in the home—refined foods, lots of saturated fat and sugar, very few fruits and vegetables, and margarine with its hidden cargo of trans-fatty acids. My first job following my training was directing the newborn nursery at George Washington University, and I saw once again that diet and lifestyle can have dramatic effects on the health of the child. This observation made me interested in the interplay between genetics and nutrition as well. Which types of food were ideally suited for a child's genetic background? How could diet help compensate for genetic defects? I found the answers to many of my questions when I went to study endocrinology and metabolism at the National Institutes of Health (NIH).

In the late 1970s and 1980s, I added another interest—food politics. Medical research alone cannot change what Americans eat. Vital research paid for with taxpayers' money remains locked in the medical journals unless it is communicated to the public and implemented by government policy. To help shape that policy, I chaired the Nutrition Coordinating Committee at the NIH for nine consecutive years and co-chaired the Interagency Committee for Human Nutrition Research at the Office of Science and Technology Policy at the White House for five years. These committees influenced nutrition and food policy throughout the federal government.

While chairing the committees, I became aware of a number of new findings about essential fatty acids and, in 1985, helped organize the first international conference devoted exclusively to this topic. Following the conference, my colleagues and I wrote a comprehensive research program focusing on essential fatty acids that was adopted by ten separate institutes of the NIH.

One of the most important findings to come out of the research program is that our bodies function most efficiently when we eat fats that contain a balanced ratio of the two families of essential fatty acids—omega-6 and omega-3 fatty acids. The ratio in the typical American diet has been estimated to be as high as 20 to 1. One of the few diets in the world to have a balanced ratio of essential fatty acids is the traditional Greek diet. Ironically, I had spent much of my medical career gaining scientific insight into the very diet on which I was raised.

When you follow The Seven Dietary Guidelines of **The Omega Diet**, you will be fueling your body with a ratio of essential fatty acids ideally suited for your metabolism. You will also be enriching your diet with fresh fruit, vegetables, legumes, and oils high in omega-3 fatty acids. A study conducted in the 1990s (the Lyon Diet Heart Study) demonstrated convincingly that this type of diet protects your cardiovascular system more effectively than any other heart diet or drug.

Although this book is focused primarily on diet, I will also be stressing the importance of physical exercise. Regular physical activity enhances your health in many of the same ways as eating the right balance of nutrients. When you combine exercise with a healthy diet, you have what Hippocrates defined as "Positive Health":

> Positive health requires a knowledge of man's primary constitution [what we now call genetics] and of the powers of various foods, both those natural to them and those resulting from human skill [today's processed foods]. But eating alone is not enough for health. There must also be exercise, of which the effects must likewise be known. The combination of these two things makes regimen, when proper attention is given to the season of the year, the changes of the winds, the age of the individual, and the situation of his home. If there is any deficiency in food or exercise, the body will fall sick.

*I have written this book with the hope that it will empower you to make healthier food choices, greatly increasing your chances of enjoying lifelong "positive health."*

# PART 1

# Your Health Is in the Balance

# ONE

# Found:
# The Missing Ingredients
# for Optimal Health

IN RECENT YEARS, medical research has shattered many of our simplistic notions about diet. For example, the popular ideas that "fat makes you fat" and that animal fat is "bad" and vegetable oil is "good" have been overturned by exciting new discoveries about fat that are helping to fight disease and promote optimal health. Similarly, the naïve notion that vitamin supplements can replace fruits and vegetables has given way to a new appreciation for the treasure trove of nutrients these wholesome foods contain, including antioxidants that are not vitamins, folate, and cancer-fighting nutrients called "phytochemicals." This book translates these new findings into a simple, delicious dietary plan that will greatly increase your chances of living a long, lean, and healthy life.

One of the main conclusions to come from the medical labs is that you don't have to give up fat to lose weight or enjoy better health. Most weight-loss diets and so-called healthy diets throw out the good fat with the bad fat, leaving you with dry, lackluster food. Very few people are able to stay on such a diet, resulting in a sense of frustration and failure. **The Omega Diet**, the breakthrough dietary plan featured in this book, replaces harmful fats with beneficial ones, *allowing you to eat from 30 to 35 percent of your calories as fat—absolutely free of guilt!* In fact, I will be urging you to eat more of certain kinds of fat. Yet studies show that you will be healthier on this new, moderate-fat program than if you were to submit yourself to a dreary succession of watery salad dressings, fat-free cheese, rice cakes, steamed vegetables, and skinless chicken breasts poached in broth.

And, no, you won't gain weight. In fact, as you will learn in later chapters, when you combine **The Omega Diet** with a program of regular exercise, you will *increase* your chances of being fit and lean. If you have a substantial amount of weight to lose (ten pounds or more), this book can help you do that as well. Chapter 13 features two weight-loss versions of **The Omega Diet**—a "fast burn" program, and a more moderate weight-loss program. Both contain the same generous percentage of fat as the regular diet. Today, you can start losing up to two pounds a week as you reap all the health benefits of the regular program.

## New Discoveries About Fatty Acids

Our new appraisal of fat comes from studying its molecular building blocks—"fatty acids." When you pour vegetable oil into a measuring cup, it looks like one uniform substance, but on a submicroscopic level, it is composed of six or more different types of fatty acids. New studies show that the individual fatty acids can have remarkably different effects on your health. Some promote cancer growth; some block it. Some increase your risk of heart attack and stroke; some reduce it. Some are more likely to be stored as body fat; others are quickly burned as fuel. Some are linked with depression and other mental problems; some foster emotional well-being. The way a given fat influences your health depends on its unique blend of fatty acids.

Unfortunately, the typical Western diet is loaded with the types of fatty acids that are linked with some of our most serious health problems, while it is markedly deficient in some that are essential for optimal health. Even if you are well informed about nutrition and very careful about what you eat, you may still be fueling your body with the wrong ratio of fatty acids. Many of the physicians, medical researchers, and even dietitians who attend my lectures discover that they are eating the same unbalanced blend of fats as the general public.

## The Bad Fats and the Good Fats

One type of fat—saturated fat—has lived up to its reputation of being a "bad" fat. Found in meat, dairy products, and some tropical oils, saturated fat increases your risk of coronary artery disease, diabetes, and obesity. Recently, another culprit has been identified— "trans-fatty" acids, manmade molecules that are produced during the hydrogenation of vegetable oil. New studies show that trans-fatty acids can be even worse for your cardiovascular system than saturated fat and may also increase the risk of breast cancer. Switching from butter to margarine was not such a good idea after all.

Some fatty acids, however, are actually *good* for your health. Monounsaturated fatty acids, the type found in olive oil and canola oil, help protect your cardiovascular system. They also *reduce* the risk of certain metabolic disorders such as "insulin resistance" and diabetes, and are linked with a lower rate of cancer. This good news is beginning to reach the general public, resulting in a newfound popularity for canola oil and olive oil, a healthy trend that is consistent with **The Omega Diet.**

But some of the most significant research about fatty acids has remained locked in the medical journals. In particular, few people know about the health benefits that come from eating the right balance of "essential fatty acids," or EFAs. EFAs are fatty acids that are necessary for normal growth and development and cannot be manufactured in your body; you must get them from your diet. There are two families of EFAs, *"omega-6"* fatty acids and *"omega-3"* fatty acids. Omega-6 fatty acids are most abundant in common vegetable oils such as corn, safflower, cottonseed, and sunflower oils. Omega-3 fatty acids are found primarily in seafood, green leafy vegetables, fish, canola oil, and walnuts. A critical finding is that your body functions best when your diet contains a balanced ratio of EFAs, yet the typical Western diet contains approximately fourteen to twenty times more omega-6 fatty acids than omega-3s.[1-7] This imbalance is now being linked with a long list of serious conditions and diseases including:

- Heart attack
- Stroke
- Cancer
- Obesity
- Insulin resistance
- Diabetes
- Asthma
- Arthritis
- Lupus
- Depression
- Schizophrenia
- Attention deficit hyperactivity disorder
- Postpartum depression
- Alzheimer's disease

To learn more about EFAs, researchers have raised lab animals on diets similar to ours that are high in omega-6 fatty acids and low in omega-3 fatty acids. Invariably, the animals have suffered. When implanted with cancer cells, for example, their tumors have grown faster, larger, and more invasive. When allowed free access to food, the animals have gained weight and developed a common metabolic disorder called "insulin resistance." When given psychological and mental tests, they've had a difficult time finding their way out of mazes, engaged in more random and self-destructive behavior, and been less willing to explore open spaces. *Evidence that I will present throughout this book* strongly *suggests that eating an unbalanced ratio of essential fatty acids is causing* the same *havoc in our own bodies as well.*

**The Omega Diet** fuels your body with an ideal balance of EFAs and other key nutrients, allowing every cell and system in your body to function more effectively. If you have a serious health problem, making these simple changes can relieve your symptoms, allow you to cut back on medications, or even save your life.

## What Is the History of The Omega Diet?

Although **The Omega Diet** is supported by cutting-edge medical research, it has its roots deep in history. Indeed, it is based on the traditional diet of the Greek island of Crete, a diet that was virtually unchanged from 4,000 B.C. until modern times. The Crete diet first came to the attention of the medical community in the 1960s when an influential fifteen-year study revealed that the men from Crete were healthier than all the other 12,000 men surveyed in seven quite different countries—Greece, Italy, the Netherlands, Finland, Yugoslavia, Japan, and the United States.[8]

The difference in health between the men from Crete and the rest of the men was remarkable. Compared to the Americans, for example, they had half the cancer death rate and an astonishing *one-twentieth* of the mortality from coronary artery disease. Compared to the Japanese, they had half the overall death rate—even though the Crete diet was a 40 percent-fat diet that contained three times more fat than the Japanese diet. Surprisingly, the men from Crete also had half the overall death rate as men from Italy, even though both groups of men were eating Mediterranean-style diets that were rich in olive oil, legumes, fruits, and vegetables. There was something unique about the Crete diet, but at that time, medical science was unable to pinpoint what it was. (The educated guess was that it had something to do with its lower saturated fat and higher olive oil content.)

## *The Missing Clue*

Two decades later, I was able to provide one of the missing clues: The traditional Crete diet has an ideal ratio of EFAs. I gathered this insight in a roundabout fashion while investigating the omega-3 fatty acid content of wild plants. As I had suspected, I found that certain wild plants contain far more omega-3 fatty acids than cultivated plants.[9] This finding helped shed new light on the Crete diet because people from Crete eat large quantities of greens and wild plants, including purslane, the plant that was the subject of one of my studies. Perhaps this hidden bounty of omega-3 fatty acids was one of the reasons for their superb health.

My suspicions were confirmed by a landmark heart study conducted shortly thereafter by two French colleagues, Serge Renaud and Michel de Lorgeril. In a carefully designed study known as the Lyon Diet Heart Study, Renaud and de Lorgeril assigned 302 heart

attack survivors to a traditional heart diet, the "prudent" heart diet
recommended by the American Heart Association (AHA).[10] A similar
group was assigned to a slightly modified version of the Crete diet.
This new diet was based on canola oil and olive oil, and it had a ratio
of omega-6 to omega-3 fatty acids of 4 to 1, much lower than the
AHA diet and the traditional Western diet. The diet was also lower
in red meat and deli meats, but higher in fish, grains, fruits, and vegetables. Overall, it contained 35 percent fat, whereas the AHA diet is
30 percent.[11]

The results of the study made medical history. Just four months
into the clinical trial, the researchers discovered there had been significantly fewer deaths in the group on the modified Crete diet than
on the AHA diet. This in itself is remarkable because no other heart
diet or drug has ever shown a lifesaving benefit until patients have
been treated for at least six months. The survival gap widened with
each passing month. When the patients had been followed for about
two years, the study was halted abruptly because the new diet was

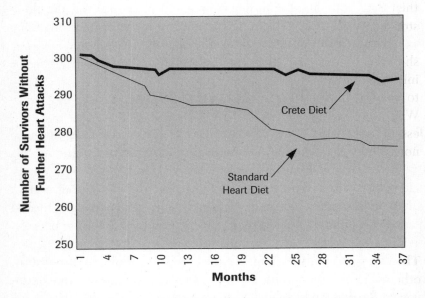

Figure 1-1. Superior Heart Protection of the Crete Diet

This graph compares the number of patients in each diet group who survived and
did not have additional heart attacks. As you can see, the patients on the modified
Crete diet fared much better.[13]

proving so superior it would have been unethical to continue the research. *Compared to those on the AHA diet, the patients on the Crete diet had an unprecedented 76 percent lower risk of dying from cardiovascular disease or suffering heart failure, heart attack, or stroke!* Remarkably, the new diet had proven more effective at saving lives than any other heart diet, drug, lifestyle program, or any combination of these elements. These results were deemed important enough to be published in three prestigious medical journals, *The Lancet,*[10] *The American Journal of Clinical Nutrition,*[11] and the *Journal of the American College of Cardiology.*[12]

**The Omega Diet** gives you the same balance of essential fatty acids and other nutrients that proved so beneficial for the French heart attack patients, *allowing you to benefit from this lifesaving research for the very first time.* So often you hear about a promising medical study, only to discover you can't take advantage of it for years to come because "more research needs to be done." Not so with the Lyon study. This book allows you to start profiting from this amazing heart research with your very next trip to the grocery store.

But **The Omega Diet** is far more than a heart diet. Studies show that this new program will also make you less vulnerable to inflammatory and autoimmune diseases. You may even be less prone to mental disorders such as depression and Alzheimer's disease. When you eat a diet that contains the right balance of fats and other essential nutrients, every system in your body will function more normally.

## The Omega Diet Is Delicious and Easy to Follow

**The Omega Diet** is a very simple program to follow. Unlike some other popular diets, you won't have to deprive yourself of fat, force yourself to eat abnormally high amounts of protein, or make sure that every bite that you eat conforms to a rigid ratio of fat, carbohydrates, and protein. Indeed, most of the "work" of the diet takes place at the grocery store. If you fill your shopping cart wisely, you will be well on your way to satisfying its Seven Dietary Guidelines.

The most important change you will be making is in eating a healthier balance of fat. A combination of olive oil and canola oil will become your primary oils. Just as important, you will be supplementing your diet with foods rich in omega-3 fatty acids while you limit your intake of omega-6 fatty acids, saturated fat, and trans-fatty acids. These changes are easier to make than you might expect. Simply using canola oil as your primary oil, for example, will satisfy most of these dietary requirements. You may be aware that canola oil is rich in monounsaturated fatty acids, but it is also an unheralded source of omega-3 fatty acids as well. The fact that it is low in saturated fat, trans-fatty acids, and lower in omega-6 fatty acids than many other oils makes it one of the healthiest foods in your kitchen.

Another change you will be making is eating more fruits, vegetables, and legumes. The current USDA guidelines recommend that you eat five or more servings of these wholesome foods every day. On **The Omega Diet** you will be eating *seven* or more servings a day, giving you added helpings of vitamins, fiber, minerals, antioxidants, and health-enhancing substances called "phytochemicals."

---

### The Seven Dietary Guidelines of The Omega Diet

1. Eat foods rich in omega-3 fatty acids such as fatty fish (salmon, tuna, trout, herring, mackerel), walnuts, canola oil, flaxseeds, and green leafy vegetables. Or, if you prefer, take omega-3 supplements.
2. Use monounsaturated oils such as olive oil and canola oil as your primary fat.
3. Eat seven or more servings of fruits and vegetables every day.
4. Eat more vegetable protein, including peas, beans, and nuts.
5. Avoid saturated fat by choosing lean meat over fatty meat (if you eat meat) and low-fat over full-fat milk products.
6. Avoid oils that are high in omega-6 fatty acids, including corn, safflower, sunflower, soybean, and cottonseed oils.
7. Reduce your intake of trans-fatty acids by cutting back on margarine, vegetable shortening, commercial pastries, deep-fat fried food, and most prepared snacks, mixes, and convenience food.

---

# Medical Proof of The Omega Diet

Understandably, the public has grown weary of books that proclaim to reveal THE secret to health and fitness, especially when the advice is so contradictory. One year, the ultimate solution to good health is to strip all the visible fat from your diet. The next year, the "revolutionary" new program is very high in protein. Just when you think it's safe to go to the store, someone tells you that you need to be eating a highly specific balance of fats, protein, and carbohydrates. What is even more confusing is that all of these diets are purported to be based on "the latest medical science."

What assurance do you have that **The Omega Diet** is not just another fad diet? Fortunately, there are ways you can judge the validity of this program, or any other diet for that matter. The most important question to ask is whether a diet has been tested in a large-scale clinical trial. If the only "proof" of a diet is one small, unpublished study; or the testimony of a select group of clients; or, worse yet, the enthusiastic claims of a celebrity promoter—"I was on this diet for three weeks and I feel terrific!"—you have no assurance that the diet will work for you.

**The Omega Diet** stands up to this scrutiny because, as I have explained, its heart-protective properties were carefully tested in the Lyon Diet Heart Study. The Lyon study was a "randomized clinical trial"—the gold standard of medical studies. In such a study, a new therapy is compared with either a placebo or a commonly accepted form of treatment. The term "randomized" means that the patients are assigned by chance to the different study groups, which prevents the researchers from biasing the results by routing healthier or more treatable patients to a particular treatment. An added precaution of the Lyon Diet Heart Study is that it was "blinded." This means that the physicians who evaluated the results did not know if a given patient had been on the Crete diet or the AHA diet, which helped them evaluate the results more objectively.

But no diet, no matter how thoroughly it's been tested, can guarantee to promote better health unless it has also stood the test of time. The medical literature is full of examples of diets and drugs that were beneficial in short-term studies but were proven to be harmful in the long term. **The Omega Diet** passes this final test as well. Based on the traditional diet of Crete, it has changed little since the time of Hippocrates. In essence, it has been "field tested" in the kitchens of generations of the world's healthiest people. But as you will learn in chapter 3, the diet has roots even deeper in history. The balance of EFAs it contains is similar to that found in wild plants and game, the type of food eaten by early humans throughout several million years of evolution. For this reason, the diet is ideally suited for our genetic makeup. In essence, **The Omega Diet** fuels our bodies with the food they "expect" to be fed.

## QUESTIONS ABOUT THE OMEGA DIET

Q: **What role does exercise play in the program?**

A: This book is focused primarily on diet, but exercise is just as vital to your health. In fact, regular physical exercise improves your health in many of the same ways as **The Omega Diet**, including reducing your risk of cancer, obesity, diabetes, and heart disease. When you combine this new diet *with* exercise, you have an unbeatable combination. I strongly urge you to exercise forty-five minutes or more *every* day.

Q: **I'm a strict vegetarian. Will The Omega Diet work for me?**

A: As a vegetarian, you are fortunate because you are probably following many of the seven dietary guidelines already. For example, it is likely that your diet is low in saturated fat and cholesterol and contains generous amounts of fruits and vegetables. You will need to make a special point to add more omega-3 fatty acids to your diet, however, because the typical vegetarian diet is high in omega-6 fatty acids and poor in omega-3s.

Q: **I'm diabetic. Is The Omega Diet a good diet for me?**

A: Yes it is. Several studies show that the combination of fats in this diet improve lipid levels, blood sugar, and insulin sensitivity. Therefore, the diet is not only safe but highly recommended. Of course, you should always seek the advice of your own physician.

Q: **I'm taking a number of heart medications. If I follow the diet religiously, can I stop taking them?**

A: Only with your doctor's advice. The men and women who took part in the Lyon study were heart attack survivors who had been prescribed a number of medications and continued to take them throughout the study. If your cardiovascular health improves a great deal, however, ask your doctor about decreasing your medications. But I must stress again, you should do so *only* with your doctor's approval.

Q. **I've heard that seafood is a good source of omega-3 fatty acids, but I'm not very fond of fish. Do I have to eat fish on this diet?**

A: The bottom line is that you need to increase your intake of omega-3 fatty acids, but as you will learn in Part II, you can get these vital nutrients in a number of ways, including taking supplements, using canola oil as your primary oil, adding flaxseeds or flaxseed oil to your diet, or eating more walnuts, legumes, and green leafy vegetables. (In many areas of the country it is also possible to buy eggs that are enriched with omega-3 fatty acids.)

Q: **Can I drink wine with this diet?**

A: Yes, you can. In Greece, people drink wine with most dinners. Also, the Lyon Heart Diet Study was conducted in France, a country of wine lovers, so moderate alcohol consumption was allowed—even encouraged. If you would like, you can drink one or two glasses of wine a day, preferably with meals.

Q: **I need to lose weight, but I find it very difficult to do. Can I get the benefits of The Omega Diet if I stay at my present weight?**

A: Unlike other heart-healthy diets, **The Omega Diet** does not require you to lose weight. The patients in the Lyon Heart Diet Study had no restrictions placed on the amount of food they ate, other than to cut back on "bad" fats. On average, their weight stayed the same, yet they reaped unprecedented health benefits. The same is likely to be true for you.

If you are considerably overweight, however, you will derive additional benefits if you shed some pounds. Among other plusses, you will look better; have more energy; relieve stress on your joints; and lower your blood pressure, triglycerides, cholesterol, and risk of diabetes. The weight-loss versions of the diet contain the same generous percentage of fat as the regular version, which will make dieting much more enjoyable.

Q: **I would like my partner to go on the diet with me, but I don't think I will get any cooperation.**

A: Ideally, **The Omega Diet** should become a family affair. But if you meet with resistance, you can accomplish a great deal behind the scenes. For example, you can switch the kind of fats that you use in your baking, with no one the wiser. You can add more vegetables to soups, meat loafs, and stews. You can serve fruit for dessert. You will learn about additional steps you can take in later chapters.

# TWO

# The Skinny on Fat

THE NOTION THAT some types of fat are essential for optimal health comes as a surprise to many people. The message they've been given is that all fats are equally bad and that they're responsible for a long list of ills, including cancer, heart disease, and obesity. For this reason, they try to eat as little fat as possible. They scrutinize food labels to find the products with the fewest fat grams per serving. They try to resign themselves to the taste and texture of low-fat cheese, ice cream, and salad dressing. They search for books and magazine articles that promise to teach them how to make low-fat food palatable. They say to each other with pride, "I eat hardly any fat at all."

This thinking is both outmoded and potentially hazardous to your health. In truth, a moderate amount of fat is essential for your physical and mental well-being. On the most basic level, fat helps form the membrane that surrounds each of your cells; without this membrane, your cells would not be able to control which elements enter and leave their domain. Fat is the raw material for hormonelike substances called "eicosanoids" that influence virtually every function in your body, from your blood pressure to your sensitivity to pain. Your brain is composed primarily of fat, including the neurons, the cells that transmit electrical messages; if you don't eat enough of the right types of fats, you are depriving your brain of a critical nutrient and risk falling prey to depression and other mental disorders. Eating too little fat can also diminish your supply of testosterone, a sex hormone that plays important roles in the health of women as well as men.[1]

Equally important, fat is essential for the absorption of vital nutrients. As just one example, tomatoes contain a cancer-fighting antioxidant called "lycopene" that has been linked with a lower risk of breast, prostate, and cervical cancer. If you eat tomatoes without any added fat, however, only a small amount of lycopene gets into your bloodstream. If you eat tomatoes along with a moderate amount of fat, your blood levels greatly increase, bolstering your nutritional barrier against cancer.[2]

Finally, as you will be learning throughout Part II, eating the right balance of essential fatty acids can reduce your risk of a number of diseases, including cardiovascular disease, cancer, diabetes, allergies, autoimmune diseases, and depression. Ultimately, fat is as essential to your health as vitamins, minerals, antioxidants, carbohydrates, and protein. Good fat is good food.

All well and good, you might say, but won't eating fat *make* you fat? No matter how beneficial certain fats may be to your health, they're reputed to be a leading cause of obesity. This widely held belief has spawned a multibillion-dollar low-fat–food industry and launched a dozen best-selling books, but, as you will see, it is *not* based entirely on scientific fact. In the remainder of this chapter, I will examine four common myths about fat and body weight, so you can have the *real* skinny on fat.

## *Myth #1: "Fat Makes You Fat"*

The most common misconception about fat is that "eating fat makes you fat." One reason so many people have been taken in by this mantra is that it has been the central theme in several best-selling diet books. Eat a high-fat diet, say a number of prominent diet doctors, and you will have a high-fat body. One has gone so far as to say: "YOU CAN'T GET FAT *EXCEPT* BY EATING FAT!"[3]

What is the scientific truth? Eating a high-fat diet *can* make you fat if you pay no attention to calories because fat is a calorie-dense food, packing in nine calories per gram. By comparison, carbohydrates and protein contain only four calories per gram. If you eat a lot of fat, therefore, you take in a lot of calories. If you consume a lot of calories and don't burn them off through normal metabolism or physical activity, you *will* gain weight. Guaranteed.

You will also have a tendency to gain weight if you eat a typical American diet and load up on "bad" fat, namely saturated fat, trans-fatty acids, and oils high in omega-6 fatty acids. These fats can disrupt your metabolism and make your cells more likely to store fat than to burn it, a phenomenon that will be discussed in more detail in chapter 7.

But, in general, the tendency of fatty foods to make you fat has been overstated. In fact, you may be surprised to learn that you can *lose* weight just as effectively on a high-fat diet as a low-fat diet, provided the two diets contain the same number of calories. A study that proves this point took place at the University Hospital in Geneva, Switzerland. One group of overweight patients was put on a succulent 45-percent–fat diet, and the other on a lean 26-percent–fat diet. (The typical Western diet is about 35 percent fat.) Both diets contained the same Spartan 1,200 calories. To guarantee full compliance, all the food was prepared and consumed at the hospital. At the end of three months of dieting, there was no difference in weight loss between the two groups. In fact, the group on the *high*-fat diet had lost a slightly greater percentage of body fat—8 percent versus 7.2 percent—proving that you *can* have your fat and lose fat, too.[4,5]

I don't want to give the impression that I am advocating a high-fat diet, however, because I am not. I believe that an ideal diet contains a *moderate* amount of healthy fat. I mention this study to make the important point that eating fat *in and of itself* will not make you fat. The primary reasons people gain weight is that they are exercising too little, eating the wrong kinds of fat, and taking in too many calories.

# *Myth #2: A Low-Fat, High-Carbohydrate Diet Boosts Your Metabolism*

A second common myth about fat and weight loss is that stripping the fat from your diet will boost your metabolism and thus help you lose weight, or as one diet doctor claims, "turn on your body's innate, hidden potential for melting off excess body fat."[3] As a result of this appealing theory, people have been heaping their plates with pasta but holding back on the cream sauce, hoping that their body furnaces will heat up and burn calories at a faster rate.

Once again, there is an element of truth to this myth. It does take more energy for your body to use the calories in carbohydrates than in fat, resulting in the generation of "waste" heat or "free" calories. But the amount of free calories you gain from this maneuver is minuscule, as was shown by a carefully controlled six-week study that took place at the Mayo Clinic. For the first part of this particular study, overweight women were fed a diet that contained a moderate amount of carbohydrates and a substantial amount of fat—in other words, pasta with lots of cream sauce. (Forty to 45 percent of the calories came from fat, more than the women normally consumed.) Two weeks later, the women were switched to a diet that contained the same number of calories but was much lower in fat and higher in carbohydrates. After a month on the low-fat diet, the researchers tested the women to see if there had been any change in their metabolic rate. Despite the fact that the women had been substituting carbohydrates for fat for a full month, their metabolic rates had not changed. More to the point, they had *not* lost any weight or body fat. According to the Mayo team, "No effect of the four-week, low-fat diet could be detected."[6] From this and other studies we now know that trying to lose weight by eating less fat and more carbohydrates *without cutting calories* is a prescription for failure.

## *Myth #3: "You Can't Get Fat Eating Carbohydrates"*

A third myth about fat that is contributing to our epidemic of obesity is that "carbohydrates cannot be converted into fat." This myth states that *none* of the carbohydrates you eat can be transformed into body fat; it's a metabolic impossibility. According to one diet guru (emphasis his), **"NOTE THAT SOME FOODS HAVE SO LITTLE FAT THAT THEY CAN BE EATEN IN UNLIMITED QUANTITIES AT ANY TIME, AS PART OF YOUR MEALS OR AS**

**UNLIMITED SNACKS."**[3] Eat all the fat-free food you want, in other words, and you cannot possibly gain weight. All those carbohydrate calories will be used as energy or simply vanish into thin air.

This wishful thinking prompted the feeding frenzy a number of years ago when nonfat cookies were first introduced. You may recall seeing ads of women chasing Snackwell delivery trucks, desperate to get their hands on the cookies before they sold out. The reason they had become so in*fatu*ated with the cookies is that they had been duped into thinking that "fat-free" means "calorie-free." They were going to be able to feast on fat-free cookies and ice cream and not gain any weight!

Not so. In fact, new research shows that eating a very low-fat diet—the express goal of millions of dieters—has the *opposite* effect: It turns your body into a fat-making machine! Just as a cow can transform low-fat grass into a generous layering of body fat and creamy milk, your body can convert fat-free food into a bulging belly and thicker thighs—and it will do so whenever your diet is very low in fat and high in carbohydrates. To add insult to injury, the type of fat that your body manufactures is *saturated* fat, specifically a type of fatty acid called "palmitic acid" that is linked with an increased risk of heart disease.

Just how efficiently your body can transform carbohydrates into saturated fat was shown in a 1996 metabolic study that also took place at Rockefeller University.[7] Healthy, normal-weight volunteers were placed on either an ultralean 10 percent–fat diet or a rich 40 percent–fat diet. Each person ate the number of calories required to maintain his or her body weight. Every ten days, the researchers measured how much new fat the volunteers were making by analyzing their fatty substances called "triglycerides." They found that the volunteers on the high-fat diet were manufacturing little or no fat. It was as if their bodies were saying, "Okay, I'm getting an adequate supply of fat in my diet, so I don't need to make any of my own." By contrast, the volunteers on the low-fat diet were producing copious amounts of saturated fat. In fact, between 30 and 57 percent of the fatty acids in their triglycerides was self-made saturated fat. Sensing that a fat famine was under way, their bodies had cranked up the machinery that converts carbohydrates into fat, one of the many built-in mechanisms that has allowed humans to survive lean times.

# Myth #4: An Ideal Way to Lose Weight Is to Eat Fat Substitutes

The food industry is betting the bank that many of the 50 million overweight people in this country will try to control their weight by relying on "fake" fats such as Olestra and Simpless. The lure is that fake fats offer the sensual pleasure of fat (what food scientists would refer to as "lubricity and organoleptic properties") without all those bothersome calories. Theoretically, people should be able to feast on potato chips fried in a fat substitute and be no worse off than if they had eaten a plain baked potato.

It is indeed true that fake fats are low or devoid of calories, and that some can even give you the illusion that you're eating real fat. In numerous tests, volunteers have been unable to distinguish between fake fat and the real thing. But even though your taste buds may be fooled, your body is not. Your body needs fat to function effectively, so it is genetically programmed to select food that contains a suffi-cient amount of this nutrient. This programming, we are now learn-ing, rejects pale imitations. In a 1996 study, volunteers were given either normal meals containing 32 percent fat or meals in which a third of the fat had been replaced with a fat substitute (sucrose poly-ester or Olestra). The volunteers were not told which meals were which. Nonetheless, on the day they were given the fat substitute, they reported feeling hungrier than usual. Furthermore, on the fol-lowing day when they were allowed to choose freely from the menu, they unconsciously selected food that was much higher in fat. In just one day of unsupervised eating, they had made up 74 percent of the fat deficit from the previous day.[8] Eating fake fat had simply deferred their fat consumption for twenty-four hours.

## The "Bulk Factor"

Amidst all the false claims being made about fat and weight loss, one claim does stand up to medical scrutiny: It is indeed true that you can "eat more and weigh less" on a low-fat diet. But there's a catch.

You have to eat very little fat and lots of bulky, complex carbohydrates—food that takes up a lot of room on your plate and in your gut. Here's how this works. Imagine for a moment that I have just served you a cabbage salad. Suppose that the salad contains one cup of shredded cabbage and one tablespoon of mayonnaise, for a total of 130 calories. As you know, the vast majority of those calories, 110 of them, are in the mayonnaise. If I were to take away the mayonnaise and replace it with 110 calories of cabbage, you would end up with a six-cup cabbage salad. My guess is that the salad would contain so much bulk (and so little flavor) you would stop eating long before you reached the bottom of the bowl. Without effort, you would be eliminating a few calories. If you continued to restrict yourself to a low-calorie, high-bulk diet, you would eventually lose weight.

But most people find it very hard to stick to an ultra-low-fat diet. They yearn for a pat of butter on their bread, a slice of *real* cheese, the occasional sirloin steak, or a piece of exquisite chocolate. Many become so desperate for "real" food that they stop dieting altogether. Others try to replace the fruits, vegetables, and brown rice with reduced-fat products such as nonfat ice cream, cookies, and cake. After all, they tell themselves, these foods are just as low in fat. But what they don't realize is that these highly refined products are missing the critical element—bulk. You can chew a nonfat cookie in ten seconds. When you swallow it, it takes up so little room in your stomach that you are not sent a "stop-eating" message. You might have to eat half a dozen cookies before you feel satisfied, burdening your body with hundreds of empty calories. It is much less likely that you would work your way through half a dozen carrots.

The tendency to eat excessive quantities of fat-reduced products has been dubbed "the Snackwell phenomenon," a phenomenon that is one of the hidden causes of our growing problem with obesity. This point is illustrated in the accompanying figure. In 1955, Americans were getting about 40 percent of their calories from fat; by 1995, the percentage had fallen to 35—a substantial drop. Yet during this same time period, the percentage of overweight adults grew from 25 percent to an alarming 40 percent.[9] The underlying problem is that we have been compensating for eating less fat by eating more calories. In fact, we are now eating more calories than at any time in this century. To make matters worse, we've become more sedentary than ever. We "rake" our leaves with gas-powered leaf blowers, drive to the corner grocery store, and spend hours each day sitting trans-fixed in front of our televisions and computer screens. Medical stud-ies have shown time and again that when people eat more calories than they burn, they pack on the pounds. Now it's being demon-strated on a national scale.

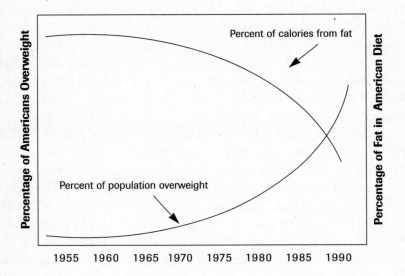

Figure 2-1. Americans Have Gotten Fatter as Our Fat Con-sumption Has Decreased[10]

---

The upward curving line shows how the percentage of overweight Americans has increased over time. The downward curving line shows the gradual drop in the amount of fat in our diet. Paradoxically, we've gotten fatter at the same time we've been cutting back on fat. The problem is that our total intake of calories has increased.[11]

What is the solution to our growing problem with obesity? First of all, we need to acknowledge that fat is more than mere fuel—it's an essential, life-giving nutrient. If we don't eat enough fat, our bod-ies will make it; if we feed our bodies fake fat, we will feel compelled to search out the real thing. The human body needs fat, and it will accept no substitute.

Second, we need to abandon the notion that we can lose weight simply by cutting back on fat. It doesn't work. As the studies have shown, ferreting out the fat grams won't jump-start our metabolism or give us a significant number of "free" calories. To maintain a healthy weight, we need to go back to basics and balance our caloric intake with our energy output. For most of us, this means eating less *and* exercising more. We need to throw away the fat-gram counters, dust off the calorie counters, and put on our walking shoes.

**The Omega Weight-Loss Diet** featured in chapter 13 will help you do just that. This novel program is carefully designed to give you the types of fats and number of calories you need to lose weight safely and effectively. It is rich in fruits, vegetables, and whole grains, foods that will fill you up before they fill you out. Meanwhile, as you lose weight and develop a sleeker and more toned body, you will also be enjoying the flavor, texture, and health benefits of good fat. This is a program you will want to stay on for life.

---

### The Bottom Line

- Contrary to popular belief, eating fat will not make you fat unless you also take in too many calories or eat the wrong *types* of fat.
- You can even lose weight on a high-fat diet—provided you cut back on calories.
- Eating a low-fat, high-carbohydrate diet will *not* boost your metabolism or give you a significant number of "free" calories.
- Eating a very low-fat diet can turn your body into a fat-making machine, and the type of fat that your body manufactures is saturated fat.
- Eating fat substitutes creates a craving for real fat.
- You can eat more food on a low-fat, high-carbohydrate diet provided you restrict yourself to bulky, high-complex carbohydrate foods such as fruits and vegetables. Low-fat or nonfat cookies, crackers, cake, and ice cream do not provide sufficient bulk to satisfy your appetite, causing you to take in too many calories.
- **The Omega Weight-Loss Diet** is high in bulk, but unlike low-fat, high-carbohydrate diets, it also allows you to enjoy the flavor and texture of healthy fat.

---

## · THREE ·

# Why We Eat
# the Wrong Fats

ONCE THE MYTHS are cleared away, there's room to explore
some exciting new discoveries about fat. One of the most
important medical findings of recent years is that eating a balanced
ratio of essential fatty acids (EFAs) brings your diet back in synch
with your genes and helps you experience optimal health. Human-
like creatures have existed on this planet for as long as four million
years, and for roughly 99 percent of this time, they were hunters and
gatherers. During this long period of evolution, human genes
became adapted to the balance of EFAs found in wild plants and
game. According to an expert in the field of evolutionary nutrition,
Boyd Eaton, M.D., from Emory University: "The principles of evolutionary adaptation suggest that if a dietary pattern is maintained
within a lineage for nearly two million years, it must be optimal."[1]

The fats eaten by early humans are just as optimal for us today
because our genes are virtually identical to theirs. Even though our
ancestral line diverged from the chimpanzees more than four million
years ago, for example, there is only a 1.6 percent difference between
chimp genes and human genes, any difference between our present
genetic makeup and that of humans who lived during the Paleolithic
era, a mere 40,000 to 15,000 years ago, is believed to be negligible.
This means that when we're sitting down to lunch, our stone-age

bodies "expect" to be fed the same types and ratios of fat that nourished our cave-dwelling ancestors. When we eat French fries cooked in partially hydrogenated vegetable oil instead of wild plants; or wolf down a fat-laden hamburger heaped with mayonnaise instead of meat from a lean, free-ranging game animal, our bodies register the insult.

## New Fats and Old Genes

One of the reasons that our bodies are so finely attuned to the types of fat in our diet is that EFAs can "talk" to our genes, sending them clear messages to make more or less of certain vital proteins.[2] For example, a recent study has shown that oils high in omega-6 fatty acids send a message to the genes to produce more of a cancer-promoting protein called "ras p21." By contrast, omega-3 fatty acids render this protein inactive, possibly reducing the risk of cancer.[3] Other studies have shown that omega-3 fatty acids send heart-protective messages to your genes instructing them to produce less of an enzyme that is essential for the production of fat.[2] As a result, you have lower levels of triglycerides in your blood, reducing your risk of cardiovascular disease.

Clearly, if you want to fight disease and enjoy optimal health, you need to be eating the ratio of EFAs that sends cancer-fighting, heart-healthy messages to your genes. The ratio that sends those messages, studies have shown, is a ratio of omega-6 to omega-3 fatty acids that is less than 4 to 1.[4] Not by coincidence, this is similar to the ratio found in our evolutionary diet. Yet today when we forage for food at the local grocery store, we are likely to bring home food that contains from fourteen to twenty times more omega-6 than omega-3 fatty acids, upsetting a critical balance that has been maintained for millions of years and putting us at greater risk for virtually all the diseases referred to as "the diseases of civilization."

## Dissecting the Paleolithic Menu

How do we know which types of fats were eaten by our early ancestors? Researchers have sought answers to this question by using a variety of strategies, including studying cave paintings, cooking artifacts, hunting implements, shells, bones, seeds, and the fossilized remains of food. With advanced technology, they've even been able to analyze the remnants of cholesterol found in the fossilized bones and teeth of early humans—the first direct evidence of the fats they were eating. This information has been supplemented with a painstaking analysis of the diets of the handful of hunter-gatherer tribes that have survived into the twentieth century. To date, ethnobiologists have determined the nutritional content of more than 320 common wild plants and game animals eaten by primitive people.[5]

One of the conclusions that has been drawn from all this work is that early humans got most of their nourishment from fish and meat, and fruits and vegetables—just two of what we now regard as "the four food groups." It has been estimated that they ate about three times more fruits and vegetables than we do today and substantially more meat and fish. The other two food groups—cereals and bread, and dairy products—played minor roles in the Paleolithic diet. Grain-based products were virtually nonexistent until the agricultural revolution because wild grains are too small and scattered to be practical to harvest. Dairy products were unknown prior to the domestication of animals approximately 10,000 years ago. According to Eaton, "Americans think of bread and milk as quintessentially 'natural' foods. This is understandable, as nutritionists have designated cereal grains and dairy products as two of the four 'essential' food groups. However, from the standpoint of genetically determined human biology, these foods are Johnny-come-latelies."[5]

The fact that our ancestors ate more greens and less grains than we do today helps explain the great difference in our intake of EFAs. Through sophisticated analysis, we have learned that the EFAs are not spread uniformly throughout the plant kingdom. Omega-3 fatty acids are concentrated in the green leaves of plants (and in a few seeds and nuts such as flaxseeds, rapeseed, and walnuts), while omega-6 fatty acids are most highly concentrated in the seeds and grains, newcomers to our diet. Our present-day reliance on grain-based products—cereal, bread, crackers, pastries, cakes, and cookies—and our minimal intake of greens is one of the reasons that we are so top-heavy in omega-6 fatty acids and deficient in omega-3 fatty acids.

# Lessons Learned from Purslane

In the early 1980s, when I was serving as chair of the Nutrition Coordinating Committee at the National Institutes of Health (NIH), few realized that green plants are a significant source of omega-3 fatty acids. Plants, as a rule, are generally low in fat, and their omega-3 content was thought to be negligible. As fate would have it, I helped revise this thinking. One of my first insights came in the spring of 1985, while I organized and co-chaired the international conference titled "The Health Effects of Polyunsaturated Fatty Acids in Seafoods." This was the first big conference devoted exclusively to omega-3 fatty acids, and it opened the eyes of the scientific community to the vital importance of these long overlooked nutrients. During the conference, I found myself thinking about a common plant called "purslane." Purslane had come to mind because I knew it had been used by traditional societies to treat many of the same health problems that were now responding to omega-3 fatty acids, including inflammation, heart problems, stomach disorders, pain, and fever. For example, Theophrastus (372–287 B.C.), the father of botany, had recommended purslane as a remedy for heart failure, scurvy, sore throats, earaches, swollen joints, and dry skin. On a different continent, northwest Indians were using purslane tea to soothe sore throats and inflammation. Tribes from west tropical Africa were using purslane as a heart tonic and an ointment for boils and burns. In the Punjab and Cashmere, purslane seeds were recommended for inflammation of the stomach and intestinal ulceration.[6]

Surely, I told myself, it was more than coincidence that purslane had so many of the healing properties now being attributed to omega-3 fatty acids. The plant *must* be a rich source of these nutrients. I convinced my friend and colleague, Norman Salem, Jr., Ph.D., also at NIH, to help me analyze its fatty acid content. But where to find purslane? I knew that it was commonly eaten in Greece, my homeland, and throughout most of Europe, Mexico, and Asia, but in the United States it was considered a noxious weed. To help control this "pest," the U.S. government had gone so far as to import the "purslane sawfly" (*Schizocerella pilicornis*), a fly that thrives on the ubiquitous plant and is capable of gnawing it to the ground.

You can imagine my delight when I found a clump of purslane growing in a highly convenient place: the cracks in the pavement outside my office at NIH. I collected the stalwart plants and submitted them for analysis. The results confirmed my hunch. Purslane is loaded with omega-3 fatty acids. One hundred grams contain 400 milligrams of the plant-based form of omega-3 fatty acids called alpha-linolenic, or LNA—fifteen times more than most commercial lettuce. As an added bonus, it is rich in antioxidants. One serving fulfills the daily requirement of vitamin E and provides significant amounts of vitamin C, beta-carotene, and glutathione.[7-9]

One of the implications of my discovery, I realized, is that purslane and similar wild plants must have contributed a substantial amount of LNA and antioxidants to the diets of early humans. Purslane, in particular, is very widespread. Ranked as the eighth most common wild plant in the world, it was also one of the first plants cultivated by early humans: Purslane seeds were found in a cave in Greece that was last inhabited 16,000 years ago.

We now know that purslane is not alone in its bounty of omega-3 fatty acids. Following my discovery, other plants were tested for LNA, revealing that they, too, contained significant amounts of this nutrient. Appreciable amounts of LNA have been found in most dark green leafy vegetables, mosses, ferns, and legumes, as well as in many herbs and spices such as mustard, fennel, cumin, and fenugreek. As the research continues, the list is likely to grow.

## What Chickens Like to Eat

My findings about purslane soon led to another discovery: The eggs of chickens that graze on wild plants are also rich in omega-3 fatty acids. I gathered this additional insight while visiting my ancestral home on the southwestern Peloponnese in Greece. My family has a large farm with olive trees, fruit trees, a vegetable garden, a goat, and a flock of free-ranging chickens. One day, as I was watching the chickens forage for food, I was surprised to see that they were seeking out grass and green plants. In my ignorance, I asked my father, a physicist and a man with encyclopedic knowledge, what was wrong with the chickens that they "had" to eat greens. Wasn't their mash giving them enough nutrients? He reminded me that greens, insects, and worms were the natural diet of chickens, and that they ate commercial cornmeal mash only because that's what we deigned to feed them. As I watched the chickens more closely, I saw that they were particularly attracted to purslane. This made me wonder if the nutritional content of their eggs was different from that of ordinary eggs. I gathered some eggs from the henhouse, hard-boiled them, and brought them back to the NIH for analysis by Norm Salem. The lab tests showed that the eggs from our free-ranging hens contained *twenty* times more omega-3 fatty acids than standard supermarket eggs. (They had a ratio of omega-6 to omega-3 fatty acids of 1 to 1, while the supermarket eggs had a lopsided ratio of 20 to 1.[10])

When I researched the literature, I found that my observations about chicken eggs held true for the flesh of free-ranging animals as well: Any grazing animal that is allowed to eat its natural diet of wild plants and greens is far richer in omega-3 fatty acids than an animal kept in confinement and fed an artificial, grain-based diet. For example, Michael Crawford found that the flesh of a wild Cape buffalo that is free to forage in its natural habitat contains one-tenth as much total fat, about half as much saturated fat, but nearly six times more omega-3 fatty acids than a similar cut of meat from a grain-fed steer.[11] It is as if they were different foods altogether.

A critical insight about the Paleolithic diet had just fallen into place. Whether early humans were eating fish, plants, or land animals, they were being nourished by omega-3 fatty acids. Today, we consume a fraction of this essential nutrient. Surveys show that one-fourth of the U.S. population eats no fish whatsoever. Meanwhile, we eat a third of the amount of green leafy vegetables as our ancestors, and the eggs and meat that we eat comes from animals whose diets are artificially low in omega-3 fatty acids. It has been estimated that we are now eating one-tenth of the amount of omega-3 fatty acids required for normal functioning. Alarmingly, 20 percent of the population has levels so low that they defy detection.[13] The admonishment to "eat a balanced diet" makes no sense when our food has been stripped of one of its most essential nutrients.

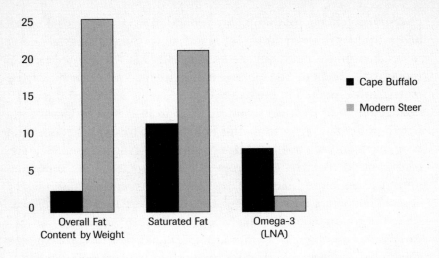

Figure 3-1. Difference in Fat Between a Wild Cape Buffalo
and a Modern Steer

Meat from a modern steer contains more total fat and saturated fat but only a fraction as much LNA as meat from a free-ranging Cape buffalo. This is further evidence that our hunter-gatherer ancestors consumed far more omega-3 fatty acids
than we do today.[12]

# Planting the Seeds of Destruction

To the same degree that our diet is deficient in omega-3 fatty acids,
it is overloaded with omega-6 fatty acids. The main reason for the
deluge is our growing reliance on vegetable oils such as corn, safflower, sunflower, and cottonseed oil, oils that had no place whatsoever in the evolutionary diet. These oils were not used by traditional
societies because they were too difficult to extract. Corn oil is a particularly good example. If you were to shuck a hundred ears of corn
and crush them under a stone wheel, you would produce a milky liquid that is only 1 to 3 percent fat, yielding, at best, five tablespoons
of corn oil. It was not practical for people to use corn oil until the
invention of sophisticated equipment in the twentieth century
designed to process tons of corn at a time, leaching out every drop of
oil through the combined persuasion of high temperature, hydraulic
pressure, and chemical solvents.

Our use of vegetable oils escalated during the 1960s and 1970s—due in large part to an aggressive campaign to lower cholesterol. An important medical finding during that era was that a diet high in saturated fat raises cholesterol, and that high cholesterol levels are linked with a high rate of coronary artery disease. Logically, heart researchers began researching cholesterol-lowering diets. One of their discoveries was that adding vegetable oils such as corn oil to the diet caused a slight drop in cholesterol levels. At the time, the ideal heart diet appeared to be one that was low in saturated fat and high in omega-6 polyunsaturated oils.[14]

Before long, thousands of volunteers in the United States and Europe were enrolled in studies designed to test this new concept. Most of the studies were short-term affairs designed to detect changes in cholesterol levels, so whether the diets actually saved lives was anybody's guess. Those few studies that lasted long enough to produce valid mortality statistics yielded disappointing results. For example, a corn-oil diet tested in England in 1965 actually *increased* the risk of dying from heart disease. The researchers concluded: "Under the circumstances of this trial, corn oil cannot be recommended as a treatment of heart disease. It is most unlikely to be beneficial, and it is possibly harmful."[15] Other diets based on omega-6 oils lowered the risk of cardiac deaths, but they *increased* the mortality rate from other causes, notably cancer, violence, and suicide. The net result was zero. Ominously, in a study that took place in a Los Angeles veterans' hospital in the 1970s, a group of men assigned to a diet high in omega-6 oils had twice the number of cancer deaths as those on a more traditional diet, making it the first large study to show a link between omega-6 fatty acids and cancer.[16]

Although these negative findings were published in medical journals, they were not picked up by the popular press. This lack of public awareness, coupled with permissive economic policies, allowed food manufacturers to develop and sell whatever oils they wished. It was highly advantageous for them to sell more omega-6 oils, because, at the time, these oils were little-used by-products of the animal feed and cotton industries. They could be sold to the general public as "heart-healthy" foods. A well-financed advertising campaign was set in motion to help grease the wheels. An ad typical of the era appeared in the September 1, 1969, edition of the *National Geographic* magazine.

The full-page ad features a smiling, middle-aged man sitting at the dinner table. His beaming wife, decked out in a shirtwaist dress and checkered apron, hovers over him as she hands him a large bowl of salad greens. The caption reads: "Tonight's the night Mrs. Ed. Flynn starts Polyunsaturating her husband . . . with a big assist from Mazola."

To a public that was not fully informed, ads such as this one were highly persuasive. Seemingly overnight, millions of people began switching from butter to corn oil margarine, from lard to all-vegetable shortening, and from bacon grease to PAM. A 1972 survey revealed that nine out of every ten people who had chosen to eat more vegetable oils had done so because of commercial advertising or the media, "not on the advice of, or even with the knowledge of, their personal physicians."[17]

Since the 1960s, our consumption of omega-6 oils has more than doubled, making Americans the world's second largest consumer of omega-6 fatty acids, topped only by the Israelis. As you will learn in later chapters, it seems increasingly likely that this glut of omega-6 fatty acids is contributing to our high rates of cancer, depression, obesity, insulin resistance, allergies, autoimmune diseases, and diabetes.

## Please Pass the Trans-Fatty Acids

Little did Americans know that along with the highly touted corn oil margarine and all-vegetable shortening came trans-fatty acids. Liquid vegetable oils present food producers with a number of problems. Corn oil can't be spread on bread, for instance, and it makes a poor pie crust. It is also prone to oxidation by light, air, and heat, especially after the refining process has robbed it of its natural antioxidants and phytochemicals. Hydrogenation was the answer. Through modern alchemy, vegetable oil could be heated, exposed to a metal catalyst such as nickel or copper, and transformed into a more plastic, less perishable fat. This fat could then be added to convenience foods, allowing them to be shipped in warm, humid weather and parked on the grocery shelf for months on end. By 1979, the American public was consuming an estimated 10 billion pounds of fat and oil per year, of which 60 percent was partially hydrogenated oil.[18]

The hydrogenation process has a number of unwanted consequences, however. One rarely discussed fact is that it reduces the essential fatty acid content of oils, both omega-6 and omega-3. Untreated soybean oil, for example, contains about 8.5 percent omega-3 fatty acids. When partially hydrogenated, its omega-3 content drops to 3 percent. Another drawback of hydrogenation is that it rearranges the molecular bonds on fatty acids, transforming them into look-alike molecules called "trans-fatty acids." Trans-fatty acids behave in many ways like saturated fat, including raising your LDL (bad) cholesterol. But they are even more destructive than saturated fat because they also lower your HDL (good) cholesterol, pushing both of these blood fats in the wrong direction. To make matters worse, they take the place of EFAs in cell membranes, interfere with their metabolism, and usurp some of the enzymes needed to create hormonelike substances called eicosanoids that are involved in many aspects of human physiology.

Today, Americans are consuming from 5 to 10 percent of their calories as trans-fatty acids. Studies show that amounts greater than 5 percent of your calories can have negative health consequences. It is alarmingly easy to reach this level because any product that has the words "partially hydrogenated" on the label contains trans-fatty acids. This includes most types of margarine, shortening, artificial cheese, deep-fat fried foods, commercial baked goods, prepared mixes, snack food, and crackers. You can reach the 5 percent level simply by eating one doughnut for breakfast, a small order of fries with lunch, a teaspoon of margarine at lunch and dinner, and two cookies for dessert.[19]

The current antifat craze has caused the final disruption in our fat consumption. Out of an irrational fear of fat, people have been avoiding healthy oils, nuts, and fatty fish, unwittingly robbing themselves of the few remaining sources of omega-3 fatty acids. Fish suppliers have been quick to capitalize on the trend. Much of the tuna now on the market is very low in fat, containing as little as 0.5 grams of fat per two-ounce serving. Full-fat tuna contains as much as 5 grams of fat. To satisfy your daily allotment of omega-3 fatty acids, you would have to eat *five* whole cans of low-fat tuna but only one half can of regular tuna! Another product to make its debut has been "fat-free" salmon patties. In addition to being "fat-free," of course, these patties are "omega-3 fatty acid" free. Eating fat-free salmon makes as much nutritional sense as buying carrots that have been stripped of their beta-carotene or oranges that have been hybridized to be low in vitamin C.

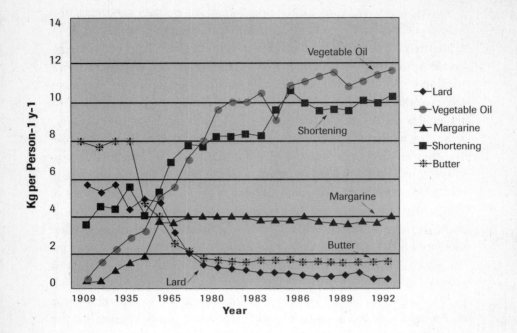

Figure 3-2. Changes in Our Consumption of Fat, 1909–1992

This graph shows the dramatic changes in oil consumption that took place between 1909 and 1992. At the beginning of the twentieth century, butter, lard, and shortening were the most commonly used fats. During World War II, rationing greatly decreased butter consumption, a trend that continued in later years as the food industry began promoting omega-6 oils, margarine, and "all-vegetable" shortening.[20]

Where do we go from here? There is such a wealth of evidence now supporting the importance of eating a balanced ratio of EFAs and restricting the intake of saturated fat and trans-fatty acids that I believe The Seven Dietary Guidelines of **The Omega Diet** will eventually replace our current dietary guidelines.[22] What's more, people will find it easy to follow the new guidelines because public opinion will have forced the food industry to awaken to the importance of eating healthy fats. In the twenty-first century, you will be able to shop at an ordinary supermarket and buy meat and eggs from animals raised on omega-3 enriched diets; the produce section will feature purslane and other vegetables that have been hybridized to be

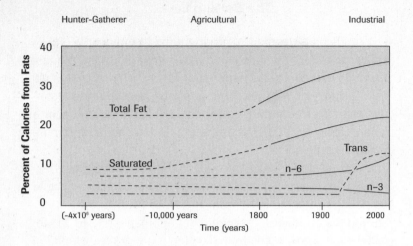

Figure 3-3. Changes in Fat Consumption Throughout
Human Evolution

This illustration shows how far we have strayed from the natural human diet, the
diet upon which our species evolved. We are eating more fat overall, more saturated
fat, more omega-6 fatty acids, and more trans-fatty acids. Meanwhile, we are eating
a fraction of the amount of omega-3 fatty acids required for optimal health.[21]

high in omega-3 fatty acids; you will be able to buy mayonnaise,
salad dressings, and snacks made from canola oil; flaxseeds and
flaxmeal will be included in many types of baked goods. To help you
select healthier foods, product labels will include information about
EFAs and trans-fatty acids.

Until that day arrives, however, you will have to take matters into
your own hands. You will need to avoid products that contain
unhealthy fats and go out of your way to find ones that contain
health-enhancing fats. Part III of this book gives you all the advice
and support you need to make these potentially lifesaving changes.

## The Bottom Line

- Our bodies are genetically programmed to thrive on a diet similar to that of the Paleolithic era. Compared to the modern diet, this diet contained more meat and fish, more greens and fruit, virtually no milk products or grains, less saturated fat, less than 2 percent trans-fatty acids (which naturally occur in some animal products), fewer omega-6 fatty acids, and more omega-3 fatty acids.
- The ratio of omega-6 to omega-3 in the Paleolithic diet is believed to have been approximately 1 to 1. Our current ratio has been estimated to be from 14 to 1 to 20 to 1.
- During the agricultural revolution of approximately 10,000 to 5,000 years ago, people began eating more grains, which increased their intake of omega-6 fatty acids. In addition, they domesticated animals and fed them an artificial diet of grains, resulting in meat and eggs that had more omega-6 and less omega-3 fatty acids than the meat from wild game.
- The industrial revolution made it practical for people to eat large quantities of omega-6 vegetable oils, further upsetting the omega-6 to omega-3 balance.
- The campaign to lower cholesterol has led to an excessive consumption of omega-6 oils.
- The widespread fear of fat has further stripped omega-3 fatty acids from our diet.
- Until government and industry recognize the importance of eating a balanced ratio of EFAs, you must take matters into your own hands.

• FOUR •

# A Fatty Acid Primer

## *What You Need to Know About Fats to Make Healthy Choices*

As YOU CAN SEE by referring back to The Seven Dietary Guidelines on page 10, you can balance the fats in your diet without knowing any more about fatty acids than you already do. Simply keep a list of which fats to select and which to avoid. Part III of the book, with its recipes and menu plans, will make your life even easier. To balance your diet, all you will have to do is follow the detailed instructions. Nonetheless, I believe you will benefit from understanding fatty acids on a somewhat deeper level. The more you know, the better you can safeguard your health and the health of those you care about.

Fatty acids are grouped into three broad, familiar categories: saturated, monounsaturated, and polyunsaturated. These designations refer to the types of bonds that hold their carbon atom chains together. **Saturated fatty acids** have single bonds between all the carbon atoms. (In this configuration, a fatty acid has all the hydrogen atoms it can accommodate, so it is said to be "saturated with hydrogen," or simply a "saturated fatty acid.") A "saturated" fat or oil is one that contains a significant amount of saturated fatty acids. Most saturated fats are solid or semisolid at room temperature. The exceptions are the tropical oils—palm oil, palm kernel oil, and coconut oil.

**Monounsaturated fatty acids** have one ("mono" = "single,"

37

from the Greek) double bond in the fatty acid chain. Olive oil and canola oil contain high amounts of monounsaturated fatty acids, 80 and 70 percent respectively, so they are classified as "monounsaturated oils." Two new oils on the market also belong in this category—"high-oleic" safflower and "high-oleic" sunflower oil. (Regular safflower oil and sunflower oil are classified as polyunsaturated oils.) Monounsaturated oils are liquid at room temperature, but may become cloudy or semisolid in the refrigerator.

**Polyunsaturated fatty acids** are fatty acids that have two or more ("poly" = "many," from the Greek) double bonds. Oils that contain a high percentage of polyunsaturated fatty acids include corn, safflower, sunflower, peanut, cottonseed, soybean, fish, walnut, and flaxseed oil. All polyunsaturated oils are liquid at room temperature and remain liquid in the refrigerator. (The more double bonds on the carbon chain, the more "unsaturated" the oil, and the colder temperatures it can withstand without congealing. Flaxseed oil and fish oil are the most highly unsaturated of all the oils.)

The following table sorts the most common fats into these three broad categories:

| Saturated Fats and Oils | Monounsaturated Oils | Polyunsaturated Oils |
|---|---|---|
| Butter Fat | Olive Oil | Corn Oil |
| Animal Fat | Canola Oil | Safflower Oil |
| Coconut Oil | High Oleic Safflower Oil | Sunflower Oil |
| Palm Oil | High Oleic Sunflower Oil | Peanut Oil |
| Cocoa Butter | Avocado Oil | Cottonseed Oil |
| Palm Kernel Oil | | Canola Oil (Note: Canola oil is high in both monounsaturated and polyunsaturated oils) |
| | | Soybean Oil |
| | | Fish Oil |
| | | Flaxseed Oil |
| | | Walnut Oil |
| | | Primrose Oil |
| | | Sesame Oil |
| | | Grapeseed Oil |
| | | Borage Oil |

In the past, nutritionists made little distinction between the various polyunsaturated oils (shown on page 38 in the right-hand column) because all of them are low in saturated fatty acids and cholesterol, and this was believed to be their most important characteristic. Thus, you were free to choose your polyunsaturated oils on the basis of cost, habit, flavor, or cooking qualities. The Food and Drug Administration and many people, even health professionals, are still locked into this antiquated point of view. But the new research shows that the various polyunsaturated oils can have dramatically different effects on your health depending on their ratio of omega-6 to omega-3 fatty acids.

Omega–3 fatty acids have their first double bond between the third and fourth carbon atoms and are therefore called omega–3s, while the omega–6 fatty acids have their first double bond between the sixth and seventh carbon atoms and, hence, are called omega–6s (see figure on page 349).The following chart shows which polyunsaturated oils are high in omega-3 fatty acids and which are high in omega-6 fatty acids, abbreviated in this book as "omega-3" oils and "omega-6" oils.

| Omega-3 Oils | Omega-6 Oils |
| --- | --- |
| Fish Oil | Corn Oil |
| Flaxseed Oil | Safflower Oil |
| Canola Oil | Sunflower Seed Oil |
| Walnut Oil | Cottonseed Oil |
| Soybean Oil (Note: Soybean oil is higher in omega-6 fatty acids than most omega-3 oils, so it belongs in both categories.) | Soybean Oil |
| | Peanut Oil |
| | Sesame Oil |
| | Grapeseed Oil |
| | Borage Oil |
| | Primrose Oil |

# Getting on a First-Name Basis

Several members of the omega-6 and omega-3 families of fatty acids are so critical to your health that I will be referring to them by their "first" names, not just their family names. The primary fatty acid in the omega-6 family is "linoleic" (lin-oh-LAY-ik) acid, or LA. The corresponding fatty acid in the omega-3 family is alpha-linolenic (lin-oh-LEN-ik) acid or, LNA. (Note the similarity in spelling between "linoleic" and "linolenic.") The typical Western diet is overloaded with linoleic acid and relatively deficient in alpha-linolenic acid, so for optimal health you will need to be eating less of the first and more of the second, a change that takes place automatically when you follow **The Omega Diet.**

When linoleic acid and alpha-linolenic acid interact with certain enzymes, they go through two transformations: They become desaturated by losing hydrogen and increasing the number of double bonds, and they become longer (add more carbon atoms). When they change in this manner, they are given new names. Linoleic acid becomes gamma-linolenic, or GLA, and then arachidonic acid, or AA. Alpha-linolenic acid becomes eicosapentaenoic acid, or EPA, and then docosahexaenoic acid, or DHA. (Note that DHA is different from DHEA. DHEA is a hormone that has been in the news in recent years because of its purported antiaging properties.)

This information is summarized in the following chart. You might want to mark the page for later reference. (For an illustration of the chemical structure of fatty acids, see page 349 of the Appendix.)

---

**FATTY ACIDS MADE SIMPLE**

**The Omega-6 Family**

**Linoleic Acid (LA)**
(Found in vegetable oils, seeds and nuts.)

*Your body converts LA into:*

↓

**Gamma-Linolenic Acid (GLA)**
(GLA is also found in borage and primrose oil.)

*Your body converts GLA into:*

↓

**Arachidonic Acid (AA)**
(AA is also found in meat.)

↓

**The Omega-6 Family of Eicosanoids**

**The Omega-3 Family**

**Alpha-Linolenic Acid (LNA)**
(Found in green leafy vegetables, flax, flaxseed oil, canola oil, walnuts, and Brazil nuts.)

*Your body converts LNA into:*

↓

**Eicosapentaenoic Acid (EPA)**
(EPA is also found in fish oil.)

*Your body converts EPA into:*

↓

**Docosahexaenoic Acid (DHA)**
(DHA is also found in fish oil.)

↓

**The Omega-3 Family of Eicosanoids**

This illustration shows how your body metabolizes linoleic acid, the "parent" molecule in the omega-6 family, and alpha-linolenic acid, the "parent" molecule in the omega-3 family. (For an illustration of LA and LNA, see page 349.)

Now that you are more acquainted with the names of individual fatty acids, the following chart will make more sense to you. It shows the fatty acid content of common fats and oils, in particular their percentage of saturated fatty acids, monounsaturated fatty acids, linoleic acid (omega-6), and alpha-linolenic acid (omega-3). Each fat or oil has a unique combination of these four elements.

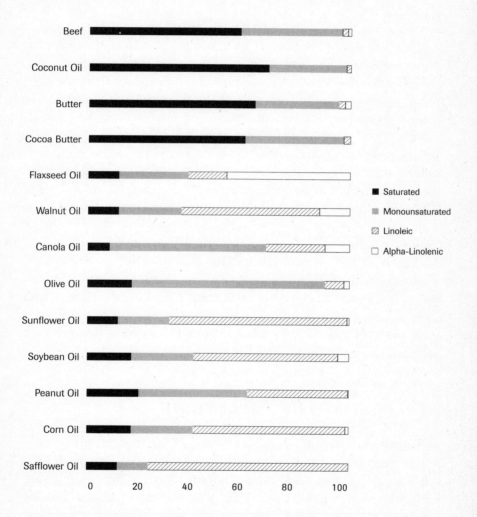

Figure 4-1. The Fatty Acid Content of Common Fats and Oils

This chart shows the percentage of saturated fatty acids, monounsaturated fatty acids, linoleic acid, and alpha-linolenic acid in thirteen commonly used fats and oils.

The main vegetable oils you will be eating on **The Omega Diet** are olive oil, canola oil, flaxseed oil, and walnut oil. You'll find them clustered together in the middle of the chart. As you can see, they share a number of characteristics. First, they are uniformly low in saturated fat. Second, they are either very low in linoleic acid (olive oil) or have a low ratio of linoleic to alpha-linolenic acid (flaxseed oil, canola oil, and walnut oil), giving them a favorable ratio of omega-6 to omega-3 fatty acids. Olive oil and canola oil are important components of the diet because they contain generous amounts of monounsaturated fatty acids. Olive oil has other virtues as well. It is rich in antioxidants and a substance called "squalene" that has anti-inflammatory properties, slows blood clot formation, and lowers cholesterol. Most importantly, eating olive oil increases the amount of omega-3 fatty acids taken up by the cells, whereas eating omega-6 oils such as corn oil and safflower oil decreases the amount. Butter, animal fat, and cocoa butter are included in the diet as well, but they are to be eaten in moderation. Although they are low in omega-6 fatty acids, they are very high in saturated fat. The only trans-fatty acids in the diet are the small amounts (approximately 2 percent) that occur naturally in butter and other dairy products.

When all the fats and oils in **The Omega Diet** are taken as a whole, the bulk of your fat calories will come from monounsaturated fatty acids, fewer than 8 percent will come from saturated fatty acids, and the ratio of omega-6 to omega-3 fatty acids will be less than 4 to 1—a blend of fats that is consistent with the evolutionary diet and has been proven to be ideal for health and longevity.

# The Eicosanoids

As I mentioned earlier, omega-3 and omega-6 fatty acids are unique in that they are the only fatty acids that are essential for your health but cannot be manufactured within your body. They must come from your diet. Essential fatty acids play a number of vital roles in your body. One key role is that they are converted into hormonelike substances called "eicosanoids" (eye-KOSS-uh-noids). The parent fatty acids for the eicosanoids are arachidonic acid (AA) from the omega-6 family and eicosapentaenoic acid (EPA) from the omega-3

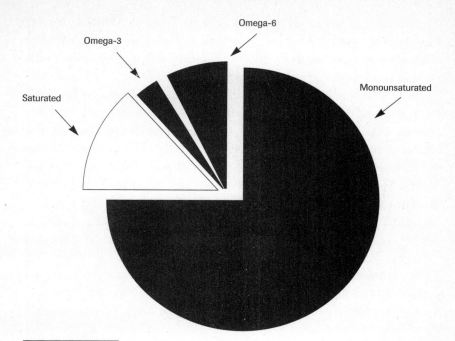

Omega-6

Omega-3

Saturated

Monounsaturated

This pie chart shows the approximate ratio of fatty acids that are featured in **The Omega Diet.** As you can see, the bulk of your fat calories will come from monoun-saturated fatty acids, and the ratio of omega-6 to omega-3 fatty acids in your diet will be less than 4 to 1.

family. The functions of the eicosanoids from these two families tend to be opposite. In other words, those from the omega-6 family oppose the functions of those from the omega-3 family.

I'm not going to discuss eicosanoids in any more detail, but there are two facts it would be helpful for you to know. First, eicosanoids are involved in every aspect of your day-to-day health. Among other vital functions, they influence your blood pressure, boost or repress your immune system, alter your perception of pain, and make you more or less prone to allergies and inflammation. Second, you can alter your body's production of eicosanoids by changing the oils in your diet because the eicosanoids produced from omega-6 fatty acids can have the opposite effect from eicosanoids produced from omega-3 fatty acids. If your diet is high in omega-6 oils, for example, your body will produce more proinflammatory eicosanoids, increas-ing your risk of asthma, allergies, arthritis, psoriasis, colitis, and other inflammatory diseases. If you follow **The Omega Diet,** however, you balance your intake of omega-6 and omega-3 oils, thereby reducing your body's production of proinflammatory eicosanoids and making you less vulnerable to these conditions.[1]

A recent study showed how effective this strategy can be. This study involved a group of young women who suffered from menstrual cramps, a condition that is caused, in part, by the overproduction of a type of proconstrictive eicosanoid called "$PGE_2$." For several months, the women were given either placebos or omega-3 fatty acid supplements. While taking the supplements, they reported a significant relief from pain, caused by a decreased production of $PGE_2$.[2]

---

## TYPES OF EICOSANOIDS

Eicosanoids are molecules that are twenty carbon atoms long. ("Eicosa" signifies the number 20 in Greek.) There are three main types of eicosanoids: prostaglandins, leukotrienes, and thromboxanes.

---

With these basic facts in hand, you will have a better understanding of the information you'll be acquiring in later chapters. Should you forget the names of the individual fatty acids or their family relationships, you can flip back to this chapter to refresh your memory. In the next section of the book, you will learn about all the health benefits that come from restoring your body's essential nutritional balance, starting with a greatly reduced risk of dying from cardiovascular disease.

## The Bottom Line

- Fatty acids are the molecular components of fats and oils. They differ from one another in their number of carbon atoms and the placement and nature of their molecular bonds.
- There are three categories of fatty acids: saturated, mono-unsaturated, and polyunsaturated.
- Polyunsaturated fatty acids are further subdivided into omega-3 and omega-6 fatty acids. These fatty acids are called "essential" fatty acids because they are essential for normal growth and development, and they cannot be manufactured by your body. They must come from your diet.
- The omega-3 fatty acid family includes alpha-linolenic acid (LNA), eicosapentaenoic acid (EPA), and docosahexaenoic acid (DHA). The omega-6 fatty acid family includes linoleic acid (LA), gamma-linolenic acid (GLA), and arachidonic acid (AA).
- Omega-3 fatty acids and omega-6 fatty acids are converted into hormonelike substances called "eicosanoids," which can have a profound influence on your health. Eicosanoids produced from omega-3 and omega-6 fatty acids have opposite functions. For this reason, you can greatly influence your health simply by choosing one type of vegetable oil over another.
- Many chronic diseases are characterized by an overproduction of eicosanoids made from omega-6 fatty acids. When you balance your intake of omega-6 and omega-3 fatty acids, you have a much lower risk of inflammatory and other diseases.
- The main oils and fats in **The Omega Diet** will give you an ample amount of monounsaturated fatty acids, relatively little saturated fat, and a ratio of omega-6 to omega-3 fatty acids less than 4. This blend of fats has been proven to promote optimal health.

# PART 2

# Fighting Disease with The Omega Diet

# FIVE

# The Genesis of a Heart Attack—and How The Omega Diet Helps You Avoid One

O F ALL THE COMMON causes of premature death—heart attack, stroke, cancer, accidents, diabetes, and infectious diseases—the odds are greatest that you are going to die from a heart attack or stroke. This is true whether you are male or female. People tend to think of cardiovascular disease as a male affliction because the symptoms show up ten years earlier in men, but women catch up after menopause. In fact, on an annual basis, more women die from heart attacks than men. *Five* times more women die from a heart attack than from breast cancer. *Whatever your gender, following* **The Omega Diet** *is one of the most important steps you can take to safeguard your health.*

Why is **The Omega Diet** so superior to other heart diets? The answer is that it attacks multiple targets. Most heart diets have one primary goal—lowering your cholesterol levels. But lowering your cholesterol is just one of a number of ways to protect your heart, and, surprisingly, it may not be the most important one. If all adults were to go on a cholesterol-lowering diet for the rest of their lives, life expectancy in the United States would increase by only three months for women and four months for men.[1] For ultimate protection, you need to reduce other risk factors as well.

For example, one risk factor of critical importance is your blood level of homocysteine, an amino acid that can injure the walls of your coronary arteries. High levels of homocysteine have been blamed for up to 30 percent of heart attacks and strokes in American men.[2] **The Omega Diet** reduces your homocysteine levels by increasing your intake of folic acid, a vitamin found in fruit, green leafy vegetables, and legumes. Fish, another key component of the plan, also lowers homocysteine levels.[3]

The diet protects your cardiovascular system in numerous other ways as well, including raising your antioxidant levels, reducing your risk of blood clots, and helping to normalize your blood pressure and heartbeat. To illustrate these multiple benefits, I'm going to describe the six steps in the genesis of a heart attack, from the first microscopic insult to your coronary arteries to the final beating of the heart. As I describe this deadly progression, I will highlight all the ways that **The Omega Diet** intervenes.

## Step #1: Minor Injury to the Wall of a Coronary Artery

For many people, the pain that heralds a heart attack seems to come out of nowhere. One minute they are tying their shoes or shoveling snow, and the next minute they are caught in the grip of a crushing pain; it is as if they were perfectly healthy one minute and knocking at death's door the next. In reality, most heart attacks are thirty or more years in the making. You may not realize that virtually all of this prolonged drama takes place in your coronary arteries, not your heart muscle. Your coronary arteries are the large vessels that deliver blood to your oxygen-hungry heart muscle. Although your heart is filled with blood, it gets all of its nourishment from the blood that flows through these vital arteries. If they become blocked, your heart muscle is starved for oxygen, triggering a heart attack.

The very first sign of coronary artery disease is minor damage to the lining of your artery walls. Some damage is unavoidable because it is caused by normal wear and tear as the blood flows through your vessels. Studies show that people as young as twenty show signs of this type of abrasion.[4] But some damage is preventable, such as that caused by high blood pressure. When you have high blood pressure, the blood flows through your vessels more forcefully, much the way that water jets out of a hose when you attach a high-pressure nozzle. The higher your blood pressure, the greater the potential damage to your arteries and the greater your risk of heart attack and stroke. A person with diastolic pressure above 105 has twice the normal risk of coronary events and nearly four times the risk of stroke. (See sidebar.)

---

### UNDERSTANDING YOUR BLOOD PRESSURE READING

Your blood pressure is expressed as two numbers, for example, "145/92." The top number, called your "systolic blood pressure," is the arterial pressure while your heart muscle is contracting. The bottom number, your "diastolic blood pressure," is the pressure when your heart is resting between beats. (These numbers are expressed in terms of millimeters of mercury, or mmHg.)

Normal blood pressure is around 120/80. Hypertension is commonly defined as having a number of consecutive blood pressure readings greater than 140/90.

---

The good news is that you can lower your blood pressure simply by choosing one type of salad oil over another. The main oils in **The Omega Diet**—olive oil and the omega-3 oils—have been medically proven to lower blood pressure. For example, studies show that taking daily fish oil supplements that contain as little as 3 grams of EPA and DHA can lower your systolic pressure by five points and your diastolic pressure by three points.[5] A shift of even this modest magnitude would reduce the number of Americans who fit the technical definition of "hypertensive" by 40 percent! LNA (the omega-3 fatty acid found in canola oil, walnut oil, and flaxseed oil) can also lower your blood pressure. A 1 percent increase in blood levels of LNA is linked with a 5 mm reduction in blood pressure.[6]

Even olive oil may help keep your blood pressure down. In a 1996 study, sixteen women with moderately high blood pressure agreed to switch to olive oil for a month. On average, their blood pressure dropped from 161/94 to 151/85 mmHg—almost a ten-point drop in both diastolic and systolic pressure.[7]

## HOW DO OMEGA-3 FATTY ACIDS LOWER YOUR BLOOD PRESSURE?

Your liver breaks down dietary fat into its individual fatty acids. These fatty acids are then converted into hormonelike substances called eicosanoids. Oils high in omega-6 fatty acids are converted into a type of eicosanoid called thromboxane $A_2$, which is a potent constrictor of your arteries. Constricted arteries force your heart to work harder to circulate blood throughout your body, contributing to "high blood pressure." Oils high in omega-3 fatty acids, on the other hand, are converted into a closely related eicosanoid called thromboxane $A_3$, which has a fraction of the potential to constrict your arteries.

In addition, new studies show that omega-3 fatty acids can increase production of an important chemical called "nitric oxide" that relaxes your arteries. In a recent study, men who were given fish oil supplements had a 43 percent increase in nitric oxide production.[8]

# Step #2: Reducing Your Risk of Arterial Inflammation

In addition to helping to prevent arterial damage, following **The Omega Diet** will make it less likely that your arteries will become inflamed, the second step in the genesis of a heart attack. Once an artery becomes damaged, it draws the attention of the body's repair crew, including platelets and white blood cells. These substances promote healing, but they can also cause clotting and inflammation. Preventing chronic inflammation is now believed to be just as effective in lowering your risk of heart attack and stroke as reducing your LDL (bad) cholesterol. A study published in 1997 in the *New Eng-*

*land Journal of Medicine* revealed that men with the highest levels of inflammation were three times as likely to have a heart attack and twice as likely to have a stroke as men with the lowest levels.[9]

The fact that aspirin helps reduce inflammation may be one of the reasons it is so protective against heart attacks. We now know that omega-3 fatty acids have similar anti-inflammatory properties. In fact, they function in much the same way as aspirin, although, unlike aspirin, they do not injure the sensitive stomach lining.[10] This is one of the reasons that fish is such a "heart-friendly" food. In a 1996 study, men who ate fatty fish on a regular basis were 42 percent less likely to die from a heart attack than men who did not eat fish.[11]

## Step #3: The Cholesterol Invasion

The third step in the decades-long buildup to a heart attack is the gradual accumulation of plaque inside your arteries. In the past, efforts to prevent this cholesterol buildup have focused on lowering blood levels of LDL cholesterol, the "bad" cholesterol that invades the arteries. Now that more is known about cardiovascular disease, the strategy has become more sophisticated—and effective. A critical insight is that LDL cholesterol is transported inside your arteries by being carried inside special white blood cells called "macrophages." But before the macrophages will engulf the cholesterol, the cholesterol must be damaged by a destructive process called oxidation. If you can keep your LDL cholesterol from being oxidized, therefore, it won't be picked up by the macrophages and carried inside your artery walls.

**The Omega Diet** slows the oxidation of your LDL cholesterol in two key ways. First, it fuels your body with monounsaturated oils such as olive oil and canola oil, which are naturally resistant to oxidation.[12] Second, it increases your intake of fruits and vegetables, raising your blood levels of antioxidants. Studies show that the more antioxidants in your bloodstream, the lower your risk of dying from cardiovascular disease.[13]

# Step 4: The Plaque Buildup

Now, we are about to enter step four in the genesis of a heart attack. In this fourth and critical step, significant amounts of oxidized cholesterol have begun to make inroads into your arteries. Having small amounts of plaque causes little harm. In fact, autopsies show that children as young as three years of age have "fatty streaks" in their arteries, the first visible signs of cholesterol invasion. The danger is in having a plaque deposit so large that it constricts or blocks a critical coronary artery. The more LDL cholesterol you have in your bloodstream, the more raw material is available for oxidation, and the greater the chances this will happen. A total cholesterol count below 200 is considered normal. If your count rises to 250, you have twice the normal risk of coronary artery disease. If it climbs to 300, your risk doubles again. If it's 350 and beyond, you have *eight* times the normal risk of having diseased and constricted arteries.[14]

Fortunately, your body has a built-in way to keep your LDL levels in check—a squadron of HDL cholesterol. HDL cholesterol is shaped like a deflated football. As it circulates through your bloodstream, it scoops up LDL cholesterol, gradually filling its pouch. It then transports the LDL to your liver, where it is grabbed by special "LDL" receptors on your liver cells, drawn into the cells, and degraded into less harmful substances. The more HDL you have on your team, the less oxidized LDL you have in your arteries.

## THE OLIVE OIL BONUS

Olive oil gives you an added bonus—it contains a substance called "squalene" (SKWAY-lean) that lowers cholesterol. In a recent study, patients who took squalene supplements for five months had a 22 percent decline in their LDL cholesterol.[15]

One of the reasons that **The Omega Diet** is so protective against heart disease is that it is based on monounsaturated oils, oils that have been proven to lower your LDL cholesterol while they maintain or even *raise* your HDL levels, the best of both worlds.[16] No other fats have this effect. Saturated fats, it has long been known, raise your LDL cholesterol. Trans-fatty acids raise your LDL cholesterol at the same time that they lower your HDL (good) cholesterol, pushing both of these blood fats in the wrong direction. (A Boston research team found that people with the highest levels of trans-fatty acids in their diet had two and a half times the risk of heart attack as those who ate the least amount of this artificial fat.[17]) Omega-6 oils lower your LDL cholesterol, but at the same time they can also lower your heart-protective HDL cholesterol.

Surprisingly, you can also upset your body's cholesterol balancing act by eating a low-fat, high-carbohydrate diet. As is true for omega-6 oils, this type of diet lowers your LDL *and* your HDL cholesterol, throwing out the baby with the bathwater. This is yet another example of how our current antifat craze is off the mark.[18] Instead of eating low fat or no fat, we need to focus on eating a moderate amount of *healthy* fat.

---

**WHAT DOES YOUR CHOLESTEROL COUNT TELL YOU ABOUT YOUR RISK OF CARDIOVASCULAR DISEASE?**

A reliable predictor of your risk of heart disease is the ratio of your total cholesterol (TC) to your HDL cholesterol, abbreviated as "TC/HDL." To find out your ratio, divide your total cholesterol count by your HDL count. The lower the number the better. If, for example, your total cholesterol count is 200 and your HDL is 50, your TC/HDL ratio is 200/50, or 4, which is about average. Ideally, you want the number to be 3.5 or lower.

---

# Step 5: The Blockage of the Coronary Artery

Let's suppose that all has gone awry and now you're at step five in this grim drama. Due to smoking, age, genetics, an unhealthy diet, a sedentary lifestyle, or, more likely, some combination of these factors, your coronary arteries have become so choked with plaque that they are squeezing off the blood supply to your heart. A deadly process that began decades ago has now reached critical mass. All that is needed for an actual heart attack to begin is for a blood clot to close off an already constricted artery, blocking the life-giving flow of blood.

Typically, an artery becomes blocked following the sudden rupture of a large area of plaque. A plaque deposit is most likely to rupture if it is large, chronically inflamed, and separated from the bloodstream by only a thin cap of tissue. Once the plaque bursts, it spews its debris into the bloodstream and triggers the formation of blood clots. Within seconds, a clot and other debris can be swept along in the current and become wedged in a coronary artery. A significant area of your heart is suddenly deprived of oxygenated blood, causing a potentially deadly heart attack.

As you can well imagine, one of the primary goals in the prevention of heart attack and stroke is to keep blood clots from blocking a critical artery. This is why people at high risk for these problems are given aspirin or more potent blood-thinning agents. A key discovery made in the early 1970s is that omega-3 fatty acids also slow the formation of blood clots. We owe this insight to two Danish researchers, H. O. Bang and Jorn Dyerberg, who became intrigued by the traditional Eskimo diet—sufficiently intrigued, in fact, to lead a twenty-team dogsled expedition to northern Greenland. Bang and Dyerberg observed that Eskimos who were eating their traditional diet of fish and marine mammals had an extremely low rate of cardiac death. In fact, when they reviewed ten years of health records at a Greenland hospital serving 2,000 people, they found not a single death caused by a heart attack. Eventually, Bang and Dyerberg were able to show that one of the primary reasons for the healthy hearts of the Eskimos was that their diet was high in omega-3 fatty acids, which, among other benefits, slowed the formation of blood clots. When Bang and Dyerberg published their findings, they made the following prophecy: "We believe that [eating more omega-3 fatty acids] could be as effective in the prevention of cardiovascular disease as the large-scale use of drugs."[19] A prophecy that **The Omega Diet** may help fulfill.

## HOW DO OMEGA-3 FATTY ACIDS
## KEEP BLOOD CLOTS FROM FORMING?

A blood clot can be likened to a creation of papier-mâché. The "glue" is provided by your blood platelets, and the shredded newspaper is provided by "fibrinogen," long strands of protein that circulate in your bloodstream. Under certain conditions, the fibrinogen becomes entangled with the platelets and other elements, resulting in a thrombus, or clot. A recent survey showed that people with high levels of fibrinogen had five times the normal risk of heart attack, recurrent heart attack, and premature death.

Omega-3 oils keep unwanted clots from forming in two ways. First, they make your platelets less "gluey," making it less likely they will stick together. Second, they decrease the production of fibrinogen.[20] The end result is a greatly reduced risk of a heart attack.

# Stage #6 : A Chaotic Heartbeat

Heart attacks are traumatic events, but they are not always lethal: You have a three out of five chance of surviving the ordeal. Whether you live or die depends to a large degree on how your heart responds to the trauma. If it begins to beat uncontrollably, an all-too-common response called "malignant arrhythmia" or ventricular arrhythmia, your chances of survival are slim. A wildly quivering heart no longer functions as an effective pump, shutting off circulation to your entire body, not just your heart. Of all your organs, your brain is most vulnerable to the lack of blood. If the blood flow to your brain is cut off for as little as four minutes, the probable outcome is either severe brain damage or death.

**The Omega Diet** helps block this sixth and most lethal step in the development of a heart attack by helping to stabilize your heartbeat. The fact that omega-3 fatty acids help prevent arrhythmia was first shown in animal studies conducted in the 1980s. In one of these experiments, eight lab animals were subjected to conditions that mimic a heart attack. All eight of the animals promptly developed arrhythmias that would have killed them had the experiment been allowed to continue. The experiment was repeated once again using a different group of animals that had been given an infusion of fish oil a mere sixty minutes prior to the test. The omega-3 fatty acids completely abolished the arrhythmia in seven out of eight animals, while the eighth animal had a mild, non-life-threatening event.[21]

Because omega-3 fatty acids have the potential to block all six steps leading up to a heart attack, including the two most deadly steps—final blockage of the coronary artery and arrhythmia —they can even save the lives of people with advanced coronary artery disease. Proof comes from the Lyon Diet Heart Study described in chapter one and also from an influential English study known as the Diet and Reinfarction Trial (DART).[22] The participants in the 1989 DART study were 2,000 men who were recovering from recent heart attacks. The men were assigned to one of three quite different diets: (1) a high-fiber diet; (2) a diet low in saturated fat and relatively high in omega-6 oils (the standard heart diet); and (3) a diet high in omega-3 fatty acids, either from fatty fish or omega-3 supplements. Relative to the other two groups, the patients who had enriched their diets with omega-3 fatty acids had a 29 percent lower death rate, which at that time was the greatest reduction of mortality of any heart diet.

As you have seen, **The Omega Diet**—with its rich supply of natural antioxidants, monounsaturated fatty acids, and omega-3 fatty acids, coupled with its low levels of saturated fat, omega-6 fatty acids, and trans-fatty acids—is the ideal prescription for cardiac health.

This chart summarizes how various fats and oils influence your cardiovascular system. The oils featured in **The Omega Diet** are in the bottom two rows.

| TYPE OF FAT | HDL (good) Cholesterol | LDL (bad) Cholesterol | Blood Pressure | Risk of Blood Clots | Oxidation of LDL Cholesterol |
|---|---|---|---|---|---|
| **Saturated Fat** Fatty meat, butter, eggs, cheese, and whole milk products. | Does not lower and may raise ☺ | Raises ☹ | May raise 😐 | May increase 😐 | Does not change 😐 |
| **Trans-Fat** Margarine, shortening, deep-fat-fried food, plus commercial pastries, snacks. | Lowers ☹ | Raises ☹ | Effect unknown ? | Does not change 😐 | Effect unknown ? |
| **Omega-6 Oils** Oils high in omega-6 fatty acids, including corn, safflower, and sunflower oil. | Lowers ☹ | Lowers ☺ | May increase ☹ | May increase ☹ | Increases ☹ |
| **Monounsaturated Oils** Olive oil, canola oil, *high oleic* safflower or *high oleic* sunflower oil. | May raise ☺ | Lowers ☺ | May lower ☺ | Does not change* 😐 | Decreases ☺ |
| **Omega-3 Oils** Fish oil, canola oil, and flaxseed oil. | May raise ☺ | May lower or slightly increase** 😐 | Lowers ☺ | Lowers ☺ | Does not change*** 😐 |

*Olive oil can decrease the risk of blood clots because it contains squalene, a substance that has anticlotting properties and can also lower cholesterol.

**Omega-3 fatty acids will lower LDL cholesterol when they replace saturated fat.

***A tendency toward oxidation can be eliminated if the diet is high in natural antioxidants. If the diet is supplemented with fish oil, however, antioxidant supplements, especially vitamin E, may be needed as well.

## The Bottom Line

• Before a heart attack or stroke can occur, a number of changes have to take place within your cardiovascular system. Some of the changes are set in motion in your twenties or thirties. The more changes you can prevent, the lower your risk of a heart attack or stroke.

• **The Omega Diet** protects your cardiovascular system in a number of ways. Specifically, it has the potential to:
  • Protect your artery linings, by reducing levels of homocysteine and blocking inflammation.
  • Help maintain normal blood pressure.
  • Lower your bad cholesterol without robbing you of your good cholesterol.
  • Slow the oxidation of LDL cholesterol.
  • Inhibit the buildup of large areas of plaque.
  • Slow the formation of blood clots.
  • Stabilize your heartbeat.

# SIX

# Taming the Savage Cell

## *Fighting Cancer with **The Omega Diet***

CARDIOVASCULAR DISEASE may be the most common killer in the world, but for many people, cancer is the more dreaded disease. When you have cardiovascular disease, you have the unhappy knowledge that your body is failing you—your arteries are clogged, your blood pressure is too high, or your cholesterol count is a cause for concern. But when you have cancer, you have to struggle with the chilling awareness that your own cells have turned against you. They have stopped responding to the instructions coded in their genes and begun transforming their energy into rampant growth.

By and large, our efforts to tame the savage cell have proven disappointing. Since 1971, the federal government has spent $30 billion on the War on Cancer. Nonetheless, the overall incidence of cancer has increased by 18 percent and the cancer death rate has risen by 6 percent.[1] Given our population increase, this means that twice as many people will be diagnosed with cancer compared with a similar time period in the 1970s, and twice as many will die. Men have a one in two chance of having cancer sometime in their lives, partly due to the high rate of lung cancer and prostate cancer in older men. Meanwhile, American women have the world's highest death rates from lung and bronchial cancer. Cancers that are more common today than they were twenty years ago include breast cancer, prostate cancer, pancreatic cancer, melanoma, liver cancer, multiple myeloma, brain cancer, non-Hodgkin's lymphoma, esophageal cancer, and chronic leukemia.

One reason we have been making so little headway is that too little effort has gone into cancer prevention. Tens of billions of dollars have been devoted to finding a cure for cancer, but a fraction of that amount has been earmarked for keeping the disease at bay. Recent discoveries about the cancer-fighting properties of fruits, vegetables, and omega-3 fatty acids may turn this around. This chapter presents a wealth of new evidence showing that following The Seven Dietary Guidelines of **The Omega Diet** may greatly lower your risk of this dreaded disease.

## Eat Your Fruits and Vegetables

A guaranteed way to lower your risk of cancer is to eat more fruits and vegetables. To date, the anticancer properties of these wholesome foods have been documented in more than 200 separate studies.[2] Taken as a whole, these studies show that if you are in the top quarter in the consumption of fruits and vegetables, you have half the usual risk of contracting cancer.

Antioxidant vitamins provide some of the cancer-fighting prowess of fruits and vegetables, but phytochemicals play just as big a role. We are now learning that the same chemicals that protect plants from viruses, bacteria, and fungi protect us from cancer. For example, people who drink green tea, which contains a phytochemical called "epigallocatechin gallate," have a lower risk of liver, lung, skin, esophageal, and urinary cancer. People who eat large amounts of cooked tomatoes, which are rich in the cancer-fighting chemical "lycopene," have a lower risk of prostate, cervical, breast, and colon cancer. Eating broccoli, cabbage and other members of the cole family offers protection against a broad array of cancers.

The fact that the phytochemicals in fruits and vegetables are potent anticancer agents helps explain why cancer studies involving vitamin supplements have had such lackluster results: The pills contain only a fraction of what the plants have to offer. Until researchers can identify and encapsulate all the myriad healing substances found in plants, it is far wiser to eat the whole foods themselves. This way, you will be getting all their known cancer-fighting nutrients—plus all those yet to be identified. On **The Omega Diet**, you will be eating seven or more servings of fruits and vegetables a day, helping to build a nutritional barrier against cancer.

---

**Cancer-Fighting Plants**

The following list shows which fruits and vegetables are thought to be most protective against specific types of cancer.

| Cancer | Type of Fruit or Vegetable |
| --- | --- |
| esophageal cancer | fruits and vegetables in general, green tea, asparagus, and mushrooms |
| prostate cancer | tomato sauce, soy products, fruits in general |
| breast cancer | asparagus, mushrooms, flaxseeds, soy products, green tea, and tomato sauce |
| lung cancer | apples, yellow and orange fruits and vegetables, cruciferous vegetables (cauliflower, broccoli, brussels sprouts), and green tea |
| cancer of the larynx | fruits and vegetables in general |
| stomach cancer | legumes, green tea, yellow and orange vegetables |
| pancreas | legumes, fruits in general |
| colon (colorectal) cancer | apples, cumin, turmeric, garlic, tomato sauce, and beans |
| bladder cancer | green and black teas, citrus fruits, cumin, fruits, garlic |
| cervical cancer | tomato sauce |
| liver cancer | green and black teas, asparagus, mushrooms, and fruits in general |
| skin cancer | green tea |

*(See page 135 for information about the phytochemical content of various fruits and vegetables.)*

---

# Eat Healthy Fats

As protective as fruits and vegetables may be, however, eating the right fats may be even more effective in fighting cancer. For decades, there has been a growing suspicion that there is a link between dietary fat and cancer, but the exact connection has been ambiguous. Some studies have shown that eating a high-fat diet increases the risk of cancer, but others have shown no connection. The source of the confusion is now becoming clear: Different fats have different effects on tumor growth. As a rule, fats high in omega-6 fatty acids promote malignant growth while fats high in omega-3 fatty acids block it. Thus, a given fat will either increase or decrease your risk of cancer depending on its fatty acid content. Ultimately, it's the *type* of fat that matters, not the amount.

This medical truth was demonstrated in a recent South African survey.[3] A research team compared the rate of colon cancer in a group of people living in a fishing village with the rate in a similar group of people living in urban Cape Town. They found that the city dwellers had six times the rate of this deadly disease. At first, this didn't make sense to the researchers because the Cape Town inhabitants seemed to have the *healthier* diet. They were eating twice as many fruits and vegetables as those living in the fishing village, for example, and their diet was richer in the very nutrients known to protect against colon cancer—fiber, calcium, and antioxidants. Lab tests provided the missing clue: The people living in the coastal village had three times more omega-3 fatty acids in their blood (primarily from the high amount of fish in their diet) and considerably less omega-6 fatty acids, giving them the ratio of essential fatty acids now proving to be highly protective against cancer. Following **The Omega Diet** will give you this same cancer-fighting balance.

## *What Tumors Like to Eat*

Researchers have been exploring the link between individual fatty acids and cancer for about twenty years.[4,5] Two people who are now pushing the frontier are Leonard A. Sauer and Robert T. Dauchy from the Cancer Research Laboratory at the Mary Imogene Bassett Hospital. Their work suggests that the American diet is a prescription for tumor growth.

Sauer and Dauchy gathered this disturbing information while trying to solve a medical mystery: They had observed that tumors grew much faster in rats that had been denied food. This was puzzling. Logically, they assumed that taking the food away from the rodents would *slow* the tumor growth. But they were stunned to see that some types of tumors would grow *four* times as fast in food-deprived rats, such an accelerated rate of growth that the researchers could actually see a visible difference in tumor size from day to day. When the rats were fed once again, the runaway tumor growth would come to a halt. In a matter of hours, the tumors would be growing at their former, stately pace. For some inexplicable reason, the tumors were better fed when the rats were starving.

Sauer and Dauchy managed to solve the puzzle. When a rat is denied food, they discovered, its body senses that a famine is under way and sends out a biochemical cry of alarm. This SOS releases fatty acids from the animal's fat stores and sends them into the bloodstream. Within half a day, the rat's blood contains five times as much fat as when the animal is freely fed. As this fat-laden blood filters through the tumor, the tumor hoards as much as half of the fatty acids for its personal use—a bonanza of nutrients that quadruples its growth. Returning food to the rat silences the internal alarm and stops the emergency forays into the fat stores. Once again, the tumor must be content with the leaner ration supplied by the regular laboratory chow, resulting in a slower rate of growth.[6]

As is often the case in science, however, answering this one question posed a number of others. Next Sauer and Dauchy wanted to know if all fatty acids had the same effect on tumor growth. This was more than an academic question. If they found that some fatty acids promote tumor growth and others do not, then it might be possible to prevent or even treat cancer by eating a specific balance of fats. To find out, they perfected a sophisticated technique that allowed them to infuse tumors growing in living animals with blood that had been mixed with known amounts of individual fatty acids. They found that the tumors responded to the fatty acids in dramatically different ways. When the tumors were infused with omega-3 fatty acids, their growth rate was greatly slowed; it was as if they had been given fat-free blood. But when the tumors were infused with omega-6 fatty acids, they were jolted into hyperdrive. Sauer and Dauchy found that the entire family of omega-6 fatty acids promote tumor growth, but linoleic acid, the "parent" fatty acid, is by far the most potent. Even a trace amount of linoleic acid makes tumors grow faster, and the more that is added, the faster they grow. Linoleic acid seems to be the preferred diet of malignant tumors.

As Sauer and Dauchy were solving their medical mystery, other cancer researchers were pursuing the same trail of evidence. The findings have been surprisingly consistent. In virtually every experiment in every research institution, feeding lab animals linoleic acid has made their tumors grow faster and become more aggressive,[7] while feeding them omega-3 fatty acids has slowed their tumor growth and made it less likely that the cancer would spread.[8]

But do fatty acids have the same influence on human cancers? Dietary surveys and tissue studies suggest that they do. In addition to the South African study already mentioned, fourteen human studies have linked omega-6 fatty acids with a higher risk of cancer and omega-3 fatty acids with a lower risk.[9] One of the consequences of our misguided efforts to add more omega-6 oils to the Western diet may have been a much higher rate of cancer.

# Evidence from Small Clinical Studies

Showing a statistical link between fatty acids and cancer, however, does not *prove* that eating certain fatty acids makes it more or less likely that you will succumb to the deadly disease. That proof must come from clinical trials. Regrettably, to date no one has conducted a large cancer study to test this hypothesis, largely due to a lack of funding. (Fatty acids are natural substances and therefore cannot be patented, greatly limiting the money available for research from industry.) A number of small studies have been conducted, though, and the results have been very promising. Three different groups have shown that omega-3 supplements can reduce the risk of colon cancer. In a study that took place in Italy, a group of patients with precancerous colon polyps were given low daily doses of omega-3 supplements. In just two weeks, there was less proliferation of cells. The therapy was well tolerated and without negative side effects. The investigators concluded: "Fish oil appears to exert a rapid effect that may protect high-risk subjects from colon cancer."[10] In 1996,

Harvard Medical School researchers conducted a similar study that confirmed these results. According to the Harvard scientists, "The fish oil supplement was well tolerated by study participants. There were no side effects, and no additional polyps were found in [any of] the patients who completed 12 months of supplementation. . . . These cases suggest that [omega-3] fatty acids may be useful chemo-preventive agents."[11]

---

### HOW DO OMEGA-3 FATTY ACIDS FIGHT CANCER?

There are a number of theories to explain how omega-3 fatty acids fight cancer. First, it has been shown that omega-3 fatty acids reduce the amount of linoleic acid that tumors withdraw from the bloodstream, denying them a much-needed nutrient. Blunting the cancer-promoting effects of linoleic acid in this manner is known as "competitive uptake."[12]

Second, omega-3 fatty acids compete with omega-6 fatty acids for enzymes that are needed for the creation of cancer-promoting metabolites.

Third, omega-3 fatty acids make cancer cells more vulnerable to free-radical attack by making their membranes less saturated. A cancer cell will die if it sustains sufficient free-radical damage.[13]

Finally, new research suggests that linoleic acid may help make cancer cells immortal by turning on a gene that prevents automatic cell death. By contrast, omega-3 fatty acids seem to *promote* the self-destruction of cancer cells, increasing their rate of die-off and thereby slowing overall tumor growth.[14]

---

## Heading Cancer Off at the Pass

Therapies that prevent existing tumors from spreading are critical to cancer therapy because most people die from tumors that colonize new areas of the body, not ones that remain in one place. It is very encouraging, therefore, that there is new evidence that omega-3 fatty acids might slow the rate of metastasis. Recently, a group of French researchers monitored 120 breast cancer patients for a period of three years. They found that women with low amounts of LNA in the fatty tissue surrounding their breasts were five times as likely to develop metastatic disease. This one factor alone was a better predictor of metastasis than all the other traditional risk factors. The researchers concluded: "These data . . . stress the need for a close evaluation of the dietary intake of this essential fatty acid."[15]

Lillian Thompson, a cancer researcher from the University of Toronto, has gone one step further and developed a pilot study to *treat* breast cancer patients with LNA. In an ongoing pilot study, she is giving flaxseeds to women recently diagnosed with the disease. (Flaxseeds are one of the richest sources of LNA.) She hopes to see a measurable reduction in tumor size in the short time between diagnosis and surgery.[16] Thompson stresses that there is no clinical proof that flaxseeds will prove effective against breast cancer. "We don't have the data yet. All that we know is that flaxseeds reduce cancer risk in animals."[17]

## HOW DO OMEGA-3 FATTY ACIDS KEEP CANCER FROM SPREADING?

In order for a cancer cell to migrate from the original tumor to form a distant colony, it must adhere to and then penetrate tough membranes called "basement membranes" that surround blood vessels and organs.

Omega-3 fatty acids make it harder for cancer cells to cling to basement membranes by blocking the expression of molecules on the cells' surface (adhesion molecules) that provide the necessary "grappling hooks."[18]

If cancer cells manage to attach themselves to the membranes, omega-3 fatty acids can interfere with the next step as well by blocking the production of an enzyme called "collagenase" that is needed to dissolve basement membranes and allow the cancer cells to penetrate the barrier.[19]

# Using Omega-3 Fatty Acids to Prevent Cancer and Boost Traditional Cancer Therapies

As you can see, there is growing evidence that enriching your diet with omega-3 fatty acids may be one of the keys to cancer prevention. Dr. S. Roy MacKintosh, an oncologist and professor of internal medicine at the University of Nevada, believes that these nutrients might reduce the risk of prostate cancer in men who show an early warning sign of the disease—a high score on a test for "prostate specific antigen," or PSA. According to MacKintosh, "There are a lot of men with an elevated PSA, but they don't have any symptoms and there is no accepted treatment. Giving them omega-3 supplements would be fairly non-toxic and inexpensive, and it just might reduce their risk."[20]

It is unlikely, however, that taking omega-3 fatty acids will cure an advanced form of cancer. Once cancer takes hold, more aggressive therapy is needed. But it might be possible for omega-3 fatty acids to *augment* traditional cancer therapy. In the words of Wayne B. Jonas, director of the Office of Alternative Medicine at NIH, "Whereas conventional medicine and patients often seek simple cures for chronic diseases, it is usually not magic bullets, but rather combination approaches that prove most useful."[21]

One appealing strategy would be to give omega-3 fatty acids to cancer patients who are about to undergo surgery, a combination therapy that has proven to be successful in rodents. In a 1996 animal study, David P. Rose and Jeanne M. Connolly from the American Health Foundation in Valhalla, New York, implanted human breast cancer cells into rodents. (This is the closest one can come to an actual human experiment.) They found that giving the animals a diet high in omega-3 fatty acids (EPA or DHA) before surgically removing the tumors slowed the eventual spread of the cancer. The more of these nutrients in the diet, the smaller the volume of the metastatic tumors.[22]

It is within the realm of reason that cancer patients who add more EPA and DHA to their diets prior to surgery will reap the same reward. During cancer surgery, cancer cells can be dislodged from the main tumor and spread throughout the circulatory system. If those cells are fortified with EPA and DHA, they may grow more slowly and be less able to establish themselves and colonize new areas of the body.

There is already good evidence that omega-3 fatty acids can help cancer patients recover from surgery. In a 1996 study, cancer patients recovering from major gastrointestinal surgery were given omega-3 supplements. The patients given the supplements fared much better than ones given the standard postoperative treatment. They had fewer digestion problems, more normal liver and kidney function, lower triglycerides, and a 50 percent reduction in the number of postoperative infections. Said a member of the research team, "Clearly, the [omega-3] group had all parameters shifted to a more favorable direction."[23]

Of all the possible ways that omega-3 fatty acids might augment traditional therapies, the most exciting may be its potential to enhance the effectiveness of chemotherapy and radiation. Ronald S. Pardini and coworkers at the Allie M. Lee Laboratory for Cancer Research at the University of Nevada have found that placing mice on a fish oil diet makes treatment with a common chemotherapy agent called "mitomycin C" ten times more effective. When mice were implanted with human breast cancer tissue, the tumors grew much larger in animals fed corn oil alone. (See the accompanying graph.) Mice fed the same amount of corn oil but with fish oil added to their diets had significantly smaller tumors. When the animals were then treated with mitomycin C, the ones on the fish-oil-supplemented diet had a tenfold greater response. As you can see, their tumors became almost undetectable.[24]

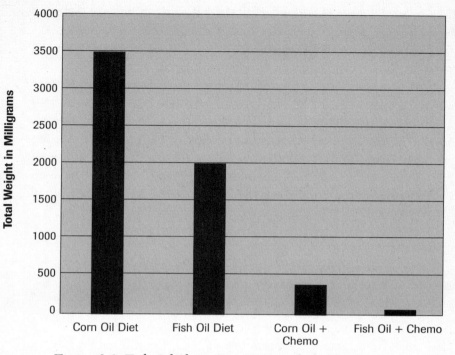

Figure 6-1. Fish Oil Slows Tumor Growth and Makes
Chemotherapy More Effective

This chart shows that omega-3 fatty acids can make chemotherapy much more
effective. The bar on the left represents the size of human breast tumors in animals
fed a 5 percent corn oil diet. The next bar shows the much smaller tumor size in
mice whose diet was also supplemented with high amounts of fish oil. The fourth
and final bar (barely visible) shows that when chemotherapy was combined with a
fish oil diet, the tumors were almost undetectable.[25]

In these animal experiments, omega-3 fatty acids do more than
make chemotherapy more effective; they also reduce its toxicity.
When Pardini and his colleagues saw the spectacular results from
the above experiment, they decided to see if these cancer-fighting
nutrients could also buffer the toxic effects of chemotherapy. To find
out, they treated mice with a common cancer drug (cyclophos-
phamide) in a dose equivalent to that given to cancer patients.
Within sixty days, 50 percent of the mice on a 5 percent corn oil diet
had died from drug toxicity, but there were no deaths in the fish

oil group.[26] "You start adding up all that omega-3 fatty acids might do for a cancer patient," says Pardini," and it becomes astounding. Yet the current protocol for physicians is to put their cancer patients on low-fat diets. And nobody cares what *kind* of fat."[27]

Meanwhile, Pardini and MacKintosh (both from the University of Nevada) are discussing plans to treat prostate cancer patients with a combination of fish oil and chemotherapy. According to MacKintosh, "At the present time, only 25 percent of the men with prostate cancer benefit from chemotherapy. We're hoping that adding fish oil will increase those odds. The combined therapy appears to have no added risks, and if it enhances the effectiveness, it will be very good news, indeed."[28]

---

### HOW DO OMEGA-3 FATTY ACIDS ENHANCE RADIATION AND CHEMOTHERAPY?

Radiation and some types of chemotherapy kill cancer cells by generating large bursts of free radicals (highly reactive molecules) that attack the cells' membranes. Once a membrane sustains enough damage, the cell will self-destruct. Omega-3 fatty acids make cell membranes more vulnerable to free-radical attack, thereby enhancing the effects of both chemotherapy and radiation.[29]

---

# Omega-3 Fatty Acids Block Wasting Syndrome

Meanwhile, researchers from Aston University in Birmingham, England, have begun to use omega-3 fatty acids to treat cancer patients suffering from "cachexia" (ka-KEX-see-a), the rapid weight loss, or "wasting syndrome," that afflicts half of all cancer patients. The lead researcher, Michael Tisdale, reports that cachexia causes an estimated 10 to 25 percent of all cancer deaths. When two patients have the same type of tumor, but one has cachexia and the other does not, the one with cachexia lives half as long.[30] Tisdale believes that finding a treatment for this debilitating condition would improve the quality of life of many cancer patients and extend their survival. His group may be closing in on a treatment. A colleague has given EPA to a small number of cancer patients with cachexia. Before starting the study, the patients were losing an average of six and a half pounds a month. Three months later, they were *gaining* more than half a pound a month.[31] Additional studies are under way.

It may be years, if not decades, before "omega-3 therapy" becomes an accepted part of cancer prevention and treatment, but you can take advantage of the new research right now simply by following **The Omega Diet.** By following The Seven Dietary Guidelines you will:

1. Reduce your intake of cancer-promoting omega-6 fatty acids.
2. Increase your consumption of cancer-fighting omega-3 fatty acids.
3. Gain the added protection of the antioxidants and phytochemicals found in fruits and vegetables.

The fact that that these dietary changes also offer you the highest possible level of protection against heart disease is all the more reason you will want to adopt this program for life.

| Effect on Cancer | Omega-6 Fatty Acids (Corn oil, safflower oil, sunflower seed oil, soy oil) | Omega-3 Fatty Acids (Fish, canola oil, flaxseeds and flaxseed oil, walnuts, walnut oil, green leafy vegetables.) |
|---|---|---|
| Growth rate of precancerous cells | Enhances ☹ | Inhibits ☺ |
| Initiation of new tumors | Enhances ☹ | Inhibits ☺ |
| Rate of tumor growth | Enhances ☹ | Inhibits ☺ |
| Spread of tumors | Enhances ☹ | Inhibits ☺ |
| Cachexia (weight loss) | ? | Inhibits ☺ |
| Chemotherapy | ? | Enhances ☺ |
| Recovery from surgery | ? | Enhances ☺ |

## The Bottom Line

- More than two hundred studies have shown that eating high amounts of fruits and vegetables lowers your risk of cancer.
- Animal studies show that oils high in omega-6 fatty acids, especially linoleic acid, speed the growth of malignant tumors and make them more aggressive.
- By contrast, omega-3 fatty acids (DHA, EPA, and LNA) *delay* the appearance of tumors in animals, make them grow more slowly, and reduce the risk of metastasis.
- At least fifteen studies show that a diet such as **The Omega Diet** that is lower in omega-6 fatty acids and relatively higher in omega-3 fatty acids than the prudent or average American diet reduces the risk of cancer.
- Several pilot studies have shown that omega-3 fatty acid supplements can decrease excessive cell growth in people with colon cancer or who have early signs of the disease.
- Flaxseeds, a rich source of omega-3 fatty acids (LNA), are now being tested as a possible addition to breast cancer therapy.
- Animal studies show that omega-3 fatty acids increase the effectiveness of a number of traditional cancer therapies, including surgery and chemotherapy.

# SEVEN

# Defeating Syndrome-X, Obesity, and Diabetes

## How The Omega Diet Normalizes Your Metabolism

MILLIONS OF PEOPLE in this country have been struggling to lose weight by adopting a low-fat, high-carbohydrate diet. A more effective strategy, we are learning, is to eat a moderate-fat diet based on monounsaturated and omega-3 oils. Such a diet lowers your risk of obesity at the same time that it protects against other metabolic disorders such as diabetes.

To understand why this is so, you need to understand a medical condition called "insulin resistance." The main job of insulin is to regulate your blood glucose, or "blood sugar." This is an essential function. If your blood glucose rises too high, you are at risk for dehydration, coma, and—in extreme cases—even death. If it drops too low, your brain is denied its primary nutrient and, once again, you face coma and death. If you have a healthy metabolic system, your glucose levels will stay within normal limits. Here's how it works. When you eat a meal, your blood sugar rises, which prompts your pancreas to release insulin into your bloodstream. Insulin sends a signal to your muscle cells that they need to take up the excess sugar. Your muscle cells either use the glucose as an energy source or store it in a slightly altered form called "glycogen" (GLY-ko-jin).

When you haven't eaten for several hours, your blood sugar starts to fall. To restore equilibrium, your pancreas pumps out a complementary hormone called "glucagon" (GLUE-ka-gone) that converts the glycogen back into glucose (or forms new glucose from protein) and then sends it back into your bloodstream. If all goes well, your pancreas produces just enough of these hormones at just the right time to keep your blood glucose within optimal levels. The system should work even if you skip a meal or eat a "lunch" that consists of three glazed doughnuts and a can of sugary soda.

Unfortunately, the system malfunctions in a large segment of the population. The most common problem is "insulin resistance," which occurs when the muscle cells do not respond adequately to insulin. As a result, normal amounts of the hormone fail to produce the desired drop in glucose levels. In other words, the muscle cells "resist" the hormonal cue. The pancreas senses that glucose levels are still high and releases more insulin. Eventually, the muscle cells respond, but it takes an excessive amount of the hormone to get the job done. As a result, you have abnormally high insulin levels, even while fasting.

Large numbers of Americans are believed to be insulin resistant, including everyone who is obese, diabetic, or has high blood pressure. In addition, this disorder plagues 25 percent of the people without these conditions. All told, as many as half of the adults in this country may suffer from some degree of insulin resistance.

## Syndrome-X

One problem with insulin resistance is that it often comes bundled with a cluster of other worrisome health problems, including high blood pressure, high LDL (bad) cholesterol, low HDL (good) cholesterol, and high triglycerides. A person with this particular set of conditions is said to have "Syndrome-X," a term coined by Stanford researcher Gerald Reaven to describe this all-too-common phenomenon.

## THE COMPONENTS OF SYNDROME-X

- Insulin resistance
- Hyperinsulinemia (high fasting insulin levels)
- High blood pressure
- Glucose intolerance
- Low HDL (good) cholesterol
- Increased very low density lipoprotein (VLDL) triglycerides

No one can say for sure that insulin resistance causes Syndrome-X, but there is solid evidence that it precedes it. For example, an eight-year study of over a thousand people found that those who began the study with signs of insulin resistance (determined by having high fasting insulin levels) were more likely to develop Syndrome-X by study's end.[1] Another study revealed that children whose parents had high blood pressure showed signs of insulin resistance years before they had weight problems or developed high blood pressure, again suggesting that insulin resistance might be a causal factor.

People with Syndrome-X are at greater risk for a number of deadly diseases. For example, a person who has high blood pressure, low HDL, high LDL, and high triglycerides is much more susceptible to coronary artery disease. A person with hyperinsulinemia is more likely to develop "adult-onset diabetes" (Non-Insulin Dependent Diabetes Mellitus, or NIDDM, also known as "Type-II" diabetes).[2,3] Thus, the inability of the muscle cells to respond normally to insulin is associated with a complex set of metabolic disorders, which, in turn, increase the risk of life-threatening disease.

# Foods That Can
# Trigger Insulin Resistance

As is true for many conditions, whether or not you become insulin resistant is greatly influenced by your genes. If close family members are obese or have hypertension, coronary artery disease, or diabetes, you are more likely to develop this disorder. But you can increase or

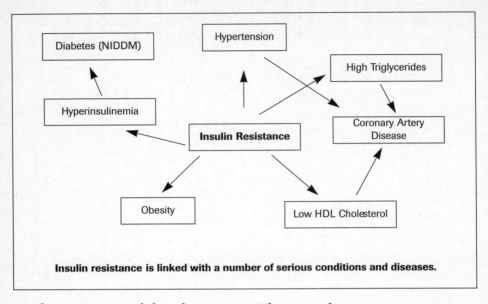

**Insulin resistance is linked with a number of serious conditions and diseases.**

decrease your risk by what you eat. There are three proven ways to *increase* the chances you will be afflicted with this disorder: (1) eat a diet high in refined carbohydrates; (2) eat a diet that is low in omega-3 fatty acids and high in omega-6 fatty acids; and (3) eat food that is high in saturated and trans-fatty acids. Living in the United States, it is easy to have all three strikes against you. Tens of millions of people in this country eat high amounts of refined carbohydrates such as candy, pastry, doughnuts, soda, white rice, and white flour. In addition, their diet has a high ratio of omega-6 to omega-3 fatty acids because they eat little fatty fish or dark green leafy vegetables and use omega-6 oils for cooking and salad dressings. Finally, they eat high amounts of trans-fatty acids and saturated fat due to their reliance on fast food and convenience food. The current food supply provides the perfect environment to foster insulin resistance—especially if you have an inherited predisposition.

# *Refined Carbohydrates and Insulin Resistance*

One of the reasons that eating a diet of simple sugars and refined carbohydrates can lead to insulin resistance is that these foods have a "high-glycemic index." This means that they cause a spike in your blood sugar level, forcing your pancreas to counterattack with a surge of insulin. If you persist in eating this type of diet, your pancreas has to pump out more and more insulin. Over time, the ceaseless demand for the hormone can exhaust the gland, culminating in adult-onset diabetes—especially in those who are genetically predisposed. A 1997 survey found that women who eat a diet high in sugars and low-fiber carbohydrates are twice as likely to become diabetic as those who eat less refined foods.[4]

---

### Glycemic Index of Common Foods

*"High-glycemic" foods produce a sharp rise in blood glucose levels. These foods tend to be low in fiber and are easily digested. "Low-glycemic" foods release sugar into your bloodstream more gradually, helping to stabilize your glucose levels.*

**High-Glycemic Carbohydrates**

- Soft drinks
- White rice, especially the instant variety
- White bread
- Honey, glucose
- French fried potatoes
- Cooked potatoes of all kinds
- Jams
- Low-fiber, sugary breakfast cereals
- Crackers
- Millet
- Corn
- Corn flakes
- Puffed Rice and Puffed Wheat
- Raisins
- Orange Juice
- Corn chips
- Bananas

**Low-Glycemic Carbohydrates**

- Sourdough bread
- Legumes, especially lentils, chick peas, split peas, kidney beans, white beans, soybeans
- Barley
- Whole-grain rye bread
- High-fiber, whole-grain cereals
- Protein-enriched pasta
- Oranges
- Peanuts
- Split peas
- Milk, skim milk, yogurt
- Fructose, lactose
- Apples
- Apricots
- Bulgur, brown rice

---

# An Imbalance of Essential Fatty Acids and Insulin Resistance

Eating a diet that is low in omega-3 fatty acids and high in omega-6 fatty acids can also contribute to insulin resistance. When lab animals are fed a diet high in saturated fat or omega-6 oils, they become insulin resistant. Supplementing their diets with omega-3 fatty acids normalizes their metabolism—even if they continue to eat the other fats.[5] This same strategy can prevent the animals from becoming obese. For example, when mice prone to diabetes and obesity are raised on a variety of high-fat diets, the fattest ones will be those fed omega-6 oils or saturated fat; the leanest will be those fed omega-3 oils. In the study illustrated in the accompanying figure, the difference in weight between the mice fed a soybean-oil diet and a fish-oil diet is comparable to the difference in weight between a 225- and a 150-pound man. Yet, both diets contained the same number of calories and percentage of fat.[6]

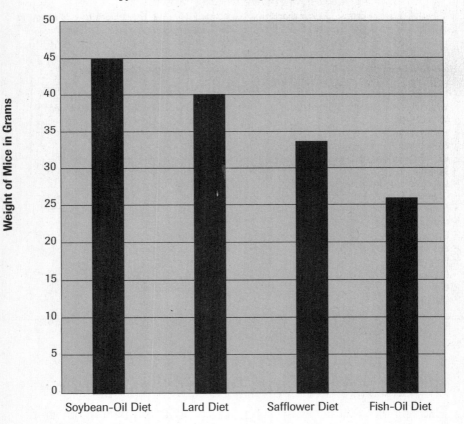

Figure 7-1. The Type of Fat in the Diet Influences the Body Weight of Mice

---

Despite the fact that the mice in this study ate the same amount of fat and the same number of calories, there was a dramatic difference in their weight.[7]

## Warning Signs and Risk Factors of Diabetes

Of the estimated 16 million people in the United States with diabetes, half don't know they have it. Below are the most common symptoms and risk factors.

- **Unusual thirst.**
- **Frequent urination.**
- **Fatigue.**
- **Unexplained weight loss.**
- **A body-mass index greater than 27.**
- **A waist-to-hip ratio greater than 0.8.**
- **Muscle cramping, especially in the calves.**
- **Numbness, tingling, or burning in the fingers and toes.**
- **Frequent infections of the urinary tract, vagina, skin, mouth, or respiratory tract.**
- **Fasting glucose levels above 126 mg/dl.**
- **A family history of diabetes.**
- **Advanced age.**

Unwittingly, Americans are being subjected to a similar experiment. The typical Western diet is low in omega-3 fatty acids and high in omega-6 fatty acids—the very recipe that causes obesity and insulin resistance in rodents. It seems to be having the same effect on us. An Australian researcher, Leonard A. Storlien, has found that people whose muscle cells contain low levels of omega-3 fatty acids (especially DHA) and high levels of omega-6 fatty acids are more likely to be insulin resistant and obese.[8] The more unbalanced the ratio, the more people weigh and the more severe their metabolic problems.

Americans are not the only guinea pigs in this unsupervised experiment. According to a recent report, Israeli Jews have a higher rate of obesity and diabetes than Americans, even though the Israelis eat fewer calories and less fat, a phenomenon that has been called "the Jewish Paradox." There is growing suspicion that their reliance on oils high in omega-6 fatty acids is partly to blame. This population consumes more linoleic acid than any other population in the world—8 percent more than Americans, and 10–12 percent more than most Europeans.[9] This preponderance of omega-6 fatty acids could be at the heart of their health problems.

As I mentioned earlier, genetics can have a major influence on whether or not you become insulin resistant. This is clearly the case for the Pima Indians. These Native Americans have captured the attention of the medical community because they have ten to twenty times the rate of insulin resistance, obesity, and diabetes of people of European ancestry. Because their diet differs little from the diets of people without these disorders, heredity, not diet, seems to be the determining factor. Storlien has a theory about how genetics might be involved. He has found that the muscle cells of the Pima Indians contain 40 percent less DHA than expected.[8] This population may have inherited a disorder that prevents DHA from taking its rightful place in their cell membranes.

## HOW MIGHT DHA INFLUENCE INSULIN RESISTANCE?

The higher the percentage of unsaturated fatty acids in your cell membranes (ones with a high number of double bonds), the more fluid they become. DHA, with its six double bonds, is the most unsaturated of all the fatty acids and results in the most fluid cell membranes. Fluid membranes have a greater number of insulin receptors and more responsive receptors, resulting in heightened sensitivity to insulin.

## *Trans-Fatty Acids Promote Insulin Resistance and Obesity*

Eating a high amount of trans-fatty acids is the third dietary factor that can make you more vulnerable to insulin resistance. Margarine, as you know, is high in trans-fatty acids, especially stick margarine. (The firmer the margarine, the greater the percentage of trans-fatty acids.) In one study, women who ate margarine four or more times per week had a higher than normal risk of having three of the symptoms of Syndrome-X: low HDL cholesterol, high total cholesterol, and high triglycerides. They also weighed, on average, five pounds more than women who used other types of fat, with no indication they were eating more food or being less active.[10] A related phenomenon has been observed in rats. When rats are fed a diet high in trans-fatty acids, they develop larger fat cells.[11] Large fat cells have fewer insulin receptors and can store considerably more fat, increasing the likelihood of obesity.

---

**THE LINK BETWEEN TRANS-FATTY ACIDS AND INSULIN RESISTANCE**

Trans-fatty acids interfere with normal fatty acid metabolism by crowding out essential fatty acids from the cell membranes and interfering with the conversion of the shorter chain fatty acids (such as LNA) into the longer ones (such as DHA). As a result, there are fewer long-chain fatty acids in the membranes. This makes the membranes less fluid and reduces the number and sensitivity of the insulin receptors.[2]

---

## The Omega Diet Increases Your Insulin Sensitivity

We now know that a diet enriched with omega-3 fatty acids can help prevent insulin resistance in humans, just as it can in lab animals. In a 1997 study, fifty-five people diagnosed with Syndrome-X were assigned to a diet that was low in "bad" fat but high in fish. A year later, lab tests showed they had become less insulin resistant. They also had lower body weight, blood pressure, and triglyceride levels.[12]

However, an even more effective diet—one virtually identical to **The Omega Diet**—was tested recently by Storlien and his colleagues. (Like the dietary program described in this book, the experimental diet was a 35-percent-fat diet that was low in saturated fat, trans-fatty acids, and omega-6 fatty acids but relatively high in monounsaturated oils and omega-3 fatty acids. The ratio of omega-6 to omega-3 fatty acids was 4 to 1.) Forty-eight people with diabetes were assigned to either this experimental diet or to a low-fat, high-carbohydrate diet. A year later, the difference in health between the two groups was remarkable. The patients eating the low-fat, high-carbohydrate diet had gotten worse, not better: they had a higher level of fasting glucose and a reduction in insulin sensitivity. Meanwhile, the patients eating the experimental diet had improved across the board: they were more sensitive to insulin, they had higher HDL (good) cholesterol, and they had lower blood pressure, fasting glucose, and triglycerides—all highly positive signs.[13] The new diet had managed to reverse all of the metabolic problems linked with Syndrome-X.

The Storlien study offers further proof that **The Omega Diet** is highly protective against disease. When your diet contains a healthy ratio of fatty acids, you have a more normal metabolism and a lower risk of Syndrome-X, obesity, and diabetes.

| Components of Syndrome-X | Low-Fat, High-Carb Diet | Moderate-Fat Canola Diet with a 4 to 1 Ratio of Omega-6s to Omega-3s. |
|---|---|---|
| Hypertension | No Change ☺ | Decrease ☺ |
| Insulin Sensitivity | Decrease ☹ | Increase ☺ |
| Fasting Glucose Levels | Increase ☹ | Decrease ☺ |
| Triglycerides | Increase ☹ | Decrease ☺ |
| HDL-Cholesterol | Decrease ☹ | Increase ☺ |

## The Bottom Line

- The primary function of insulin is to help regulate your blood sugar levels.
- When a normal amount of insulin does not cause the expected drop in glucose levels, a person is said to be "insulin resistant." People who are obese, hypertensive, or diabetic are likely to have this metabolic disorder. It also afflicts approximately 25 percent of the adult population who do not have these problems.
- Heredity has a significant influence on whether or not you become insulin resistant.
- Insulin resistance is commonly linked with a number of health problems, including hyperinsulinemia, high blood glucose, high blood pressure, low HDL (good) cholesterol, and high triglycerides. A person with this cluster of conditions is said to have "Syndrome-X." It is not known whether or not insulin resistance causes Syndrome-X, but it often precedes it.
- A person with Syndrome-X has an increased risk of becoming obese, diabetic, or having coronary artery disease.
- What you eat can either increase or decrease your risk of insulin resistance. You increase your risk if your diet is: (1) high in sugar and refined carbohydrates, (2) has a high ratio of omega-6 to omega-3 fatty acids, and/or (3) contains relatively high amounts of trans-fatty acids. The typical Western diet has all three of these drawbacks.
- **The Omega Diet** contains the types and ratios of fat that have been proven to increase insulin sensitivity and lessen the severity of many of the conditions linked with Syndrome-X.

# EIGHT

# Food for Thought

*The Surprising Connection Between Dietary Fat,
Intelligence, Mental Disorders, and Mood*

O NE OF THE MOST intriguing new discoveries about fat is that it
is inextricably linked with your state of mind. The kind of mayonnaise you spread on your sandwich and the type of dressing you
pour on your salad may influence your moods, stress level, impulsiveness, feelings towards others—even your ability to learn.

One reason that fat has such a profound effect on your mind and
moods is that your brain is largely made up of fat. Fifty to sixty percent of its solid matter is fat, making the term "fathead" an apt
description of human physiology. Furthermore, the fat in your brain
is not "depot" fat, the kind you pack around your middle and thighs
to ward off famine, but "structural" fat, the kind that forms your cell
membranes and plays a vital role in how your cells function.

Another unique feature about the brain is that your neurons, the
cells that transmit chemical messages, are unusually rich in omega-3
fatty acids. There is a lot more DHA in your neurons than in your red
blood cells.[1] If you are eating a typical Western diet that is deficient in
DHA and other omega-3 fatty acids, you are depriving your brain of a
critical component, which could be impairing your ability to learn and
remember. One of the first animal studies showing a link between fat
and intelligence was published in 1975. In this experiment, one group

of rats was raised on a safflower oil diet, an oil that is very high in omega-6 fatty acids and has only trace amounts of omega-3 fatty acids. Another group was raised on a diet that contained an appreciable amount of LNA. When tested in a simple maze, the rats raised on safflower oil made the right choice only 60 percent of the time, compared with a 90 percent success rate for rats whose diet contained an adequate amount of omega-3 fatty acids.[2]

A second group of researchers conducted a test that had the potential for life-or-death consequences. A colony of mice was divided into groups and raised on diets that were either high or low in omega-3 fatty acids. During one experiment, the mice were placed into a tank of water that had one safe haven—a small platform submerged just below the surface of the water. The researchers timed how long it took each mouse to reach the platform, then tested them again on subsequent days. Consistently, the mice with the omega-3-enriched diet reached the platform in less time than the mice whose diet had been low in this nutrient. On the second day, for example, the omega-3-enriched mice reached safety in an average of forty-two seconds, while the deficient mice floundered for eighty-one seconds.[3]

## Brain Food

Do omega-3 fatty acids help humans learn and remember? Evidence from the nursery suggests that they might. Human breast milk contains DHA, but infant formulas do not. (U.S. manufacturers of baby food are not yet required to add DHA to their products.) As a result, breast-fed babies have more DHA in their brains and retinas than bottle-fed babies.[4] Breast-fed babies also have better visual acuity than bottle-fed babies, and, years later, score higher on standardized tests of reading, visual interpretation, sentence completion, nonverbal skills, and math.[5] The superior performance of breast-fed babies could be due to any number of factors, however, including the fact that women who breast-feed their babies tend to be of a higher socioeconomic class. But careful studies show that DHA plays a key role in cognitive development. Researcher Ricardo Uauy has compared the brain and visual function of three groups of infants: breast-fed babies; babies fed a standard (omega-3-deficient) infant formula;

and babies fed the same formula enriched with fish oil. One test he uses measures "visual evoked potential," which is the way the brain responds to a changing sequence of black-and-white patterns displayed on a video monitor. He has found that breast-fed babies and those supplemented with fish oil have similar scores, while those given a standard infant formula have significantly lower scores.[6]

Premature babies who have been given omega-3 supplements for only a few months have performed better on tests of infant intelligence a year later. In a study conducted at the Department of Pediatrics at the University of Tennessee, preterm infants were given either a standard infant formula or a formula that had been enriched with DHA. Two months past term, all the babies were fed a standard (DHA-deficient) infant formula. At one year of age, the infants were given the Fagan Test of Infant Intelligence. The results showed that the babies who had been given the DHA processed information more rapidly than those fed the standard formula. The researchers noted that "because supplementation was stopped at two months and the effects were seen at 12 months, this study demonstrates for the first time that a relatively short period of DHA supplementation can produce significant effects on later visual attention."[7]

### INTELLIGENCE AND BREAST-FEEDING

The longer infants are fed breast milk, the more DHA accumulates in their brains. Studies show that infants breast-fed for at least four months score as well on vision tests as infants that have been breast-fed throughout infancy. Babies that nurse for a shorter period of time have lower scores. According to one group of researchers, "the data indicate a need for a continuous supply of [omega-3 fatty acids] from breast milk for at least the first four months of life."[8]

There is also some intriguing new data about school-aged children. Recently, researchers at Purdue University measured the essential fatty-acid levels of one hundred boys between the ages of six and twelve. They found that the children with the highest levels of omega-3 fatty acids had the fewest learning problems.[9]

There is new evidence that taking omega-3 supplements might enhance the mental abilities of adults as well. A certain type of brain wave called "p300" is linked with learning and memory. The faster the rate of transmission, the more efficiently the brain is functioning. The rate declines with age and is noticeably slower in people with dementia. To see if omega-3 fatty acids influence this particular brain function, twenty-six normal adult volunteers were hooked up to electrodes and given a test that determined their p300 rate. Immediately after taking the test, they were given supplements of either DHA or EPA (two omega-3 fatty acids). Two hours later, their brain waves were measured once again. This time, the p300 rate was significantly faster in people given the DHA. Said the researchers, "DHA, therefore, appears to be an exciting drug which can improve brain function . . . in healthy persons."[10]

Supplementing your diet with DHA (one of the main constituents of fish oil) might also reduce your risk of dementia. Ernst Schaefer from Tufts University has found that the amount of DHA in your blood at age sixty-five is a possible predictor of whether or not you will become senile in old age. Schaefer determined the amount of DHA in the plasma of 1,137 healthy older adults. Over

---

### The Link Between Omega-3 Fatty Acids and Learning

A new theory has been proposed to explain how omega-3 fatty acids might enhance the ability to learn. The process of learning and remembering involves the transmission of various chemicals from one nerve ending to another. These chemicals are stored in tiny packages called "synaptic vesicles." The more synaptic vesicles in a nerve ending, the more chemicals that can be transmitted.

In a study of learning ability, rats were raised on either a diet that was deficient in omega-3 fatty acids or one that was nutritionally complete. Initially, both groups of rats had similar numbers of synaptic vesicles. After a month-long learning program, however, the omega-3 enriched rats had considerably more vesicles in their nerve endings and also performed markedly better on the tests.[11] This study suggests there may be a direct connection between the amount of omega-3 fatty acids in your diet, the number of synaptic vesicles in your neurons, and your ability to learn.

the next nine years, 64 of these subjects developed dementia. Those who had the lowest levels of DHA at the beginning of the study had a 160 percent greater chance of becoming senile.[12] Schaefer's finding supports an earlier Dutch survey of fifty-one elderly men. In this study, researchers found that the men who were eating the most fish were the least likely to be senile, while those whose diets were highest in omega-6 fatty acids were the most likely to be demented.[13]

Will giving demented patients omega-3 supplements improve their mental state? Perhaps so. In a pilot study conducted in Japan, eighteen older patients (ages fifty-seven to ninety-four) with clear signs of dementia were given 700 to 1,400 milligrams of DHA every day for six months. Seventy percent of those with a type of dementia caused by insufficient blood flow to the brain (cerebro-vascular dementia) showed significant signs of improvement. Meanwhile, all of the Alzheimer's patients were "slightly improved." Although the response was more modest in the Alzheimer's patients, the researchers noted that a wide range of symptoms had improved, including mood, gait, and the ability to carry on a conversation. The research team concluded, "These results suggest that DHA-rich oil is useful for the improvement and prevention of both cardiovascular and Alzheimer's dementia."[14]

## Is Your Diet Depressing You?

Two researchers from the National Institutes of Health, Joseph Hibbeln and Norman Salem, have spent years exploring the connection between EFAs and depression. One finding that prompted their research is that people who eat a lot of fish have low rates of depression. In Japan, Taiwan, and Hong Kong, for example, fish consumption is high and the rate of depression is low. The Japanese are a striking example. The traditional Japanese diet contains about fifteen times more omega-3 fatty acids than the American diet.[15] Careful studies show that the Japanese people have one-tenth the rate of depression of Americans.[16] The difference is even more pronounced between members of the older generations. Approximately 44 percent of the American elderly have symptoms of depression, compared with only 2 percent of the Japanese elderly. The very lowest rates of depression in

Japan are found in fishing villages. In 1995, a team of psychiatrists interviewed all the older inhabitants living in a Japanese fishing community, yet did not find a single case of clinical depression.[17]

The balance of EFAs in the diet also seems to influence the severity of depression. Australian mental patients whose blood was relatively high in omega-6 fatty acids and low in omega-3 fatty acids were more likely to be severely depressed than those with a more balanced ratio.[18]

Hibbeln and Salem suggest that the epidemic of depression in the United States might be linked to our increasingly unbalanced diet. In the past fifty years, Americans have been eating more omega-6 fatty acids and less omega-3 fatty acids. During this same time period, we have witnessed a steadily rising rate of depression. People born after 1945 are as much as twenty times more likely to have episodes of depression than those born before 1934.[19] Furthermore, depression is hitting people earlier in life. An estimated 500,000 grade-school children are now taking antidepressants. In the teen years, this high rate of depression translates into a tragically high number of suicides and attempted suicides. The teen suicide rate has increased threefold since 1960, making it the third leading cause of death among adolescents.[20]

## Eat Fish, Be Happy

Hibbeln and his colleagues are now conducting a study to see if omega-3 supplements can *relieve* depression. A group of depressed patients are being given either placebos or two grams of DHA per day. During the course of the study, they are being closely monitored for changes in mood and serotonin levels. (Serotonin is the "feel good" neurotransmitter that is boosted by antidepressants such as Prozac and Zoloft.)

While we await the results of this and other studies, we can glean some insights from doctors who have already treated patients with omega-3 fatty acids, including a physician named Robert Burdon who practiced more than 300 years ago. Burdon's standard practice for treating depression was to put his patients on a diet that was low in ordinary types of fat but rich in fish oil. If a patient was severely depressed, he would recommend a two-week diet of cow brains. Cow brains, it turns out, are an excellent source of DHA.[21]

In Italy, researchers are continuing the long tradition by treating depressed patients with an extract of cow brains called "phosphatidylserine." In a pilot study, ten elderly depressed women were given the extract for thirty days. By study's end, the women were less depressed, more sociable, less anxious, less irritable, and scored higher on tests of long-term memory.[22] Salem suggests that the active ingredient in this new antidepressant is DHA. "By weight, 40 percent of phosphatidylserine is DHA," he says. "The Italian studies may, in reality, be a test of the mood-elevating effects of omega-3 fatty acids."

One of the first American physicians to treat patients with omega-3 fatty acids is Donald O. Rudin, former director of the Department of Molecular Biology at the Eastern Pennsylvania Psychiatric Institute. In the early 1980s, he set up an uncontrolled experiment in which he gave flaxseed oil to 44 people with mental disorders. (Flaxseed oil is a concentrated source of LNA.) The dose varied from two to six tablespoons a day. Incredibly, he reports that within two hours of taking the supplement, "mood is improved and depression is lifted" in some patients.[23] One of his chronically depressed patients had a pronounced mood shift in just a few days. "Three days after starting on 6 tablespoons of [flaxseed oil] daily, she developed a marked sense of increased physical energy and unique exuberance." The woman claimed that taking the flaxseed oil "gave me the only feeling of real joy I have known in life."[23] Within six to eight weeks, the majority of his patients slept better, had more energy, and felt less anxious and depressed. When he switched the patients to supplements high in omega-6 fatty acids or took them off the supplements altogether, their symptoms returned. Rudin found that flaxseed oil had such a profound mood-elevating effect on some patients that large doses made some of them manic, giving them racing thoughts, insomnia, and feelings of grandeur. Cutting back on the dose, he reports, brought them safely back to earth.[24]

Case histories such as these are intriguing, but they are not regarded as scientific proof. Although Hibbeln believes there's a reasonable chance that omega-3 fatty acids might indeed relieve depression, he warns people not to jump to any conclusions. "As a physician, I cannot recommend that anyone take omega-3 fatty acids to treat any mental disorder. Not enough trials have been done to prove their effectiveness. The evidence so far is suggestive and provocative, but it is far from conclusive. There's no harm in taking them—but it's like oat bran. Everyone jumps on the bandwagon before we know what the truth is. In a few years, we will be in a much better position to judge."

That said, like virtually all researchers in the field, he has taken steps to enrich his own diet with omega-3 fatty acids. "I eat a lot of fish," he reports.

# Alcoholism

Alcoholism and depression go hand in hand. Between 16 and 50 percent of all alcoholics suffer from depression, and the rate climbs as high as 70 percent in chronic, heavy drinkers. Given the relationship between booze and bad moods, it is significant that alcohol is one of the few substances that leaches DHA out of the brain. "Your brain is reluctant to part with DHA," according to NIH's Salem. "It is tenaciously retained, even when you're not getting any from your diet. We can put rats on low-fat diets for as long as a year—that's half their life span—and they end up with the same amount of DHA in their brains as when the experiment began." But give them a single drink of alcohol, he has found, and their brains lose DHA within a matter of hours. The same is true for cats. "We've given cats one small drink of alcohol a day," he reports, "and they lose a significant amount of DHA from both their brains and retinas." In another experiment, rhesus monkeys were given free access to alcohol for a period of three years. Although the monkeys were more restrained in their drinking than many humans, their brains were still robbed of DHA.

Salem is another one of the researchers whose work in the field of EFAs has compelled him to change his diet. "I have increased my intake of omega-3 fatty acids, selecting fish and poultry when I can. I also stay away from omega-6 oils. I won't use corn oil or safflower oil, for instance"—changes that are central to **The Omega Diet.**

# Postpartum Depression

Immediately following childbirth, women have six times the normal risk of serious mental disorders, a risk that remains high for the next two years.[25] Hormonal changes and the stresses of parenting are two possible causes, and a third one may be a deficiency of omega-3 fatty acids.

Omega-3 fatty acids are essential for the normal development of the unborn baby's brain, especially during the final three months of gestation when the size of its brain increases threefold. If the mother fails to get enough of these nutrients in her diet, the fetus will pirate what she has stored in her tissues—including her brain. Lab tests show that new mothers have half the normal blood levels of omega-3 fatty acids.[26] (It was common practice decades ago for women to take cod liver oil during pregnancy.) Women who breast-feed their babies have even lower levels of DHA because they are continuing to supply the baby's need for omega-3 fatty acids. If a woman does not replenish her store of these essential elements following the birth of a child, she will have lower and lower levels with each additional child.[27] Some people suggest this is why firstborn children score higher on intelligence tests. Until now, people have attributed the well-documented mental superiority of firstborn children to the fact they spend more one-on-one time with a parent. It is now being suggested that their greater cognitive abilities may also be due to a more generous supply of maternal DHA.

To date, no one has conducted a study to see if omega-3 fatty acids can reduce the risk of postpartum depression. However, the fact that these nutrients are essential for fetal development is reason enough for pregnant women to ensure that they get an adequate supply. A group of investigators from the Mayo Clinic go one step farther and recommend that women balance their diets *before* conception: "The mental apparatus of the coming generation is developed in [the womb] and the time to begin supplementation is before conception. A normal brain cannot be made without an adequate supply of omega-3 fatty acids, and there may be no later opportunity to repair the effects of an omega-3 fatty acid deficiency once the nervous system is formed."[26]

# Ain't Misbehaving

One of the consequences of growing up deficient in omega-3 fatty acids may be a higher risk of "attention-deficit hyperactivity disorder," or ADHD (also referred to as attention deficit disorder, or ADD). Five out of every 100 schoolchildren are diagnosed with ADHD, making it the most common of all childhood behavioral problems. (In recent years, hundreds of thousands of adults have been diagnosed with the disorder as well.) Symptoms include hyperactivity, impulsiveness, and difficulty concentrating and planning. Children with ADHD are the ones who are continually urged to "Calm down and pay attention!" and "Think before you act!" The accepted treatment is to give them stimulant drugs such as Ritalin, but one day they may be prescribed fish for dinner instead.

Researchers found a link between fatty acids and ADHD when they discovered that boys with ADHD have significantly lower levels of both EPA and DHA than those without the disorder. The boys with the most abnormal behavior have the lowest levels of DHA.[28] In particular, they are more likely to be hyperactive, impulsive, anxious, prone to temper tantrums, and bothered by sleep disorders, including difficulty going to sleep and getting up in the morning.[29] A pilot study is now under way at Purdue University to see if omega-3 supplements can relieve some of these troubling symptoms.

# Impulsive, Violent Behavior

A deficiency of omega-3 fatty acids has also been linked with abnormal adult behavior, including impulsiveness and aggression. Blood tests of a group of violent criminals showed that they had lower levels of DHA than people without a history of violence.[30] A similar phenomenon has been observed in primates. Feeding male monkeys a diet with a high ratio of omega-6 to omega-3 fatty acids (33 to 1) has resulted in more slapping, grappling, pushing, and biting.[31]

Now there is evidence that giving normal people omega-3 fatty acids can help reduce the low-level hostility that comes from the stresses of daily life. A team of Japanese investigators gave placebos or omega-3 supplements to a group of college students. The study began in the middle of summer vacation, a time of low stress, and continued through the harrowing week of final exams. During exam week, the students who had been given placebos scored higher on hostility tests, while those taking the omega-3 supplements sailed through the ordeal with their goodwill toward others intact.[32]

Omega-3 supplements may also relieve some physical manifestations of mental stress. A group of men with hypertension were hooked up to blood-pressure-monitoring equipment and then subjected to a stressful test of math and verbal skills. As expected, all of the men responded to the mental challenge with a sudden spike in blood pressure. For the next two weeks, the men were given either placebos or daily supplements of flaxseed oil (60 ml, or approximately four tablespoons). At the end of this period, the men were tested once again. This time, the ones who had been taking the flaxseed oil had a noticeably smaller rise in blood pressure. As an unexpected bonus, they also had lower levels of triglycerides, total cholesterol, and LDL (bad) cholesterol, but higher levels of HDL (good) cholesterol.[33]

## The Hostile Heart

A number of years ago, heart disease was thought to be more common in people with so called "type-A" behavior—competitiveness, perfectionism, impatience, time urgency, and hostility. Now only hostility—type "H" behavior—is believed to be a contributing factor. In a recent survey, medical students who scored high on the hostility scale were nearly seven times as likely to be dead by age fifty as their more docile classmates.[34] The difference in longevity was largely due to an increased incidence of heart attacks.

Depressed people are also more likely to suffer heart attacks. In fact, a person who has experienced at least one serious bout of depression has four times the normal risk. In an attempt to explain the connection between hostility, depression, and coronary artery disease, some researchers have suggested that the stress hormones produced during depression or anger are the ultimate source of the problem. Others have proposed that hostile and depressed people are more likely to engage in self-destructive behaviors such as drinking, smoking, and neglecting to take their heart medications. Now a third explanation has been proposed. In a recent article, Hibbeln and Salem have suggested that a deficiency of omega-3 fatty acids might underlie all three conditions—coronary artery disease, hostility, and depression.[17] It is possible that mood disorders don't *cause* heart disease, in other words, but may result from the same underlying deficiency of omega-3 fatty acids.

## Making Life More Bearable for Schizophrenics

Schizophrenia is a devastating mental disorder that tends to strike early in adulthood. New antipsychotic drugs have helped many schizophrenics function minimally in society, but they have failed to relieve all of the troubling symptoms. Recently, three independent groups of researchers have found that schizophrenics have abnormally low levels of DHA. Prompted by these findings, a fourth group treated twenty schizophrenic patients with fish oil. The therapy was well tolerated and relieved both types of symptoms commonly seen in schizophrenics: "positive symptoms," such as delusions and hallucinations, and "negative symptoms," such as social withdrawal and lack of emotions. Some patients also got relief from abnormal involuntary movements called "tardive dyskinesia," which are a common side effect of prolonged drug treatment. The investigators concluded that omega-3 fatty acids present "novel and exciting therapeutic possibilities."[35]

These investigations into the relationship between EFAs and the brain have opened up a new and promising area of research. At this stage, there is more promise than proof. Yet the data are compelling enough that anyone who wants to experience peak mental performance and enjoy life to the fullest would be wise to follow the guidelines of **The Omega Diet.** In the prophetic words of Hippocrates, "Food that is good for the heart is likely to be good for the brain."

## The Bottom Line

- The types of fat in your diet may influence your memory, moods, response to stress, and learning ability.
- Your brain contains a high percentage of fat. This is "structural" fat, the kind that helps form your cell membranes and plays a vital role in how your brain cells function. Your brain is unusually rich in the omega-3 fatty acid DHA.
- Human breast milk contains DHA, but in the United States and some other countries, infant formulas do not. Breast-fed babies score higher on many types of standardized tests than bottle-fed babies. DHA has improved brain function in infants, adults, and the elderly.
- Depression is linked with low blood levels of DHA.
- Alcohol leaches DHA out of the brain. Between 16 and 50 percent of alcoholics suffer from depression, as do up to 70 percent of chronic, heavy drinkers.
- If a pregnant woman does not have enough omega-3 fatty acids in her diet, the fetus will rob the fatty acids from her tissues. If a woman has additional children and does not replace the missing EFAs, a woman will have lower levels of DHA with each subsequent child. A lack of DHA has been linked with postpartum depression.
- Blood tests show that children with attention deficit hyperactivity disorder, or ADHD, have abnormally low levels of omega-3 fatty acids. This is correlated with temper tantrums, impulsivity, sleep disturbance, and an inability to concentrate.
- A number of studies have shown that adult violent offenders have unusually low levels of omega-3 fatty acids.
- Depressed, angry, or hostile people are more likely to have heart attacks. A deficiency of omega-3 fatty acids may underlie both the mood problems and the heart problems.
- Schizophrenics as a group have abnormally low levels of DHA. In a small study, omega-3 supplements relieved a number of key symptoms.

# NINE

# How The Omega Diet Fine-tunes Your Immune System

## Creating a "Smart" Immune System

PEOPLE SPEND MILLIONS of dollars each year on vitamins, herbs, and hormones that promise to boost their immune system. What they may not realize is that many health problems are caused by a *hyperactive* or misguided immune system, not a sluggish one, including such diverse conditions as allergies, asthma, diabetes, atherosclerosis, rheumatoid arthritis, Crohn's disease, lupus, multiple sclerosis, Parkinson's disease, Alzheimer's disease, shingles, psoriasis, bronchitis, and colitis. Clearly, the solution is to have not just a strong defense system but a "smart" one—one that knows when to attack, what to attack, and when to hold back. Eating the balance of essential fatty acids found in **The Omega Diet** will help you achieve just that.

## What the Eskimos Taught Us

Medical researchers have known for some time that omega-6 fatty acids can provoke inflammation. When you eat oils high in these

EFAs, your body speeds up production of a number of substances that can cause fever, pain, irritation, and swelling.[1] These substances play a key role in many of the "itis" diseases— rheumatoid arthritis, bursitis, colitis, dermatitis, gingivitis, and bronchitis. In an effort to block these aggravating elements, people resort to taking nonsteroidal anti-inflammatory drugs (NSAIDs) such as aspirin or ibuprofen or more potent steroid drugs.

It may be possible to find relief from a safer and more natural remedy—omega-3 fatty acids. There was little awareness that omega-3 fatty acids can tame a hyperactive immune system until the 1970s when researchers began exploring the health of Greenland Eskimos. A key observation was that the Eskimos were rarely troubled by immune disorders such as diabetes and asthma. Their seafood diet, with its bounty of omega-3 fatty acids, was believed to be one of the reasons why. This theory triggered a number of other surveys, which ultimately revealed that people with a high intake of fish have a lower risk of arthritis, asthma, emphysema (chronic obstructive pulmonary disease), bronchitis, Crohn's disease, multiple sclerosis, and psoriasis.

Today, medical researchers have gone one step further and are beginning to *treat* immune disorders with omega-3 supplements. The results have been encouraging—in some instances, lifesaving. This is very good news, because the drugs used to treat immune-related illnesses can have some serious side effects. Steroid drugs, for example, can increase your risk of infection, raise your blood pressure and blood sugar, influence your moods, disrupt your sleep, and cause fluid retention. Frequent users of NSAIDs are three times as likely to have "severe adverse gastrointestinal events," that is, bleeding, perforation, or other events that result in hospitalization or death. The UVB light therapy commonly used to treat psoriasis makes people more vulnerable to melanoma, a deadly type of skin cancer. Judging by the findings you will read about in this chapter, eating a more balanced ratio of essential fatty acids may allow many people to reduce the dose of NSAIDs.

# Quenching the Fire
# of Chronic Inflammation

Inflammation was first described by Hippocrates as a condition marked by redness (rubor), heat (calor), pain (dolor) and swelling (tumor). Because inflammation does indeed involve rubor, calor, dolor, and tumor, most people view it as an unwelcome event. But in reality, it is a necessary part of the healing process. Let's suppose that you have a sliver in your finger that has gotten infected. Unbeknownst to you, nearby immune cells detect the presence of the bacteria and release substances called histamines, which increase blood flow to your finger by relaxing your small blood vessels. All you know is that your finger is beginning to feel hot and tender. As the blood vessels expand, they become more permeable, which allows white blood cells to penetrate the walls and migrate to the site of the infection. Along with the white blood cells comes a clear fluid, flooding the infected area and diluting any harmful substances. As soon as the white blood cells arrive on the scene, they engulf and then destroy the offending bacteria by zapping them with noxious molecules called "free radicals." In their zeal, they continue to absorb more and more bacteria until they become so bloated that they burst. The resulting cell debris mixes with the clear fluid, becoming the viscous substance known as "pus." Once the bacterial invasion is subdued, the swelling goes down, your finger cools off, and life returns to normal. Thanks to the inflammatory response, an infection that could have spread throughout your body has been quarantined and vanquished.

In some people and under some circumstances, however, inflammation can become more of a problem than a cure. For example, too many white blood cells can congregate on an infected area, generating so many free radicals that healthy tissue gets damaged by friendly fire. Or the white blood cells can remain active long after the enemy is subdued, causing chronic inflammation. Or your immune system can overreact to relatively harmless substances such as mites, ragweed pollen, or cat dander, burdening you with all the discomforts of inflammation without any benefit.

To some degree, the vulnerability to inflammatory diseases is inherited. African Americans, for example, are more prone to allergies and chronic inflammation. It has been proposed that their immune systems become hyperactive because they are designed to combat the bacteria and parasites that are more prevalent in Africa.

We now know omega-3 fatty acids can apply the brakes to an immune system that has gotten out of control.[2] One way they do this is by slowing the recruitment of white blood cells. When an area of your body becomes infected, bacteria-fighting white blood cells need to be directed to the area. To help show the way, your body produces a chemical "scent" trail. Omega-3 fatty acids can make that trail less attractive, reducing the number of white blood cells that descend upon the scene.

## HOW DO OMEGA-3 FATTY ACIDS SLOW THE RECRUITMENT OF WHITE BLOOD CELLS?

A key substance that the body uses to recruit white blood cells is called "leukotriene $B_4$," or $LTB_4$. $LTB_4$ is produced from arachidonic acid, or AA. The more AA in your body, the greater your production of $LTB_4$. Most chronic inflammatory diseases are characterized by an overproduction of $LTB_4$.

Omega-3 fatty acids are converted into a related substance called "leukotriene $B_5$," or $LTB_5$. It, too, can attract white blood cells, but it is thirty times less effective. If you eat more omega-3 fatty acids and less omega-6 fatty acids, therefore, you are replacing a strong recruiter of white blood cells with a weaker one, reducing your risk of chronic inflammation.

Omega-3 fatty acids can block inflammation in another way as well, and that is by sending a message to your genes to slow down production of an important signaling protein called interleukin-1, or IL-1. An overproduction of IL-1 is involved in a great number of diseases, including all those pictured in the accompanying illustration. Supplementing your diet with omega-3 fatty acids can lower your IL-1 levels by as much as 50 percent, a degree of suppression similar to that caused by some steroid drugs.[3]

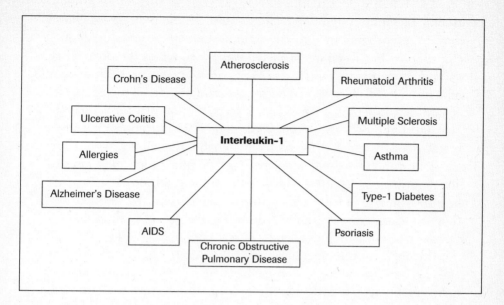

Figure 9-1. Interleukin-1 Is Linked with Many Inflammatory Diseases

All of the diseases shown in this illustration are characterized by high levels of the signaling molecule IL-1. Omega-3 fatty acids slow your body's production of IL-1.

# Autoimmune Diseases

Having an autoimmune disease can be likened to being attacked by a misguided missile. Instead of assaulting the enemy, your immune system has turned around and begun destroying your own healthy cells. The kind of disease that develops depends on the type of cells being besieged. If your immune system attacks the sheaths that surround your neurons, for example, you develop multiple sclerosis. If it destroys the insulin-producing cells in your pancreas, you develop Type-1 diabetes; if it assaults the cartilage and bones in your joints, you become arthritic.

The culprit in many autoimmune diseases is a type of white blood cell known as an "auto-reactive T-cell." Normal T-cells are among the most important cells in your immune system because they are preprogrammed to mount an instant attack on a highly specific target. One T-cell might be tailor-made to attack the polio virus; another, hepatitis B; a third, the AIDS virus, and so on. Each of your billions of T-cells has its own target. As soon as a T-cell recognizes its "mark," a complex chain of events is set in motion that turns that one cell into hundreds of thousands of clones. Within hours there is a battalion of customized T-cells ready to battle the enemy.

Unfortunately, some of your T-cells come preprogrammed to attack your own healthy cells. This is true in all individuals, even healthy young children. Unless these rogue cells are weeded out, they can cause an autoimmune disorder. The job of culling them is assigned to your thymus gland. T-cells continuously filter through the thymus, and the ones that have the potential to destroy healthy cells are given orders to self-destruct. This essential safeguard is deficient in people with autoimmune diseases: Auto-reactive cells enter the thymus and come out the other end intact. An important new finding is that omega-3 fatty acids may speed up the destruction of misguided T-cells.[4]

In the pages that follow, I will describe a number of diseases that may be prevented or improved by eating a more natural balance of essential fatty acids. Chances are great that the information will be helpful to you or someone close to you.

## *Rheumatoid Arthritis*

There are two kinds of arthritis—osteoarthritis and rheumatoid arthritis. Osteoarthritis is caused by wear and tear of your joints as you age. Rheumatoid arthritis (RA) is a chronic inflammatory disease that damages connective tissue and bone throughout your body, especially your joints.

RA afflicts more than six million Americans, three times as many women as men, with most people showing the first signs of the disease in middle adulthood. The underlying problem is that the immune system manufactures antibodies that attack an important protein (IgG). When the antibodies attack the protein, large complexes are formed that cause a hypersensitivity reaction, resulting in chronic inflammation. For a number of reasons, the inflammation targets the joints. Aspirin and similar over-the-counter drugs are the mainstay of RA therapy because they relieve both pain and inflammation. In severe cases, immune-suppressing drugs are needed as well.

More than a dozen studies in the past ten years have shown that omega-3 fatty acids can help alleviate some of the symptoms of arthritis, including morning stiffness, fatigue, pain, and the number of inflamed joints.[5,6] Some people who have taken omega-3 supplements have been able to eliminate traditional drugs altogether. For example, in a 1995 study, arthritis patients who were taking standard anti-inflammatory drugs were given omega-3 supplements. After several months, the anti-inflammatory drugs were replaced with look-alike placebos. A significant number of the patients were able to stay off their prescription drugs without experiencing a flare-up of the disease.[7]

Omega-3 fatty acids can also be used as a topical treatment for inflammation. Flaxseed oil is the same thing as "linseed oil," which has been used as an anti-inflammatory agent in animal husbandry for hundreds, if not thousands, of years. In fact, the word "liniment" is derived from the word "linseed." Flaxseed oil has also been a mainstay in folk medicine. In Old World medicine, people made poultices of flaxseeds and flaxseed oil, heated them, and applied them to strained muscles. The seeds retained the soothing heat and the oil helped reduce the inflammation.

Recently, Australian researchers reported great success in treating an arthritis patient with a liniment made from four parts flaxseed oil and one part rubbing alcohol.[8]

## *Asthma*

Fourteen million American children are plagued with the wheezing, chest tightness, and breathlessness that characterize asthma—twice as many children as in the 1980s. Asthma can range in severity from mild wheezing to respiratory collapse. Five thousand people die from asthma every year.

A recent survey showed that children who eat oily fish are less likely to develop asthma than children who eat no fish or eat only lean fish.[9] A study of a large number of adults showed that those who eat fish at least once a week have better lung function than those who do not.[10]

Just as encouraging is the fact that omega-3 supplements can help reduce the symptoms of asthma in some people. In a year-long study, asthmatics who took one gram of omega-3 fatty acids a day (three or four commercial fish oil pills) had a greater improvement in lung capacity than those who took placebos.[11] Shorter studies have shown little or no effect, however, suggesting that the nutrients must be taken for a significant amount of time before they become effective.

---

### HOW OMEGA-3 FATTY ACIDS HELP FIGHT ASTHMA

When people are experiencing an asthma attack, their bodies produce up to three times as much of an inflammatory substance called leukotriene $B_4$, or $LTB_4$. Steroid drugs block the production of $LTB_4$. Omega-3 fatty acids block them, too, but by a different mechanism. These essential fatty acids cause the immune system to produce less $LTB_4$ and more of a competing leukotriene called "$LTB_5$." The more $LTB_5$ that is produced, the less severe the asthmatic response.[12]

---

A note of caution: There is some indication that high doses of omega-3 supplements cause a slight *decline* in lung capacity in some asthmatics.[12] Consult your doctor before taking them.

## Alzheimer's Disease

Although few people realize it, Alzheimer's disease is, in part, an inflammatory disease. Autopsies show that the brains of Alzheimer's patients contain unusually high amounts of a proinflammatory element called "interleukin-1B" (IL-1B), and the IL-1B is most concentrated in the areas of the brain that are heavily damaged by the disease. Another clue that inflammation is involved is that anti-inflammatory drugs have been proven to increase the mental performance and mood of Alzheimer's patients.[13] There is additional evidence that anti-inflammatory drugs can help prevent the disease or delay its appearance: In a study of elderly twins, the twin who took more anti-inflammatory drugs had a lower risk of developing Alzheimer's.

Eating a healthy balance of fatty acids may provide a similar degree of protection. Dutch researchers surveyed the eating habits of 900 elderly men and found that the men whose diets were highest in linoleic acid were most likely to be demented. Meanwhile, those who ate the most fish had the best mental function.[14] By following **The Omega Diet**, you will be decreasing your intake of linoleic acid and supplementing your diet with fish or other sources of omega-3 fatty acids, which may help you hold on to your cognitive ability as you age.

## *Chronic Obstructive Pulmonary Disease*

Chronic obstructive pulmonary disease (COPD) is a term that encompasses three serious breathing disorders—emphysema, chronic bronchitis, and asthma. Seventeen million Americans suffer from COPD, making it the most common of all chronic lung diseases. Surveys show you are more likely to have COPD if you smoke, have allergies, or suffer from frequent respiratory infections. Smoking is by far the biggest risk factor. Inhaling cigarette smoke, whether "first-hand" or "second-hand," damages your breathing passages in a number of ways, including interfering with the action of the hairlike structures (cilia) that line your airway passages, promoting inflammation, and increasing mucus production. Symptoms of COPD typically appear in middle age. Common early warning signs are a reduced tolerance for exercise, a phlegmy cough, and a "gravelly" voice. The symptoms worsen as the disease progresses, and can lead to disability, respiratory failure, and even death.

To explore the possible link between essential fatty acids and COPD, an international group of researchers examined the diets of 8,960 smokers or former smokers. They found that the more fish in a person's diet, the lower the risk of COPD. People who ate the most fish were 40 percent less likely to have chronic bronchitis and

60 percent less likely to have emphysema. The researchers noted that, "Although most of the anti-inflammatory benefits of omega-3 fatty acids have been demonstrated with dietary supplements that provide doses much higher than the average intake in this study, very small increments in intake may have health benefits, possibly the result of a cumulative effect."[15] Eat fish two or three times a week, in other words, and you are less likely to have a serious pulmonary disorder—even if you smoke. One researcher went so far as to say, "Supplemental fish oil and/or heavy consumption of fish may be considerably more protective [against COPD] than any other single measure."[16]

# Crohn's Disease

Crohn's disease, a painful inflammation of the gastrointestinal tract, is most common in people aged twenty to forty. Its symptoms include pain (primarily in the lower right quadrant, which is why it can be confused with appendicitis), cramping, tenderness, weight loss, weakness, depression, nausea, fever, bleeding, and diarrhea. In severe cases, sections of the bowel are removed.

Like many immune disorders, Crohn's disease is characterized by flare-ups and periods of remission. In a randomized, clinical trial, omega-3 supplements were given to patients who were in remission from Crohn's disease but who had a high risk of relapse. No additional medications were given. At the end of a year, 59 percent of the patients taking the fish oil supplements were still in remission, compared with only 26 percent of those taking placebos.[17]

Medications commonly used to treat Crohn's disease can have serious side effects, including bone marrow suppression, metabolic bone disease, growth retardation, and an increased risk of cancer. This is especially troubling given the fact that the disease tends to strike young to middle-aged adults who may have to take the medications for decades. It is highly encouraging that simply eating more fatty fish or taking omega-3 fatty acids might reduce the dose or even the need for these drugs.

# Ulcerative Colitis

Many people confuse ulcerative colitis with Crohn's disease, but they are distinct conditions. Ulcerative colitis is a chronic inflammation of the large intestine. Severity ranges from a mild, localized inflammation to a perforated colon and fatal infection of the lining of the abdominal cavity. The disease occurs primarily in young women and is more prevalent in persons of Jewish ancestry.

In a study conducted by researchers at a St. Louis hospital, eighteen patients with active ulcerative colitis were treated with either omega-3 supplements or a placebo. The omega-3 supplements allowed the patients to cut their steroid medications in half. During the placebo period, the patients had to *increase* their medications.[18]

# Gingivitis

Gingivitis is an inflammation of the gums, characterized by redness, puffiness, bleeding, and gum detachment from the teeth (periodontal pockets). If the inflammation intensifies, it can advance into a more serious stage, periodontitis, which can lead to tooth and bone loss.

French researchers have shown that omega-3 fatty acids can reduce the inflammation and severity of gingivitis. In an unusual (and not likely to be repeated) study, thirty-seven healthy volunteers were divided into two groups. Half of the volunteers were given olive oil supplements, and the other half omega-3 supplements (1.8 grams of EPA plus DHA per day). Both groups were instructed to practice intensive oral hygiene for a period of two weeks. For the next three weeks, they were asked to stop brushing and flossing their teeth altogether, setting up the preconditions for gingivitis. Signs of gingivitis were much less evident in the group taking the omega-3 supplements, showing once again that these nutrients can be highly protective against inflammation, wherever it occurs.[19]

# IgA Nephropathy

This life-threatening disease with the unwieldy name is most common in people forty and older, especially those with high blood pressure. IgA nephropathy (nuh-FROP-a-thee) is a disorder of the main filtering elements of the kidneys, the glomeruli. The disease can be deadly. Five or more years after diagnosis, 20 to 40 percent of patients will die from the disease.

Presently, there is no effective treatment for IgA nephropathy, although many drugs have been tested, including steroid drugs, anticoagulants, and antiplatelet drugs. This makes it all the more noteworthy that omega-3 supplements have been shown to reduce the severity of the disease and even save lives. In a recent study conducted by Mayo Clinic investigators, 110 patients with IgA nephropathy were randomly assigned to either placebos or a high dose of omega-3 supplements (12 grams of fish oil a day). Four years later, careful measurements showed that the patients taking the fish oil had better kidney function than those who did not take fish oil. Far more important, only 10 percent of them had died or developed end-stage kidney disease, compared with 40 percent of those in the placebo group. Because of this remarkable difference in survival, the researchers believe that fish oil benefited the patients in a number of ways in addition to reducing inflammation. They suspect it might also have increased blood flow through the kidneys, reduced the risk of clotting, and lowered the risk of heart attack and stroke.[20]

# Lupus

Systemic lupus erythematosus (SLE), or "lupus," is an immune disorder that can range in severity from a mild rash to a fatal assault on the brain, kidneys, and other organs. The typical American diet, with its surplus of omega-6 fatty acids, may *worsen* lupus. To see if lowering the intake of this nutrient might be of benefit, Swedish researchers advised nineteen lupus patients to stop eating omega-6 oils and replace them with saturated fat. At the end of a year, the number of patients with active cases dropped from eleven to three. Just as important, most of the patients were able to cut back on their steroid medications.[21]

The first indication that adding omega-3 fatty acids to the diet can help control lupus came from animal studies. In one revealing study, mice with a lupuslike condition were given fish oil or beef fat. Eighty-five percent of the mice fed a fish-oil diet were still alive at nineteen months of age compared with only 2 percent of the mice fed a beef-fat diet.

Two pilot studies show that fish oil pills can help human sufferers as well. In one study, patients with active lupus were given either placebos or 20 grams of fish oil a day. While taking the omega-3 supplements, 82 percent were judged to be markedly improved. When they were switched to placebos, only 28 percent showed any benefit.[22] In a study conducted in India, a much smaller daily dose of omega-3 fatty acids (300 milligrams of EPA plus DHA) was given to ten consecutive patients with newly diagnosed SLE. All ten patients went into remission, some for as long as three years. They remained in remission at the time the study was written. Remarkably, they were able to discontinue all other medications and had no negative side effects from the omega-3 fatty acids.[23]

## Menstrual Pain (Dysmenorrhea)

The painful cramps that some women experience before and during menstruation are linked with an overproduction of an inflammatory agent called prostaglandin $E_2$, or $PGE_2$. Aspirin and similar drugs short-circuit the production of $PGE_2$, which is one of the reasons they relieve menstrual pain. Fish oil also blocks $PGE_2$, so it is not surprising that women who eat fish on a regular basis are less likely to be troubled with cramps.[24] Adding omega-3 fatty acids to the diet has been proven to be an effective therapy. Forty-eight young women suffering from menstrual cramps were given either placebos or small (1.8 grams) daily doses of EPA and DHA. After two months of treatment, the young women taking the fish oil pills had significantly less pain than those taking placebos.[25]

# *Psoriasis*

Psoriasis is a chronic skin inflammation marked by patches of red, bumpy, and scaly skin. The condition can cause pain, itching, and emotional discomfort. Like many autoimmune and inflammatory diseases, psoriasis flares and recedes, triggered by stress, hormones, changes in the weather (especially a drop in temperature), and various unknown factors.

The underlying cause of psoriasis is uncontrolled cell growth. The life cycle of a healthy skin cell is about twenty-eight days. It takes fourteen of those days for the cell to develop fully and move from the lower to the topmost level of skin. It takes another fourteen days for the cell to die and slough off. A psoriatic skin cell has a greatly speeded-up life cycle, migrating to the surface in just four days. This is not enough time for it to mature and therefore results in an abnormal appearance. Due to the rapid growth, cells crowd the surface and form a thick, flaky upper layer.

No permanent cure exists for psoriasis. To relieve the pain and itching and help soften the scales, the skin is exposed to sunlight or artificial UVB light and treated with petroleum or tar-based ointments. But there is new concern about the use of UVB light because patients who undergo a large number of treatments have nine times the normal risk of developing melanoma, a deadly skin cancer.[26]

Several studies have shown that omega-3 supplements can bring relief to psoriasis sufferers. In a double-blind study, people with active psoriasis were given daily doses of EPA or placebos. When examined two months later, the patients taking the omega-3 supplements had less itching, scaling and redness, and the affected area had grown smaller.[27] Applying omega-3 fatty acids directly to the skin may be just as helpful. In a small study, fish oil was added to petroleum jelly (the resulting unguent was 10 percent fish oil) and spread on the skin. Eight of eleven patients showed a marked improvement.[28]

# *Osteoporosis*

Throughout life, our bones are subject to the actions of two different types of cells—osteoblasts, which rebuild them, and osteoclasts, which tear them down. As we age, the osteoclasts tend to outpace the osteoblasts, making our bones less dense—and more breakable. Osteoporosis—literally "porous bones"—afflicts tens of millions of Americans, resulting in short- and long-term disability and billions of dollars of medical costs.

There is growing evidence from animal studies that following a diet such as **The Omega Diet** that is rich in antioxidants and omega-3 fatty acids may help preserve bone density. (Antioxidants help protect bone and cartilage from free radical damage, and omega-3 fatty acids lower production of $PGE_2$, $LTB_4$, and various pro-inflammatory interleukins, factors known to promote bone loss or "resorption.").[29] Much work needs to be done in this area, but there is preliminary evidence that people whose diets are relatively rich in omega-3 fatty acids and low in omega-6 fatty acids have a low rate of osteoporosis, even if they consume less than optimal amounts of calcium.

## Essential Fatty Acids and Inflammation

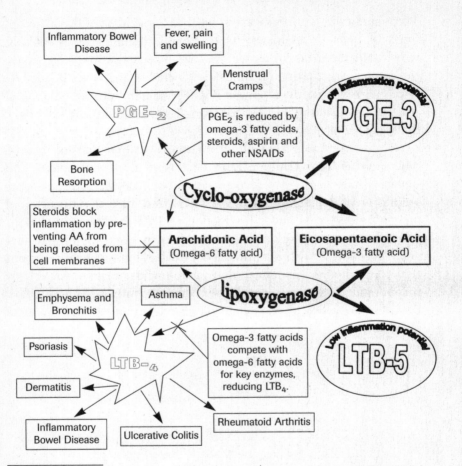

In the center of this diagram are two key fatty acids, arachidonic acid (AA), the omega-6 fatty acid derived from linoleic acid; and eicosapentaenoic acid (EPA), the omega-3 fatty acid derived from alpha-linolenic acid. Both AA and EPA interact with the same two families of enzymes, the lipoxygenase family and the cyclo-oxygenase family. When AA interacts with these enzymes, it forms inflammatory elements, in particular prostaglandin $E_2$ ($PGE_2$) and leukotriene $B_4$ ($LTB_4$). These two elements are linked with a variety of inflammatory and immune disorders, including those shown in the illustration.

When EPA interacts with these same enzymes, however, it forms closely related but less inflammatory elements—$PGE_3$ and $LTB_5$. Thus, eating a diet such as **The Omega Diet**, which is lower in omega-6 fatty acids and relatively higher in omega-3 fatty acids than the typical U.S. or Western diet replaces inflammatory eicosanoids with less inflammatory eicosanoids, decreasing the risk of chronic inflammation.

## The Bottom Line

- Inflammatory and autoimmune diseases are linked with a hyperactive immune system.
- Current treatments for blocking inflammation include steroid drugs, aspirin, ibuprofen, and other NSAIDs. All of these drugs can have serious side effects.
- Adding omega-3 fatty acids to your diet can reduce your body's production of a number of proinflammatory substances, including IL-1 and $LTB_4$, which are linked with a long list of autoimmune and inflammatory diseases.
- Decreasing your intake of omega-6 fatty acids as you increase your intake of omega-3 fatty acids can lower the risk and/or lessen the severity of a number of inflammatory and autoimmune diseases, including:
    Rheumatoid arthritis
    Asthma
    Alzheimer's disease
    Chronic obstructive pulmonary disease (COPD)
    Crohn's disease
    Ulcerative colitis
    IgA nephropathy
    Systemic lupus erythematosus (SLE), or lupus
    Dysmenorrhea (menstrual pain)
    Psoriasis
    Osteoporosis
    Gingivitis

# PART 3

# Putting The Omega Diet into Action

# TEN

# Your Health Is in the Balance

*Realizing the Seven Guidelines of The Omega Diet*

IN THIS THIRD SECTION of the book, you will be learning how to restore a natural balance of essential fatty acids and other key nutrients to your diet. The goal is to give your body what it "expects" to be fed—the types of foods that are consistent with millions of years of genetic programming and that also have been medically proven to increase your chances of living a long, lean, and healthy life.

So, what does your body "expect" to be fed? To refresh your memory, take another look at The Seven Dietary Guidelines of **The Omega Diet:**

1. Enrich your diet with omega-3 fatty acids.
2. Use monounsaturated oils such as olive oil and canola oil as your primary oils.
3. Eat seven or more servings of fruits and vegetables every day.
4. Eat more vegetable proteins, including peas, beans, and nuts.
5. Avoid saturated fat by choosing lean meat over fatty meat and low-fat over full-fat milk products.

6. Avoid oils that are high in omega-6 fatty acids.
7. Reduce your intake of trans-fatty acids.

These guidelines are quite different from the ones advocated by the Department of Health and Human Services and the U.S. Department of Agriculture. The DHHS/USDA Food Guide Pyramid in the accompanying illustration below is a low-fat, high-carbohydrate diet. The broad base of the pyramid is reserved for carbohydrates—you are advised to eat six to eleven servings of bread, cereal, rice, and pasta each day. Fat is relegated to the top of the pyramid—along with sweets, suggesting that both fats and sweets are forbidden foods. Remarkably, no distinction is made about what *types* of fat you should be eating. There is no hint of the health benefits of monounsaturated and omega-3 fatty acids, and no indication that your intake of trans-fatty acids, saturated fat, and omega-6 oils should be carefully monitored and reduced.

The Food Guide Pyramid is also vastly different from the evolutionary diet. Cereals and grains were first eaten in quantity only 10,000 years ago, a blink of the eye in terms of evolution. For this

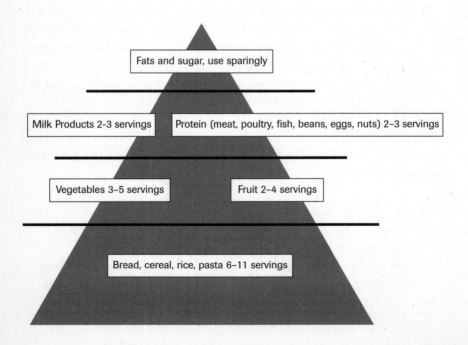

Fats and sugar, use sparingly

Milk Products 2-3 servings     Protein (meat, poultry, fish, beans, eggs, nuts) 2-3 servings

Vegetables 3-5 servings     Fruit 2-4 servings

Bread, cereal, rice, pasta 6-11 servings

reason, a diet high in carbohydrates is at odds with our genes, placing us at greater risk for obesity, insulin resistance, high glucose, high insulin, low HDL, high triglycerides, and diabetes.

When represented in graphic form, **The Omega Diet** assumes a very different shape—that of a Greek column.[1]

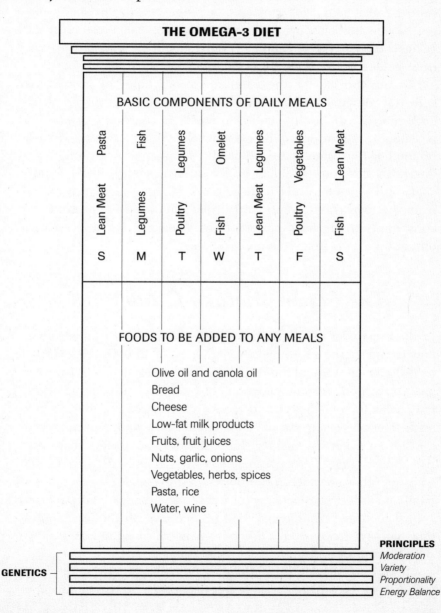

Unlike the widely publicized food pyramid, **The Omega Diet** is consistent with your genetic inheritance. The items in the lower half of the column are foods that can be added to any meal because they are rich in antioxidants and minerals and contribute to a balanced ratio of omega-3 and omega-6 fatty acids. (The only restriction, of course, is that your caloric intake should not exceed your energy output; along with balancing all the nutrients in your diet, you must also balance the energy equation.) Salads should be eaten daily, and fruits at least two or three times a day.

In the top half of the column, various types of protein are spread throughout the lunch and dinner meals, with the emphasis on legumes, fish, poultry, and lean meat. As you can see, fatty fish is eaten three or more times a week. (If you don't like fish, remember that you can take omega-3 supplements or enrich your diet with flaxseeds and flax oil.) Margarines high in trans-fatty acids and vegetable oils high in omega-6 fatty acids are absent from the food plan. Sweets, soft drinks, and hard liquor are to be consumed on special occasions only. Wine can be enjoyed with dinner on a daily basis—in moderation.

## *The Seven Dietary Guidelines*

In the remainder of this chapter, I will give you practical advice on how to realize the seven dietary guidelines of **The Omega Diet**. I believe that all seven of the guidelines are important, but if I were to give you just one recommendation, it would be to add more omega-3 fatty acids to your diet and to reduce your intake of omega-6 fatty acids. This one change would compensate for a glaring imbalance in the Western diet. By making these changes, you may reduce your risk of heart attack, stroke, cancer, obesity, diabetes, depression, and a host of other unwanted conditions and diseases. Presently, government and industry are looking for ways to add omega-3 fatty acids to animal food and commercial food products. Until they accomplish that goal—which may take decades—you will need to take positive steps on your own.

If you are striving for *optimal* health or fighting disease, however, I urge you to follow all seven guidelines. If you ignore even one, you will be denied the full benefits of **The Omega Diet.** For example, let's suppose you were to add omega-3s to your diet but continue to eat foods high in trans-fatty acids. If so, the omega-3s would have to compete with this manmade fat for vital enzymes and space in your cell membranes, diminishing their health-enhancing properties. Or let's suppose that you ate all the right kinds of oil but skimped on the fruits and vegetables. In this case, your diet would be deficient in vitamins, minerals, fiber, antioxidants, and phyto-chemicals. Even leaving out the lowly legumes would compromise your health. Beans are high in protein and contain some omega-3s, but they are very low in saturated fat and cholesterol. They are also rich in fiber and give you two additional ingredients—L-glutamine and L-arginine—which help regulate your blood pressure. To top it off, many beans are high in folic acid, which lowers blood levels of homocysteine, further reducing your risk of cardiovascular disease. Given the importance of following all the guidelines, I am devoting the rest of this chapter to helping you achieve a perfect "7."

At the same time that I urge you to adopt **The Omega Diet** in its entirety, however, please be aware that the guidelines are not rigid rules; unlike some other programs, you will not have to scruti-nize every meal and snack that you eat to make sure you are in com-pliance. Think of the guidelines as goals and make an effort to come closer to fulfilling them with each passing week.

If you are the kind of person who likes a structured program, you can follow one of the **3-Week Omega Diets** featured in chap-ters 12 and 13. These give you detailed instructions for every snack and meal for a three-week period. You won't have to make deci-sions, count calories, or think about balancing your nutrients—the work has been done for you already. At the end of those three weeks, you will have set in motion all the key changes required to enjoy the full benefits of this new program: You will have stocked your kitchen with essential ingredients, become familiar with a few new foods and ingredients, experimented with some new recipes, and developed healthier eating habits that will help you lay the foundation for optimal health.

# 1. Enrich Your Diet with Omega-3 Fatty Acids

Only 40 percent of Americans eat enough omega-3 fatty acids to meet the dietary recommendations. Twenty percent have such low levels that they defy detection. How do you know if you're eating enough of these nutrients? One indicator is your weekly fish consumption. Unless you're eating *fatty* fish two or more times a week (or taking omega-3 supplements), you are likely to be deficient in both DHA and EPA. Note that I said "fatty fish." Lean seafood, including cod, sole, flounder, crab, and shrimp, have about one-tenth the amount of omega-3s as oily fish. Fish sticks and deep-fat fried fish contain even less. Typically, these products are made from lean fish such as halibut, cod, or pollock, and the little oil that they do contain is squeezed out during processing. (When a colleague and I analyzed the fatty acids in a commercial fish patty, we found *no trace* of omega-3 fatty acids.) Fish that has been coated in cornmeal and then deep-fat fried in partially hydrogenated vegetable oil will contain more omega-6 fatty acids and trans-fatty acids than omega-3s.

---

### DON'T BE PUT OFF BY THE TERM "FATTY FISH"

Even though some types of fish contain ten times more fat than others, they are still relatively lean. The "fattest" fish has about the same amount of total fat as the leanest cuts of beef.

---

As I mentioned in chapter 3, Why We Eat the Wrong Fats, even eating tuna fish on a regular basis might leave you deficient in omega-3 fatty acids because most of the tuna now available is low in fat. Compare the labels on cans of water-packed tuna fish the next time you go shopping, and you'll see that the fat content of a standard two-ounce serving ranges from 0.5 to 5 grams—a tenfold difference! If you buy the full-fat variety, one half of a six-ounce can will satisfy your daily quota. Make sure that the tuna you buy is water-packed, not oil-packed. If it's packed in oil, the amount of fat listed on the label will include some of the fat from the vegetable oil, making it impossible to determine how much fat is in the tuna itself. Also, the oil is likely to be soybean oil, which has a ratio of omega-6 to omega-3 fatty acids of 12 or 13 to 1, tipping the nutritional balance in favor of omega-6 fatty acids.

The accompanying chart lists the omega-3 content of various types of fish. Ideally, you should be getting 7 grams of EPA plus DHA per week. Given the wide range of fat content, you could satisfy that requirement by eating two generous portions of salmon or twenty servings of sole! (You will find a more complete fatty acid table in the Appendix.)

| Fatty Fish | EPA + DHA/100 grams | Lean Fish | EPA + DHA/100 grams |
|---|---|---|---|
| Regular tuna fish | 1.3 grams | Low-fat tuna fish | 0.2 grams |
| Chinook (king) salmon | 1.4 grams | Fresh water bass | 0.3 grams |
| Atlantic salmon | 1.2 grams | Pacific halibut | 0.4 grams |
| Pacific herring | 1.7 grams | Flounder | 0.2 grams |
| Anchovy | 1.4 grams | Atlantic cod | 0.3 grams |
| Lake trout | 1.6 grams | Whiting | 0.1 grams |
| Mackerel | 2.5 grams | Sole | 0.1 grams |
| Dogfish | 1.9 grams | Snapper | 0.2 grams |
| Sablefish | 1.4 grams | Catfish | 0.3 grams |
| Lake whitefish | 1.3 grams | Crab | 0.3 grams |
| Bluefish | 1.2 grams | Shrimp | 0.4 grams |

Note: The chart above lists the total amount of EPA plus DHA per 100 grams. One hundred grams is a little under a half cup, which is a small serving.

**IF YOU ARE CONCERNED ABOUT CHOLESTEROL, SHOULD YOU EAT SHRIMP?**

The traditional advice for people with high cholesterol or a family history of high cholesterol is to avoid shrimp, oysters, lobsters, and other seafood high in dietary cholesterol—advice that may now be outdated. In a recent study, volunteers ate ten ounces of shrimp each day for three weeks. Although the diet did raise their LDL (bad) cholesterol by 7 percent, it caused a 12 percent increase in their HDL (good) cholesterol, more than canceling out the rise in LDL. The shrimp diet also lowered their triglycerides by 13 percent.[2]

**TAKING DHA AND EPA SUPPLEMENTS.** Another way to balance the essential fatty acids in your diet is to take omega-3 supplements. These products are now available in ordinary grocery stores, pharmacies, mail-order catalogues, and natural food stores.

Regrettably, they are called a bewildering variety of names including "Omega III Essential Fatty Acids," "Omega-3s," "Fish EPA," Omega-3 EPA," "Fish Body Oil," "Fish Oil Supplements," and even vitamin "F" (for "fatty" acids). To clarify matters, what you are looking for are two particular omega-3 fatty acids: *"eicosapentaenoic acid"* (EPA) and *"docosahexaenoic acid"* (DHA). (Remember that DHA and DHEA are entirely different substances. DHEA is a hormone, not an essential fatty acid.) The amount of EPA plus DHA per 1,000 milligram capsule can vary from 325 to 825 milligrams. Some labels list the amount of EPA plus DHA for more than one capsule, so don't be fooled. As a rule, the high-potency capsules cost more per milligram, but the trade-off is that you don't have to swallow so many pills.

**WHAT'S THE BEST BUY?**

To find the most cost-effective omega-3 supplements, use this formula: Add up the amount of EPA plus DHA per capsule, multiply by the number of capsules in the bottle, and divide by the cost. This will give you the cost per milligram.

To find out the cost per gram, which is the recommended daily dose, multiply by 1,000. (Or move the decimal point three spaces to the right.)

Some people supplement their diet with another type of fatty acid—gamma-linolenic acid, or GLA. GLA, a longer chain version of linoleic acid, is found in both primrose and borage oil. I recommend that you take DHA, EPA, and LNA (instead) because omega-3 fatty acids have been studied more extensively and have more proven benefits. Also, GLA is an omega-6 fatty acid, and we already have a surfeit of these nutrients in our diet. Finally, at least one study has shown that GLA promotes tumor growth in animals.[3]

I don't recommend that you use cod liver oil as a primary source of omega-3 fatty acids. As its name states, cod liver oil comes from the *liver* of the cod, an organ that accumulates high amounts of vitamins A and D. Normally, you would welcome these vitamins. (In fact, that's why parents used to dose their kids with cod liver oil. When these vitamins were synthesized and became available on the market, this practice came to a halt.) But vitamins A and D are fat-soluble, which means that whatever you don't use will be stored in your tissues. In order to get enough EPA and DHA from cod liver oil, you would exceed the recommended doses of these vitamins. Buy plain fish oil supplements instead.

As a general rule, I advise people to get about one gram of EPA plus DHA each day. This amount can come from food, food supplements, or a combination of both. People with certain health problems such as arthritis, depression, cancer, high blood pressure, and coronary artery disease might want to take more. There is no set time of day to take the supplements, but I recommend to take them with meals, since omega-3s were always part of our food. Some people burp up a mild fishy aftertaste; others don't. If you are troubled by fishy hiccups or other mild gastrointestinal complaints, take the supplements last thing at night. (A new product just introduced to the market eliminates these problems and also increases absorption of these nutrients. See page 363.)

Some people claim that taking omega-3 supplements does not give you the same health benefits as eating fish. This does not appear to be the case. In most of the studies mentioned in this book, supplements were used, not fish. Also, in the DART heart study mentioned earlier, the patients had the option of eating more fatty fish or taking omega-3 supplements. A careful analysis showed that both groups derived equal benefits. In addition, cancer studies in animals have proven that it is the EPA and DHA in fish oil that protect against cancer, suggesting, once again, that fish oil supplements should be just as effective as eating fish.[4]

Is it safe to take omega-3 supplements? In carefully monitored clinical trials, these nutrients have been given to pregnant women, nursing mothers, infants, premature infants, children, adults, cancer patients, people recovering from surgery, and very old people—with no notable side effects. In one study, patients took *six* grams of EPA plus DHA on a daily basis for seven years. The supplements were "without apparent side-effects over seven years of medication." Meanwhile, the patients enjoyed a multitude of "positive side effects," including a reduction in triglycerides and fibrinogen (a clotting agent), and an increase in HDL (good) cholesterol.[5]

A minority of people who have taken high doses of omega-3 fatty acids (3 grams a day and more) have complained of diarrhea, but similar complaints have come from the people who have taken placebo oils. In some studies, people taking omega-3 supplements have had an increased bleeding time (indicating a slower rate of blood clot formation), but this has never resulted in a serious clinical problem, not even when people have been taking high doses of fish oil plus aspirin (another blood thinner) and then had emergency coronary bypass surgery.[6]

That said, there are some people who should be cautious about taking more than one gram of omega-3 fatty acids per day:

1. People with asthma should take them only under close supervision by their doctors. While these nutrients have been highly

beneficial for some asthmatics, they have *increased* bronchial sensitivity in others.[7]

2. People with diabetes should take no more than 3 grams per day because higher amounts might disrupt glucose regulation.

3. People with clotting disorders or who are taking very potent blood thinners should *not* take omega-3 fatty acids unless prescribed by a physician. Omega-3 fatty acids also slow clotting time, and there is no way of predicting the net effect.

**ADDING LNA TO YOUR DIET.** In addition to getting an adequate supply of EPA and DHA, you also want to increase your intake of the plant-based form of omega-3 fatty acids—alpha-linolenic acid, or LNA. If you foraged your food from the wild, it would be impossible to be deficient in this nutrient because it would be present in virtually everything you ate. Now that LNA has been stripped from the food supply, you need to restore it to your diet systematically.

How much LNA do you need on a daily basis? Two grams is generally considered adequate. But you'll need to consume several times this amount if you don't eat fatty fish (or take omega-3 supplements) because the LNA will be your primary source of this entire family of nutrients. (Your body can convert LNA into the longer chain molecules, EPA and DHA, but it takes about ten grams of LNA to yield one gram of EPA and DHA.)

Flaxseed oil is the richest source of LNA, one tablespoon containing approximately *seven* grams. This unusual oil has three times more omega-3 fatty acids than omega-6 fatty acids. Flaxseed oil is highly unsaturated, making it more prone to oxidation by heat, light, and air. For this reason, it should not be heated above 210 degrees. Add flaxseed oil to salad dressings or soups and sauces just before serving. Store the oil in your refrigerator and use within a couple of months. (You will find flaxseed oil in the refrigerator case at the store.) Flaxseed oil is intensely flavored and can be somewhat "fishy" tasting. If you like, you can mix it with juice and glug it down like medicine, or stir it into flavored yogurt or cottage cheese. If you can't tolerate the taste, consider taking flaxseed oil capsules.

Flaxseeds, of course, are also a rich source of omega-3 fatty acids, providing 3 grams of LNA per tablespoon. One tablespoon also contains 3 grams of fiber. They have a subtle, nutty flavor, so you can grind them into a fine meal and add them to breads, muffins, pancakes, waffles, cereals, and cakes with little change in texture or flavor. Plan to use about one to two tablespoons of flaxseed meal or "flaxmeal" per cup of flour. (Place the flaxmeal in the bottom of the measuring cup and then add the flour.) You can grind your own flaxmeal in a food grinder or coffee grinder, or you can buy them preground. (Look in the vitamin supplement section of your natural food stores or see mail-order information on page 360.) Store flaxmeal in the refrigerator or freezer to preserve its freshness and use within two or three months.

Another way to add LNA to your diet is to use canola oil and canola mayonnaise on a daily basis. (Soybean oil also contains LNA, but only half the amount found in canola oil. More important, the ratio of omega-6 to omega-3 fatty acids in soybean oil is quite high—13 to 1. The ratio in canola oil is 2 to 1.) One tablespoon of canola oil yields approximately 1.5 grams of LNA.

So what's the bottom line on enriching your diet with omega-3 fatty acids? Ideally, you should be eating fatty fish three or more times a week. If not, supplement with fish oil pills. Pills that supply one gram of EPA plus DHA per day should be adequate for most people. Also, if possible, buy omega-3 enriched eggs. To increase your intake of LNA use canola oil and canola-oil-based products on a regular basis; add walnuts to salads and baked goods or eat a few each day as a snack; and eat dark green leafy vegetables every day.

| Type of Food | Amount of Alpha-Linolenic (LNA) per tablespoon |
|---|---|
| Flaxseed oil | 7 grams |
| Flaxseeds | 3 grams |
| Flaxseeds (ground) | 2 grams |
| Canola oil | 1.5 grams |
| Canola oil mayonnaise | 1 gram |
| Walnut oil | 1.2 grams |
| Walnuts (chopped) | 0.7 grams |

For even more LNA, eat approximately one to two tablespoons of flaxseeds or flaxmeal a day. (You can add them to cereal and baked goods or take flaxseed oil or flaxseed oil supplements. If you are a strict vegetarian, flaxseed products are highly recommended because you are not getting omega-3 fatty acids from fish or fish oil.) The recipes and menus featured in later chapters will help you adopt these potentially livesaving changes.

## 2. Use Canola Oil or Olive Oil as Your Primary Oil

If you have already made the switch from omega-6 oils to olive oil or canola oil, consider yourself lucky: You are already enjoying some of the health benefits of **The Omega Diet.** If not, you're overdue for an oil change. Throughout the text, I've mentioned that both olive oil and canola oil are desirable oils, each with its unique benefits, as indicated by the arrows in the chart that follows.

Canola oil gives you both monounsaturated fatty acids and LNA, the plant form of omega-3 fatty acids. Since it is also low in omega-6 fatty acids, saturated fat, and trans-fatty acids, it fulfills five of the seven **Omega Diet** guidelines. The people who took part in the Lyon heart study described in the first chapter used canola oil and canola margarine (specially formulated to be low in trans-fatty acids) as their primary fats, which is an indication of just how beneficial this one oil can be. (The canola oil was supplied to take the place of the LNA that the Greeks get from walnuts, purslane, and other wild plants.)

You need to be a careful shopper, however. Recently, a hybridized form of canola oil has come on the market with half the usual amount of omega-3 fatty acids. There is nothing intrinsically wrong with the oil, except that it contains half the normal amount of LNA. You can spot these hybridized oils by reading the label and looking for words like "good for high-heat cooking," or "lasts longer on the shelf." These are giveaways that it has been depleted of some of its LNA.

Olive oil, of course, is a wonderful oil—provided you can afford it and like its rich flavor. (Many people crave it.) The men from Crete were getting 30 percent of their calories from olive oil, and their superb health is a testimony to its life-enhancing properties. But keep in mind that if you use olive oil as your primary oil, you will need to

| Olive Oil | Canola Oil |
|---|---|
| → High in monounsaturates | → High in monounsaturates |
| Low in omega-3 fatty acids | → Relatively high in omega-3 fatty acids |
| → Contains cholesterol-lowering squalene | No squalene |
| Expensive | → Inexpensive |
| → Lowest in omega-6 fatty acids | → Low in omega-6 fatty acids |
| → Low in saturated fat | → Lowest in saturated fat |
| Rich flavor | Little flavor |

get your omega-3s elsewhere, either from fish, large amounts of green leafy vegetables, walnuts, flaxseeds, flax oil, or omega-3 supplements.

One way to get the benefits of both oils is to blend them together. This way you have an affordable oil that is high in monounsaturates and gives you both omega-3 fatty acids and squalene. You'll also be able to enjoy the flavor of olive oil. There is a commercial product called "canolive" that incorporates these two oils.

There are two more oils worth mentioning: "high-oleic" safflower and sunflower oil. The key words here are "high-oleic." As I've already stated, regular safflower oil and sunflower oil are very high in omega-6 fatty acids and very low in omega-3 fatty acids, making them undesirable oils. They are also low in monounsaturates. "High-oleic" oils are entirely different. Through hybridization, they have been transformed into oils that are high in monounsaturates and low in omega-6 fatty acids. They are light-tasting oils that can stand up to high-heat cooking. Use high-oleic oils if you wish, but like olive oil, they contain very little omega-3 fatty acids. You will need to get these essential nutrients from some other source.

## 3. Eat Seven or More Servings of Fruits and Vegetables Each Day

One of the reasons that people in Mediterranean countries have traditionally enjoyed such good health is that their mild climate allows them to grow fruits and vegetables year round. Thanks to the efficiency of U.S. farmers and a healthy import business, we, too, now have exotic fruits and vegetables 365 days of the year. All we have to do is eat them. Regrettably, the average American adult eats only 3.5 servings a day. Five out of ten teenagers and seven out of ten younger children eat only one serving a day.[8]

The U.S. government has launched a "Five a Day" campaign aimed at getting Americans to eat five servings of fruits and vegetables a day. This is a laudable effort, but it doesn't go far enough. For optimum health, you need to eat *seven* or more servings a day. Here are ten suggestions to help you reach the "Seven a Day" goal.

1. Eat fruit for breakfast every morning.
2. Follow the European tradition and snack on fresh fruit, not chips or crackers.
3. Take dried fruit with you to work.
4. Eat at least one green salad every day.
5. Have two vegetables at dinner.
6. Have fresh fruit for dessert, or at the very least, serve desserts that are based on fruit, such as single crust apple or berry pies, or apple cake.
7. Eat soups that contain more vegetables than meat or noodles.
8. Grill vegetables along with the meat.
9. Set aside thirty minutes each weekend to prepare fruit and vegetable snacks for the coming week. Store them in see-through refrigerator containers so they will be more tempting.
10. At restaurants, order a salad and one or two vegetables to go along with the main course. Or make the main course vegetarian.

Getting kids to eat more fruits and vegetables—especially vegetables—is an even bigger challenge. Here are some suggestions.

## Twelve Ways to Get Your Kids to Eat Their Vegetables

1. **Cater to their whims.** Find out which vegetables your kids like best and serve them the way they like them. Serve peas three times a week if that's what they'll eat.
2. **Allow them to pass on strong-tasting vegetables**. If your kids turn up their noses at strong-flavored vegetables such as turnips, broccoli, brussels sprouts, and onions, don't make them eat them. Meanwhile, as their palates mature, show them how much *you* enjoy these vegetables.
3. **Let them eat cake!** Carrot cake, that is. (For a recipe, see page 290). And don't forget chocolate zucchini cake, pumpkin bread, pumpkin pie, and sweet potato pie. The sugar and fat add calories, but they don't cancel out the beta-carotene.
4. **Don't be cowed by children who would rather eat pizza than peas.** Although you don't want to force your kids to eat vegetables, don't let them force *you* to take them off the menu. If you let some kids call the shots, it will be pizza, hot dogs, and hamburgers—period.
5. **Make single servings of the main dish**. If your kids want seconds, their only choice will be fruits and vegetables.
6. **Catch them in a moment of weakness.** Serve the salad separately at the beginning of the meal, when they are most hungry. Have celery or carrot sticks at hand when they come home from school.
7. **Dress up the vegetables.** Some kids don't like plain peas, but they'll take second helpings of creamed peas. Serve melted cheese on the broccoli and cauliflower. Add toasted almonds to the string beans. Dress up the carrots with toasted sesame seeds and a little soy sauce. Serve sliced hard-boiled eggs on the spinach. Serve pasta with pesto. Make spanakopita (Greek spinach pie).
8. **Buy a juicer and let them make their own vegetable concoctions.** Give them an array of fruits and vegetables and let them experiment. Ninety percent of the antioxidant content of fruits is in the juice—the "juicers" have been right all along.

9. **Grow a vegetable garden.** It's the rare person, child or adult, who can resist peas, beans, corn, beets, tomatoes, and carrots fresh from the garden. If the children help with the garden, the vegetables will be even more prized.

10. **Order pizza with vegetables.** True, most children would rather eat pepperoni or sausage pizza. But you're paying, so *you* get to order. Request the vegetables they like best, and chances are good they'll eat it.

11. **Bring on the catsup.** Tomatoes contain a potent antioxidant (lycopene) that is more "bioavailable" when the tomatoes are cooked and fat is added to the meal. Catsup and tomato sauces in general are the richest sources. Look for a low-salt variety.

12. **Serve cantaloupe, apricots, and mangos**. You're right. These aren't vegetables, but they are unusually high in beta-carotene, which is one of the chief vitamins in orange and yellow vegetables.

| Know Your Colors | | |
|---|---|---|
| Color of fruit or vegetable | Phytochemicals | Found in |
| Green | Thiocyanates, indoles, lutein. zeaxanthin, sulforaphane, isothicyanates | Cabbage, beet greens, collard greens, arugula, broccoli, brussels sprouts, kale, mustard greens |
| Yellow | Limonene | Lemons and other citrus fruits |
| Orange | Carotenes | Mangos, carrots, apricots, cantaloupe, peppers, squash, sweet potatoes, yams, pumpkins |
| Red | Lycopene | Tomatoes, watermelons, pink grapefruit |
| Purple, orange, red | Resveratrol, ellagic acid, cyanidin, quercetin | Red wine, grapes, grape juice, strawberries, raspberries |
| Brown | Genistein, phytosterols, saponins, protease inhibitors | Soybeans, mung beans, peanuts, dried beans |
| White | Allium, allyl sulfide, quercetin | Chives, leeks, scallions, garlic, onions, apples |

## 4. Eat More Peas, Beans, and Nuts

Peas and beans, once considered a meat substitute for people on tight budgets, have come into their own. They have so much to offer—vitamins, protein, fiber, minerals, cancer-fighting phytochemicals, folic acid, and LNA. Meanwhile, they are low in cost, low in calories, and free of saturated fat and cholesterol.

Soybeans are especially rich in LNA, and they also contain genistein, a cancer-fighting phytochemical. Years ago, manufacturers of vegetable burgers boasted that their products "contain no soy." Now savvy shoppers seek out these products precisely because of their soy content. There are a number of frozen soy patties on the market that are quite tasty. Buy several brands and see which one you like best. If you keep some in the freezer, along with hamburger buns, you can make a healthy meal in a matter of minutes. Experiment with tofu. It's practically tasteless, so you get to add all the flavor.

If you look for other opportunities to add beans to your diet, you'll find them. Add a spoonful of kidney beans or chickpeas (garbanzo beans) when you are at the salad bar. Serve hummus (recipe on page 270) as an hors d'oeuvre. Add black beans to salsa (p. 266). Make bean, pea, and lentil soups (pp. 260, 263); Provençal casserole (p. 273); and black bean quesadillas (p. 264).

If eating beans makes you a social outcast, there are two remedies. First, use canned beans or soak dry beans overnight before you cook them. The more thoroughly beans are cooked, the more of their carbohydrate is converted into sugar, easing the burden on your digestive system. You can also try "Beano," a commercial product that contains an enzyme that helps digest the starch. Some people say that it helps.

---

### WALNUTS LOWER YOUR CHOLESTEROL

To study the effects of walnuts on cholesterol, a group of men were placed on a standard cholesterol-lowering diet (the American Heart Association Step 1 Diet, the most frequently recommended heart diet). Later, some of the fat was replaced with walnuts. When the men were getting some of their fat from walnuts, they had lower LDL (bad) cholesterol and an improved ratio of LDL to HDL (good) cholesterol.[9]

---

**NUTS.** The term "health food nut" has more validity that it may first appear. Nuts are an excellent health food. Their main virtue is that they provide unadulterated oil—oil that has not been wrenched from its seed casing, exposed to air, bleached, deodorized, heated, degummed, and stripped of its antioxidants.

In order, the nuts with the largest amounts of LNA are butternuts (also referred to as "white" walnuts), English walnuts, and black walnuts. Butternuts are commonly eaten in Greece, which is another reason the people on Crete had such high levels of heart-protective LNA in their blood. Relatively little LNA is found in almonds, cashews, macadamia nuts, filberts, pine nuts, or pistachio nuts. (See chart on page 138 for a comparison.)

Like all foods rich in omega-3 fatty acids, nuts spoil rapidly (especially when shelled), so buy the amount you plan to use in one or two months and store them in a covered container in your refrigerator or freezer. Discard any nuts that have an "off" flavor. They're rancid.

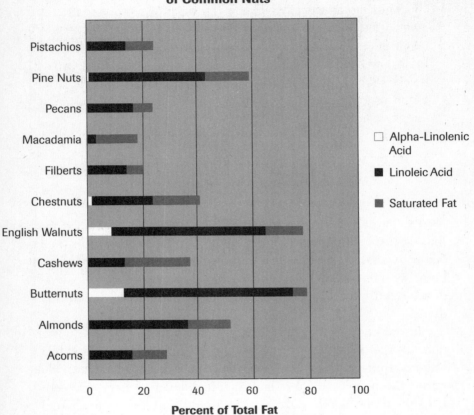

**Fatty Acid Content
of Common Nuts** [11]

Percent of Total Fat

Alpha-Linolenic Acid

Linoleic Acid

Saturated Fat

# 5. Eat Less Saturated Fat and Cholesterol

You've heard this advice before. Heart researchers have known since the 1950s that a diet high in saturated fat and cholesterol increases the risk of cardiovascular disease, particularly in those with a family history of heart disease. For this reason, most dietary guidelines recommend that you keep your daily intake below 10 percent of your total calories. On **The Omega Diet,** you will be eating less than 8 percent of your calories as saturated fat, an added measure of safety. (If you eat 2,000 calories a day, for example, you should be eating no more than 160 calories, or 18 grams, of saturated fat a day.)

But as researchers have tightened their focus from fats in general to fatty acids in particular, they've discovered that all saturated fatty acids are not alike in terms of raising cholesterol. For example, stearic acid, the type of saturated fatty acid found in meat and chocolate, does *not* raise your LDL cholesterol. (But it may increase the risk of blood clots.) The saturated fatty acids that seem to do the most harm to the cardiovascular system are myristic acid (found in dairy products) and palmitic acid, which is the type of fat your body manufactures when you eat a very low-fat diet. Low-fat and nonfat milk products are good for you, however, because they provide B vitamins, protein, and calcium.

For some people, cutting back on butter can be quite difficult— especially now that margarine has been discredited due to its high trans-fatty acid content. If you like some form of fat with your bread, consider olive oil. Many people who sit down to dinner now ask "please pass the olive oil" instead of "please pass the butter." A growing number of restaurants serve a dish of olive oil along with the basket of bread.

If you want a more buttery spread or if you want to bake a cake or pastry that requires a more malleable fat, try a fifty-fifty blend of olive oil and butter, or canola oil and butter. These spreads are very easy to make. (See page 238.) The canola/butter spread tastes like a light, less salty butter. Some people say they like it as well as butter. The olive oil/butter blend is rich with both flavors, which can be a refreshing change. Both of these butter blends are a perfect spreading and baking consistency right from the refrigerator. A commercial canola/butter has recently arrived on the market, although at the present time it is found only in natural food stores or the health food section of large supermarkets. The main difference between the store-bought kind and the homemade variety is that the commercial product costs more and contains an added (and unnecessary) stabilizer.

Although cheese is a full-fat milk product, it may not be as harmful to your cardiovascular system as butter or cream. (The reason is that cheese is especially high in calcium, and calcium links with saturated fatty acids to keep much of them from being absorbed.[12]) This is why you are allowed up to one ounce of full-fat cheese a day on **The Omega Diet**.

Tropical oils—coconut oil, palm oil, and palm kernel oil—should be used sparingly, if at all. Unlike most vegetable oils, they contain high amounts of saturated fat. These oils are commonly used in Asian countries, but they cause little harm because the overall diet is so low in other forms of saturated fat. When westerners eat tropical oils, they add them to a diet that is already high in butter fat, animal fat, and trans-fatty acids—a potentially deadly combination.

Chicken skin, turkey skin, and beef fat are to be avoided, particularly if you have coronary artery disease. In addition to contributing to heart disease, these types of fat have been linked with an increased risk of colon and prostate cancer. When you buy beef, buy the leanest cuts—round tip, top round, eye of round, top loin, tenderloin, sirloin, and extra-lean and lean ground beef. The leanest cuts of pork are tenderloin, top loin chop, center loin chop, and loin roast. Lamb has more omega-3 fatty acids than other meats.

On **The Omega Diet**, you can eat lean meat two or three times a week. A meal that contains lean meat, a salad, and one or more vegetable dishes is a nutritionally balanced meal. You might also explore some alternatives to beef. There is a growing market for "exotic" meats such as buffalo, beefalo (a cross between cattle and buffalo) and emu (an ostrich-type bird) because they are relatively low in saturated fat. For example, a buffalo steak has only 6 grams of saturated fat per 100 grams of meat, compared with 20 grams for a similar amount of beef or pork. (For information about buying exotic meat, see page 361.)

Eggs are less harmful to your health than once thought. If you have normal cholesterol levels, you can eat an egg a day without any harm. Eggs have a number of virtues. High in protein, they slow the emptying of your stomach, helping to level out your blood sugar from breakfast to lunch.[13]

If you have high cholesterol levels, however, or a family history of high cholesterol, you would be wise to use egg whites only, egg substitutes, or limit yourself to one or two egg yolks a week. But this caveat does not apply to eggs that are high in omega-3 fatty acids. A number of egg producers are now using a mash that has been enriched with omega-3 fatty acids, either from fish meal or flaxseeds.

| Saturated Fats to Avoid | Saturated Fats to Eat in Moderation |
|---|---|
| Chicken skin | Chocolate |
| Full-fat milk products except cheese | Cheese and yogurt |
| Fatty cuts of beef, lamb, or pork | Butter/canola or butter/olive oil blends |
| Tropical oils | Eggs (Look for omega-3 enriched eggs) |
| | Lean cuts of beef, pork or lamb |
| | Chicken (Look for chickens fed a diet enriched with omega-3 fatty acids) |
| | Wild game |

(Brand names include The Country Hen, Born "3," and Pilgrim's Pride's EggsPlus.) In small studies, eating two omega-3 enriched eggs a day has not caused a rise in LDL cholesterol. In addition, it has lowered triglycerides and raised HDL (good) cholesterol.

What about eggs from chickens advertised as being "free-ranging," "free-roaming," "naturally nested," or "uncaged"? Unless the chickens have been free-ranging on grounds that are rich with insects and green plants, their eggs will contain no more omega-3 fatty acids than regular eggs. Undoubtedly, it's good for the chickens' psyche to "free-roam" on a dusty barn floor, or to "free-range" on a picked-clean chicken yard, but it won't make a bit of difference in the nutritional content of their eggs.

## 6. Avoid Oils High in Omega-6 Fatty Acids

In order to eat a balanced ratio of essential fatty acids, you may need to lower your intake of omega-6 fatty acids, particularly linoleic acid. Although your body requires a minimum amount of this EFA, you will get all you need, about 3 to 4 grams a day, from canola oil, flaxseed oil, and olive oil. (All fats and oils contain some linoleic acid. Canola oil, for example, has twice as much linoleic as alpha-linolenic acid. The linoleic content of olive oil is around 6 to 10 percent.)

To keep your linoleic intake at a healthy level, avoid oils that are especially high in this nutrient, including corn oil, safflower oil, peanut oil, soybean oil, sunflower seed oil, and cottonseed oil. You will also want to avoid products made from these oils, such as mayonnaise and salad dressing. Of the lot, safflower oil has the most linoleic acid and the least alpha-linolenic acid, giving it the most unfavorable ratio of omega-6 to omega-3 fatty acids—200 to 1! For comparison, canola oil has a ratio of 2 to 1. As you know, you want to keep your ratio of omega-6 to omega-3 fatty acids below 4.

## 7. Avoid Trans-Fatty Acids

It is difficult to live in the United States and avoid trans-fatty acids because they have infiltrated the entire food supply. Anytime you see the words "partially hydrogenated" on a label, trans-fatty acids lurk within. Take the time to go through the supermarket aisles and read the labels on baked goods, snack foods, and mixes. Virtually every one contains trans-fatty acids.

> "If one does not want to read labels to avoid trans-fat one should avoid boxed and packaged foods, and eat whole unrefined foods."— *Clinical Pearls News,* May 1997

### Food High in Trans-fatty Acids

- Biscuit mixes and dough
- Cakes and cake mixes
- Cinnamon rolls
- Cookies and cookie mixes
- Corn chips
- Crackers
- Doughnuts
- Granola
- Frozen desserts (not ice cream)
- Muffin mixes
- Pastries in general
- Pie crusts and pie crust mixes
- Popcorn (flavored)
- Potato chips
- Shortening
- Tortillas and tortilla chips

A few canola-based products are beginning to appear in regular supermarkets. (Make sure, however, that the oil has not been partially hydrogenated.) Natural food stores, meanwhile, offer an abundant supply of healthy convenience food, including canola-based tortillas, salad dressings, mayonnaise, mixes, granola, tortillas, crackers, cookies, cakes, and potato chips.

When you buy salad dressings, look for ones made from canola oil or olive oil. But don't be fooled. An "olive oil" dressing may have soybean oil as the primary ingredient. I also encourage you to make your own salad dressings. It need not be difficult. In Greece, we dress our salads at the table with olive oil, a squirt of lemon, salt, and pepper. Sometimes, vinegar is used instead of lemon. Try this at home. Or make the following simple and delicious vinaigrette.

---

### THREE-MINUTE OLIVE OIL VINAIGRETTE

Mix together:

$1/2$ cup of extra-virgin olive oil

2 tablespoons plus 1 teaspoon of wine vinegar

$1/4$ teaspoon salt

$1/4$ teaspoon dried mustard

1 clove fresh garlic (finely minced or pressed through a garlic press)

Freshly ground black pepper, to taste

(Vary by adding paprika, tarragon, dill, or basil.)

---

There is only one type of margarine I can currently recommend and that is canola margarine that is sold in a squeezable container— the softer the margarine, the lower the trans-fatty acid content. One manufacturer sells a tub margarine made from canola oil that is free of trans-fatty acids, but it cannot be used in cooking. There are several other brands of soft canola margarine on the market, but, unfortunately, the manufacturers do not reveal their trans-fatty acid content. Ideally, a margarine should contain less than 2 percent trans-fatty acids, which is the amount that naturally occurs in butter, for example. (Some fatty acids are converted into trans-fatty acids in a cow's digestive system.) Stick margarines can be as high as 30 percent trans-fatty acids. Don't buy margarine made from oils other than canola oil, even if they are advertised to be low in trans-fatty acids, because they will contain an excessive amount of omega-6 fatty acids.

The beauty of **The Omega Diet** is that you can make all these changes to your diet without sacrificing flavor. In fact, you may find that you need to *add* more fat to your diet to satisfy The Seven Dietary Guidelines. For example, it is healthier to have a tomato sauce that includes olive oil than a fat-free tomato sauce because the fat helps you absorb more of the nutrients. It is better to eat one slice of toast spread with canola/butter than two slices of dry toast because you will have a better balance of carbohydrates and fat. It is better to eat a salad with an olive oil or canola oil vinaigrette than a fat-free dressing because, once again, you will be absorbing more nutrients. On **The Omega Diet**, good nutrition *tastes* good.

# ELEVEN

# The Omega Shopper

*Stocking Your Pantry with Essential Nutrients*

As I MENTIONED at the outset, most of the "work" of **The Omega Diet** takes place at the grocery store. If you fill your shopping cart wisely, you will be well on your way to satisfying all of The Seven Dietary Guidelines. A large supermarket will have most of what you need, especially if it has a health food section. But if you live in an area without a large supermarket, you will need to do some of your shopping at a natural food store.

If you live in an area of the country that does not have such a store, you may need to shop by mail. You will find mail-order information on pages 360–63.)

**COOKING AND SALAD OILS.** Let's start with the basics. First, I suggest that you rid your kitchen of unhealthy or rancid oils. Throw out all the oils high in omega-6 fatty acids (especially corn oil, safflower oil, and sunflower oil) as well as any canola oil or flaxseed oil that has been kept unrefrigerated for a week or longer.

Then you can begin restocking your kitchen with healthy oils. First on your list should be canola oil and olive oil, both good sources of monounsaturated fatty acids. Buying canola oil is a simple matter because the flavor and quality vary little from brand to brand. The only significant difference is in the way the oil is processed. Ideally, you want "cold-pressed" or "unrefined" canola oil, which means that the oil has been extracted at a low temperature without chemicals, helping to preserve its antioxidants and flavonoids. Make sure you are buying *regular* canola, not hybrid canola oil that has been stripped of some of its omega-3 fatty acids. (You will know if it's a hybrid oil if the label contains words like "better for high heat cooking," or "longer shelf life.") Also, check to make sure you are not buying a canola oil/corn oil blend. Corn oil is one of the things you are trying to *eliminate* from your diet. Buy the amount of oil that you think you will use in about two months' time and store it in your refrigerator.

Buying olive oil can seem more daunting—akin to selecting a good bottle of wine—but it needn't be difficult if all you want is a good, affordable olive oil. If so, go to your local supermarket and buy any of the major brands of *extra-virgin* oil. "Extra-virgin" means that the oil comes from the first pressing of the olives and has a low level of acidity. Extra-virgin oil also has the highest amount of monounsaturated fatty acids, the most omega-3 fatty acids, and the least omega-6 fatty acids, making it the healthiest of all the various kinds.

Olive oil, unlike wine, does *not* improve with age, so buy the amount you expect to use in three or four months' time. Olive oil is more resistant to oxidation than other oils (which is one of the reasons it slows the oxidation of your LDL cholesterol), so you don't need to keep it in the refrigerator. But do store it in a cool place that is out of the light, especially if the oil comes in a clear bottle. (Some purists wrap the bottle with aluminum foil.) Light, air, and heat speed up oxidation.

If you want to venture beyond supermarket olive oil, read on. Most of the olive oil on the market is extra-virgin. Extra-virgin olive oil comes from the first pressing of quality olives, making it low in acidity. One of its many virtues is that it is not heated, bleached, deodorized, or degummed, so it still retains the unique flavor of the olives from which it was made. Professional olive oil tasters can identify as many as thirty-two separate olive oil flavors, including "grassy," "buttery," "fruity," "chocolate" and "peppery." Don't be intimidated by the experts, however. As with wine, what matters is what you like and what you can afford.

The second grade, "virgin" oil, is actually harder to find. It, too, may come from the first pressing, but it is allowed to have a slightly higher degree of acidity. The third grade, referred to simply as "olive oil," comes from later pressings or from lesser quality, older, or bruised olives. Typically, it is treated with heat and chemicals to extract more of the oil and to remove undesirable flavors. At the end of this process, a small amount of extra-virgin oil is added to enhance the flavor. Unless indicated otherwise, store-brand olive oil and the most inexpensive brand names are of this lesser grade.

Some olive oil in the supermarkets is described as "light" or even "extra-light" olive oil. Light olive oil is *not* lower in calories than regular olive oil. "Light" refers to the fact that it has been highly refined to yield a milder flavor than regular olive oil. Light olive oil is for people who feel they "should" use olive oil but aren't wild about the taste. It still retains all the beneficial monounsaturated fatty acids, but some of the antioxidants and flavonoids have been sacrificed in the refining process.

Some terms you find on olive oil bottles are meaningless. "Pure" has no accepted definition. Nor does "premium" or "all-natural." These words are used to give the *illusion* of quality, but they tell you nothing about the actual nature of the oil.

Like wine, the aroma, color, and flavor of olive oil are influenced by a host of factors, including climate, region, soil, type of fruit, and processing technique. One notable difference between wine and olive oil is that the oil does *not* have to come from the country or area designated on the label. For example, both Spain and Greece produce large quantities of olive oil that are shipped to Italy, where it is bottled and sold as Italian olive oil. The reason for this subterfuge is that "Italian" olive oil has a better reputation with consumers and can therefore command a higher price.

The flavor of olive oil is also influenced by the ripeness of the olives. Green olives picked early in the season yield an oil that is golden-green in color and tends to be sharp, grassy, earthy, or spicy. Ripe olives produce a golden oil that is more "buttery," and, some would say, "bland." (As a rule, people who are knowledgeable about olive oil tend to prefer the younger, spicier oils that most people would find too sharp. According to some Europeans, the best olive oil leaves a "kick" in the back of the throat that lasts from lunch through naptime.) To find out which oil *you* like best, you might go to an olive oil tasting (sponsored by specialty stores or natural food stores) or buy small bottles of several varieties. You can also order a high-end olive oil sampler by mail order. (See page 363.)

---

### MONEY-SAVING TIP

One reason that olive oil is so expensive is that the trees grow very slowly, and the fruit is often picked by hand.

If you find the cost prohibitive, shop at a natural food store that sells olive oil in bulk. You'll get a good quality oil for a much lower price.

---

**FLAXSEED OIL.** Flaxseed oil is the most concentrated source of LNA commonly available. You will find it in the refrigerator case of the health food section of your supermarket or natural food store. The taste varies greatly from brand to brand. Some have a sharp, unpleasant flavor. Some people would argue that *all* brands of flaxseed oil have an unpleasant flavor. Brands that many people prefer are Omega Nutrition and Barlean's, because they have a milder, nuttier flavor than others. (See ordering information on pages 360–362.)

Flaxseed oil spoils more readily than all other oils due to its high omega-3 content, so buy the amount you plan to use in three months' time and *always* store it in the refrigerator. Some brands come with special labels telling you the date the oil was pressed and the latest date it should be used, which is very helpful information.

Recently, a new type of flaxseed oil has come on the market that contains both flaxseed oil and a lignan extract, giving you more of the benefits of whole seeds.

**MAYONNAISE.** Most mayonnaise is made from soybean oil. Soybean oil has more omega-3 fatty acids than most other seed oils, but its ratio of omega-6 to omega-3 fatty acids is still unacceptably high—12 to 1. A healthier choice is canola oil or olive oil mayonnaise. Presently, these types of mayonnaise are hard to find. Some supermarket brands are made from canola oil, but they won't say so on the front of the bottle. You'll have to read the fine print on the back. At least one manufacturer makes a "light" canola oil mayonnaise that is lower in calories. This is a reasonable choice if you're trying to lose weight, but remember that it contains fewer omega-3s per tablespoon than regular canola oil mayonnaise. You can lighten up regular canola oil mayonnaise yourself by mixing it fifty-fifty with low-fat plain yogurt. If you can't find canola oil mayonnaise, make your own. (See page 240 for an easy and delicious recipe.)

Some people are very particular about what kind of mayonnaise or salad dressing they eat. If your household is wedded to a particular brand (and it's not made from canola oil or olive oil), try blending it fifty-fifty with canola oil mayonnaise.

**FLAXSEEDS.** Flaxseeds have been part of the human diet for at least 10,000 years. Hippocrates extolled their virtues, and Pliny the Elder (23–79 A.D.) noted that the Greeks added flaxseed flour to their wheat flour when making bread. In Europe, flaxseeds still play a dominant role in the diet. The Germans, for example, consume 60,000 tons annually in breads and cereals. We eat so little in the United States that no one has bothered to measure our consumption.

> "Wherever flaxseeds become a regular food item among the people, there will be better health."
>
> Mahatma Gandhi

It's time we changed our ways. Flaxseeds are an ideal source of LNA, soluble and insoluble fiber, and a cancer-fighting substance called lignan. I suggest that you have some on hand at all times. You will find these shiny, coffee-brown, sesame-sized seeds in a natural food store or the health food section of your supermarket. They are very inexpensive. A month's supply can cost less than three dollars. Save some to use as whole seeds and grind the rest in a coffee grinder or similar device. (You can't grind them in a food processor or blender—they just bounce around.) You can purchase them preground (flaxmeal) in the supplement section of some natural food stores, or you can order them through the mail. (See page 360). Store your flaxseeds and flaxmeal in the refrigerator or freezer and use within two to three months. Sprinkle on your breakfast cereal and add to muffins, bread, cakes, pancakes, and waffles.

## A NOTE OF CAUTION

To be on the safe side, you should eat no more than three to four tablespoons of raw flaxseeds or flaxmeal a day. Flaxseeds, like lima and cassava beans, contain a chemical called cyanogen that your body converts into another chemical called thiocyanate (SCN). If you have high amounts of SCN in your blood for long periods of time, it can keep your thyroid gland from taking up enough iodine, increasing your risk of goiter. Cyanogen is inactivated during cooking, however, even if the flaxseeds are added to baked goods such as cookies or muffins that are cooked for only twelve to fifteen minutes.[1]

Flaxseed oil does not contain cyanogen, so you need not restrict your intake. Most brands of oil lack lignan, however, so there's a trade-off.

**FRESH GARLIC.** Many of the recipes in this book call for fresh garlic. Garlic contains a number of nutrients that help fight cancer, lower cholesterol, and may even lower your blood pressure, making it an essential "neutraceutical" (a food with medicinal properties). Buy it fresh and use it often. Look for heads of garlic that are firm and fill up their papery wrapper. Soft or shriveled garlic is past its prime. Garlic salt and dried garlic are often stale and off-flavored.

**FISH.** Most large supermarkets carry a dozen or more different kinds of seafood regardless of the time of year. The problem is that it's not always fresh. Fish spoils more rapidly than flesh from land animals precisely because of its high omega-3 content—all those double bonds on the omega-3 fatty acid molecules make them more vulnerable to oxidation or "spoiling." Many clerks will insist that all of their fish is impeccably fresh, but experience will tell you otherwise. Consider the fate of an Alaskan salmon. Once caught, it might spend two days in the hold of a ship, one day in the processing plant, one day in transit to the airport, one day in transport to the central distributor, and then one more day getting from the distributor to your local store. That's six days out of the water. At best, the salmon will have one or two days left before it goes bad.

Fish is more likely to be fresh if you buy it from a specialty store, a fish market, or a supermarket that has a very active fish department. One indication of fish quality is the manner in which fish are displayed. Ideally, whole fish should be packed *in* crushed ice, and fish fillets should be kept *on* crushed ice. There should be plenty of ice and little odor.

Once you've selected a store, get to know the employees. Let them know that you want the freshest fish available. Ask about their delivery schedule. If fish is delivered on Tuesday and Friday, you'll know not to shop on Monday and Thursday. Ask strategic questions. If you simply ask, "Is the salmon fresh?" the answer is going to be "yes." But if you ask, "Which day was the salmon delivered?" you might get more helpful information. The best way to ensure you'll be getting the freshest fish, however, is to go to the store without having a specific type of fish in mind. Say, for example, that you want either trout, tuna, or salmon—whichever is freshest. This gives the clerk a lot of leeway. He or she can then recommend the newly arrived tuna without having to acknowledge that the salmon and trout have been sitting in the case for days.

Finally, learn to be your own judge of freshness. A truly fresh fish has a number of characteristics you will come to recognize. If the fish is whole, it will be moist, but not slick or tacky. The scales will be firmly attached. The gills will be moist, shiny, and dark red (never light-colored or brown). The color will be uniform from head to tail. (Any change in color is an indication of spoiling.) Most important, it will not smell "fishy." All you'll detect is the aroma of a sea breeze. If you poke a freshly caught fish with your finger, its flesh will spring right back. If you make a dent, the fish is too old.

Fish can spoil in thirty minutes in a hot car, so get home quickly. Put the fish in the coldest part of your refrigerator or, better yet, pack it between two packages of crushed ice. (Fresh fish keeps best at about 32 degrees, and most refrigerators are ten degrees warmer.) Since you've gone to so much trouble to buy fresh fish and keep it fresh, eat it as soon as possible.

**BUYING FROZEN FISH.** Because the journey from sea to market may take a week, frozen fish can be fresher than "fresh" fish. As with buying fresh fish, however, it helps to be armed with information. First of all, you need to know the difference between the similar-sounding terms "fresh frozen" and "fresh from frozen." "Fresh frozen" means that the fish has been frozen as soon as possible after being caught. This is the common practice in modern trawlers, which are literal factories at sea. The fish is cleaned and blast frozen within hours of leaving the water and is then stored in subzero freezers on the ship and during land transport.

The term "fresh from frozen" means that the fish has been frozen and then thawed, a common practice that the industry refers to as "slacking." The fish may look fresh, but its taste and texture have been compromised to some degree by having been frozen. Once thawed, it can languish in the store for several days. If so, you have a worst-case scenario—a fish that has been altered by freezing and then has been kept in the display case long enough to go bad. Don't refreeze "fresh from frozen" fish because you will further undermine its quality.

There are many ways to freeze fish commercially. The best is a process called "nitrogen freezing," a procedure that freezes the fish so rapidly that the individual cells don't have a chance to break down and release their moisture. When you thaw a fish that has been treated in this manner, the flesh will be plump and moist and won't be sitting in a puddle of water.

---

### THE LABEL SAYS "SALMON"— BUT DOES IT HAVE ANY OMEGA-3s?

Read the label carefully when you buy salmon patties or sausages—the good fat may have been entirely removed. You'll get the same amount of protein but little of the flavor and none of the omega-3 content.

---

Buy a "fresh frozen" fish while it is still frozen. Pick a package that is buried deepest in the freezer. Reject packages that show signs of thawing such as water drainage or ice crystals. Also, don't buy fish with white patches, an indication of freezer burn. If you plan to use the fish at a later date, put it in your freezer immediately. Each time that fish is thawed and refrozen, it loses flavor and texture. If you plan to use the fish that day or the next, let it thaw in the refrigerator.

---

### WATCH OUT FOR SODIUM TRIPOLYPHOSPHATE

Before freezing, some processors treat fish with sulfites or a related chemical called "sodium tripolyphosphate," substances that cause the fish to retain water. The fish will look plump and firm when it is frozen (and will weigh more, thus benefiting the seller), but when it is thawed and cooked the water leaches out, leaving the fish dry and shrunken.

A retailer is not required to tell you if a fish has been treated in this manner. However, if a fish is free of added chemicals, the retailer will want to advertise that fact. Natural food stores and fish markets are most likely to sell untreated fish.

---

**FARMED FISH.** Much of the salmon and trout on the market today is farmed fish. Farmed fish are fish that have been raised in a hatchery and then transported to large cages in a saltwater bay. Because the fish are confined, they are dependent on their keepers for food, and their nutritional value is strongly influenced by what they are fed. If they're fed a grain diet instead of fish meal, they'll be abnormally high in saturated fat and linoleic acid and lower in omega-3 fatty acids—not what you want. (Interestingly, fish that are fed a diet too low in omega-3 fatty acids tend to develop cardiovascular disease.) A point in the favor of farmed fish, however, is that they are handled very efficiently. They are cleaned immediately after being killed and quickly shipped to market. Another benefit is that they are available year round and are likely to be less expensive than wild fish. As the demand for fatty fish grows, more and more of the fish being sold the world over will be farmed fish.

As any fisherman will tell you, farmed fish does not taste the same as fish caught in the wild. Wild-caught salmon needs nothing more than salt, pepper, and a squeeze of lime or lemon. Farmed fish benefit from more elaborate sauces and seasonings.

**CANNED FISH.** Americans eat more canned tuna fish than any other type of fish—about 800 million pounds a year. Canning subjects fish to high heat for long periods of time, altering its flavor and texture, but it does not destroy a significant amount of its omega-3 fatty acids. There is about the same amount of DHA and EPA in three ounces of canned tuna as there is in three ounces of fresh tuna.

Canned tuna varies in quality and price. "Solid white tuna," considered top-of-the-line, comes from albacore tuna. "Chunk light" tuna may contain irregular pieces of albacore, or it may come from yellowfin tuna or skipjack tuna. (Some people prefer the flavor of light tuna over solid white tuna.) "Flake" and "shredded" tuna, the least expensive varieties, are made from darker cuts of tuna or from irregular pieces. Dark tuna is considered less desirable because it is not as delicately flavored as light-colored meat.

Most tuna is packed in water or soybean oil, although you can now find tuna packed in olive oil or canola oil. Generally, I recommend buying tuna packed in water. When the tuna is packed in water, the fat content listed on the nutritional label reflects only the amount of oil in the fish (not any added canning oil), giving you precise information about the fat content of the fish itself. Also, soybean oil, the most commonly used oil, has a ratio of omega-6 to omega-3 fatty acids of 12 to 1, tipping the nutritional scale in favor of the omega-6 fatty acids. Tuna can be more flavorful when packed in oil, however. If you find this to be true, go to a specialty store and look for tuna packed in olive oil or canola oil. (In a recent taste test sponsored by the *New York Times,* Progresso Light Tuna in Olive Oil was the clear favorite. Chicken of the Sea Solid White Tuna in Spring Water topped the common store brands.[1])

Out of habit, you may be tempted to look for canned tuna with the lowest fat content. With fatty fish such as tuna, however, you want to buy the one with the *highest* amount of fat, because fat is its most important virtue. (But once again, make sure you are buying *water*-packed tuna.) The fat content can range dramatically—from 0.5 to 5 grams per serving.

For variety, buy canned salmon or mackerel and use it in all the ways you customarily use tuna, from sandwiches to salads. Don't overlook canned sardines and herring. They contain the most omega-3 fatty acids of all the fatty fish. Many Europeans eat a daily snack of sardines. (Look for those packed in olive oil, canola oil, mustard, or tomato sauce.)

## Get to Know Your Greens

Eating seven or more servings of fruits and vegetables a day is a vital component of **The Omega Diet.** These wholesome foods give you fiber, iron, magnesium, calcium, folic acid, antioxidant vitamins, and phytochemicals. Dark green leafy vegetables contain LNA as well.

Most Europeans eat far more greens than we do. Greeks eat vast quantities of greens, which they refer to generically as *"horta."* The Italians have a special term, *"mangia-foglia,"* which means "to eat green leaves." An American visitor to a European open-air market will see dozens of green leafy vegetables, most of them unfamiliar. In addition to this wide selection, many Europeans delight in foraging for wild greens in the countryside.

Until very recently, spinach was the only dark green vegetable most Americans would eat. This left out a long list of nutritious greens, including arugula, beet greens, broccoli raab, chard, chicory, dandelion greens, collard greens, endive, kale, mustard greens, purslane, romaine, turnip greens, and watercress. These greens have been slow to catch on because many of them have a slightly bitter or peppery flavor, which can be a bit of a shock to people who are used to iceberg lettuce.

Now, greens are coming into their own, partly due to the new-found popularity of salads made from mixed greens. Called *mesclun* in France and *saldini* or *misticanza* in Italy, this type of salad is a medley of greens, often accented with spicy greens such as arugula, watercress, basil, and radicchio. Some restaurants serve mesclun as their standard salad, throwing in a few edible flowers for added color. Mesclun has become so popular that some supermarkets carry prewashed mixed greens packaged in plastic wrap, a great convenience for busy people. They may be labeled as "European greens," "baby greens," or "spring greens." To make a great salad, all you have to do is pop open the wrapper, dump the greens into a salad bowl, and sprinkle with olive oil, lemon or vinegar, salt, and pepper. It takes just a few minutes.

Below is a brief introduction to some lesser known greens. If you are hesitant to venture into this verdant territory, begin with young plants and add them sparingly to salads made from milder and more familiar greens.

**ARUGULA (a-ROO-guh-luh).** You will recognize arugula by its dark green, deeply lobed leaves that resemble oak leaves. Arugula has a peppery taste akin to watercress and can be found in the produce section of most large supermarkets, typically in the herb section.

Arugula is commonly used as a salad ingredient or as a colorful bedding for meat or bean dishes. Large leaves can be quite bitter, but if you select young and tender ones (two to four inches long), they are mild enough to be the primary greens in a salad. Some specialty stores feature arugula that has been grown hydroponically (in a water solution, not soil), resulting in especially mild-flavored leaves. Other names for arugula include "rocket," "rocquette," and Italian cress. Arugula is great to grow in your garden because it grows rapidly (thus the name rocket?) and is frost-resistant. In some areas of the country you can have fresh arugula all year long.

**CHICORY.** The name "chicory" encompasses a large family of plants that range in color from green to red. The kind with a pale heart and green furled leaves is "curly endive." Add chicory to salads to give them more color and spice. They can also be served as a cooked vegetable.

**COLLARD GREENS.** Collard greens have large, leathery leaves with cream-colored veins and taste like a cross between cabbage and spinach. The southern tradition is to boil them for long periods of time, but you can also steam them for ten to fifteen minutes and eat them while they still have some of their crunch and more of their nutrients.

**KALE.** Kale, a member of the cabbage family, is one of the most nutritious of all vegetables. There are two basic varieties, "Russian" kale, which has a purple-green color and smooth, relatively tender leaves, and "regular" kale, which is gray-green and has tightly curled leaves. Both are excellent sources of antioxidants, phytochemicals, vitamins, calcium, magnesium, and iron. For a quick and easy vegetable dish, chop kale into bite-sized pieces and steam until tender. (Discard thick stems or cut them up and sauté them for a few minutes before adding the more tender leaves.) Toss with olive oil and lemon. Salt and pepper to taste.

Kale is also a good addition to soups and stir-fry dishes.

**MUSTARD GREENS.** You're probably more familiar with the seeds of the mustard plant—which are ground up to make the mustard that you put on your sandwiches—than its succulent, nutritious leaves. You'll be reminded of mustard when you eat the leaves, especially the spicy leaves from more mature plants.

**PURSLANE.** Purslane, once considered a weed, is now regarded as a "power plant." Among other virtues, it contains more LNA than any known green leafy vegetable. Look for purslane in farmer's markets and grocery stores with large produce departments. Until this delicious vegetable becomes better known, you might have to grow your own. (See page 363.)

When you first try purslane, serve it raw tossed with olive oil, lemon juice, salt, and pepper. Delicious. Once you've gained appreciation for its delicate flavor and unique texture (kind of a cross between tender pea pods and a buttery lettuce), add it to mesclun, toss it in soups, or sauté briefly in butter and serve with a light cream sauce. You might also consider this recipe from *Forme of Curye*, a collection of recipes from pre-fourteenth-century England:

> *"Take persel, sawge, grene garlec, oynouns, leek, borage, myntes, porrettes, fenel, and toun cressis, rew, rosemarye, purslarye; laue and waische hem clene. Pike hem. Pluk hem small with thyn honde and myng hem wel with rawe oile; lay on vyneger and salt, and serve it forth."*

Rough translation:

> *"Take parsley, sage, green garlic, chiboles (scallions), leeks, borage, mint, poretts (leeks), fennel, and garden cress, rue,*

*rosemary, purslane; wash them clean. Pick (the nasty bits) from them. Pluck them small with your hand, and mix them well with oil; add vinegar and salt, and serve it forth."*

**SWISS CHARD.** Swiss chard comes from the beet family, and is in fact a type of beet that is grown for its leaves rather than its roots. It comes in two main varieties, red and green. Red Swiss chard is a memorable sight with its blood red veins and dark green, puckered leaves. Swiss chard is milder than some other greens and can substitute for spinach in many dishes, including omelets and meat pies. Add young and tender leaves to mesclun. (You'll find a recipe for Swiss Chard with Walnuts and Raisins on page 268.)

**WILD GREENS.** As a rule, wild greens contain even more nutrients than cultivated greens, mainly because the American taste runs to mild-flavored plants. (Mild-tasting plants tend to have fewer phytochemicals.) You might start with dandelion leaves. Yes, these are the same noxious greens that invade your lawn. If you pick the leaves early in the spring before they have a chance to bloom, they make a spicy addition to your mesclun. Of course, *never* use dandelions that have been sprayed with chemicals or that you think *might* have been so treated. To venture beyond dandelions, look for a book on edible wild plants at your bookstore or take a class on edible wild greens. Cow parsnip, dock, fiddlehead ferns, and nettles are commonly eaten wild plants.

# TWELVE

# The 3-Week Omega Diet

THIS CHAPTER FEATURES the **3-Week Omega Diet**, a landmark program designed to launch you into a new, healthier, and more natural way of eating. The detailed, twenty-one-day menu gives you an ideal balance of essential fatty acids plus all the vitamins, antioxidants, minerals, phytochemicals, and other nutrients proven to be essential for optimal health. At the end of three weeks, you will have begun to replace much of the fat in your body with healthier fat, enriched your cells with vital nutrients, and begun to enjoy all the health benefits of **The Omega Diet.** Meanwhile, your pantry will be stocked with wholesome ingredients, and you will be developing new shopping and eating habits that will stand you in good stead for the rest of your life.

The 2,000-calorie menu detailed in this chapter is designed for people who want to maintain their present weight. If you want to lose weight, you can follow the weight-loss menus featured in the next chapter. (Before turning to chapter 13, however, please read the following introductory comments.) All three menus satisfy the seven dietary guidelines of **The Omega Diet.** They also contain the same balanced ratio of protein, fat, and carbohydrates—20:35:45. The primary difference is portion size. If one member of your household is on the maintenance diet and another on a weight-loss version, you can eat the same food, just differing amounts.

The menus are based on three main meals a day, plus two healthy snacks. You can eat the snacks at any time of day you wish, or combine them with a main meal. The goal is to keep from feeling overly hungry—a sure way to sabotage any diet plan. Each meal is described first in general terms ("6 ounces of skinless chicken") and is then followed by a specific recipe in italics ("*Yogurt Chicken, p. 284*"). This gives you the flexibility to improvise your own recipes or use the ones described in the book.

All the breakfasts, lunches, snacks, and dinners are grouped together so that you have a broad range of choices at a glance. You will be able to select the meal that looks the most appealing to you, matches your schedule, or uses the ingredients you have on hand. If you want to, of course, you can follow the meals in sequence, matching Breakfast #1 with Lunch #1, and Dinner #1, and so on.

If you find a meal that you like very much, have it as often as you like—provided it's not one of the few meals that has relatively high amounts of saturated fat. In other words, don't eat eggs every morning for breakfast, or cheese every day for lunch, or steak seven nights in a row. Also, make sure that you are eating fatty fish at least twice a week or that you are enriching your diet with omega-3 fatty acids in some other reliable way.

You will notice that the meals differ slightly in calorie count. If you are making a special effort to maintain your weight or lose weight, you will need to keep track of your daily caloric intake. The two daily snacks offer an easy way to adjust your calorie count upwards or downwards. If you've chosen meals relatively low in calories, you can increase the portion size of your snacks. If you've chosen meals that are relatively high in calories, you can skip a snack or eat smaller portions. The snacks, as you will see, are mainly low-fat dairy products, fruits, and vegetables. This is far healthier than snacking on chips, cookies, or crackers. The snacks will also help you reach your "Seven a Day" fruit and vegetable quota.

Desserts, other than fresh fruit, are not included on the menu. Add them if you wish, provided they don't overload you with calories. I recommend the dessert recipes in this book because they are low in bad fat and contain a significant amount of fruit. Sorbet, frozen yogurt, and low-fat ice cream are also wholesome desserts.

If you skimp on milk products, supplement your diet with calcium tablets. Taking other vitamins or minerals won't be necessary as long as you are eating seven or more servings of fruits and vegetables every day. If not, take antioxidant and vitamin supplements. If you are taking fish oil or flaxseed oil supplements, I recommend that you also take at least 100 IU of vitamin E each day. Pregnant women and nursing mothers should take the nutritional supplements prescribed by their doctors.

If you are a vegetarian, you will be replacing the meat with vegetable protein, something you know how to do already. Since there are relatively small amounts of meat in this diet, you may find this easier to do than with some other programs. But make sure that you are eating an adequate supply of omega-3 fatty acids. One survey showed that vegetarians have one-half the amount of omega-3s in their tissues as omnivores[1]—in the United States that means one-half of far too little! Supplement your diet with fish oil or flaxseed oil supplements and be sure to use canola oil, canola oil mayonnaise, flaxseeds, and flaxmeal whenever possible.

Some people like to have their meals spelled out for them in detail; others like to be more spontaneous. If the idea of following a menu seems too restrictive to you, use The Seven Dietary Guidelines on page 10 as a guideline and create your own menu.

**SPECIFIC COMMENTS ON THE MAINTENANCE PLAN.** Two thousand calories will not be the right number to satisfy everyone's maintenance requirements. A large-framed, young, or physically active person may need considerably more calories, while a small-boned, older, or inactive person might need far less. You might know if 2,000 calories is right for you simply by scanning the menus. If not, follow the program for a week and see if you gain or lose weight, then adjust accordingly. If you need to alter the calorie count, eat larger or smaller portions of the listed items rather than eliminating a food altogether or adding a different type of food. (Adding three cookies at the end of the day won't give you the same nutritional value as eating a little more vegetables, fruit, legumes, and lean meat.) If your caloric requirement is low, consider following the 1,500-calorie menu in the next chapter. For you, it will be a maintenance diet, not a weight-loss diet.

# 21 Breakfast Menus—
# 2,000 Calorie Plan

### Breakfast #1
▪   ▪   ▪   ▪   ▪

- 2 slices of whole-grain toast
  (1 large slice *Honey Flax Bread, p. 249*)
- Tomato slices
- 1½ oz. mozzarella or other cheese, melted
- 1 slice honeydew or other melon
  *approximate calories: 375*

### Breakfast #2
▪   ▪   ▪   ▪   ▪

- 1 bagel
- 2 oz. lox (cold-smoked salmon)
- 2 T. low-fat cream cheese or 3 T. low-fat cottage cheese
- Tomatoes, sliced onions, or capers
- 8 oz. juice
  *approximate calories: 462*

### Breakfast #3
▪   ▪   ▪   ▪   ▪

- 1 cup nonfat yogurt
- sprinkle with ½ cup granola
  (*Canola Granola, p. 245*)
- 1 cup sliced berries
  *approximate calories: 350*

## Breakfast #4

• • • • •

- 2 slices whole-grain toast
  (*Honey Flax Bread, p. 249*)
- 1 t. canola/butter (p. 238)
- 1 T. jam or honey
- 1 poached or boiled egg
- Fruit
  *approximate calories: 360*

## Breakfast #5

• • • • •

- 3 pancakes
  (*Cottage Cheese Pancakes, p. 247*)
- 4 T. maple syrup, jam or honey
- 2 t. canola/butter (p. 238)
- ½ grapefruit
  *approximate calories: 575*

## Breakfast #6

• • • • •

- Smoked Salmon Omelet
  (*2 t. canola oil, 2 eggs or 1 egg and 2 egg whites, 1 oz.
  smoked salmon or lox*)
- 1 slice whole-grain toast
  (*Honey Flax Bread, p. 249*)
- ¼ cantaloupe
  *approximate calories: 375*

## *Breakfast #7*

■  ■  ■  ■  ■  ■

- 1 slice of whole-grain toast
  *(Honey Flax Bread, p. 249)*
- 1 t. canola/butter (p. 238) or low-fat cream cheese
- 1 T. honey or jam
- 1 egg
- Fruit
  *approximate calories: 325*

## *Breakfast #8*

■  ■  ■  ■  ■  ■

- ⅔ cup canola or nonfat granola
  *(Canola Granola, p. 245)*
- 1 cup low-fat cottage cheese, yogurt, or skim milk
- 1 cup berries
  *approximate calories: 425*

## *Breakfast #9*

■  ■  ■  ■  ■  ■

- 3, 5-inch buttermilk pancakes
  *(Buttermilk Flaxjacks, p. 242)*
- 2 t. canola/butter (p. 238)
- 3 T. maple syrup or honey
- ½ cup sliced strawberries or other berries in season
  *approximate calories: 610*

## Breakfast #10

∎ ∎ ∎ ∎ ∎ ∎

- 1½ cups cereal sprinkled with ground flaxseeds
- ⅔ cup nonfat milk
- fruit
  *approximate calories: 360*

## Breakfast #11

∎ ∎ ∎ ∎ ∎ ∎

- 1 slice banana or other quick bread
  *(Banana Bread, p. 244)*
- 1 cup low-fat yogurt, cottage cheese, or skim milk
- Fruit
  *approximate calories: 400*

## Breakfast #12

∎ ∎ ∎ ∎ ∎ ∎

- 1 cup low-fat yogurt
- ½ cup granola
  *(Canola Granola, p. 245)*
- 1 cup fruit
  *approximate calories: 383*

## Breakfast #13

∎ ∎ ∎ ∎ ∎ ∎

- Vegetable Omelet
  *1 cup fresh vegetables sautéed in 1 t. canola or olive oil, 2 eggs*
- 2 slices whole-grain toast
  *(Honey Flax Bread, p. 249)*

- 1 t. canola/butter (p. 238)
- Juice
  *approximate calories: 425*

## Breakfast #14
■ ■ ■ ■ ■ ■

- 1 large bran muffin
  *(Flaxbran Muffin, p. 248)*
- 1 oz. cheese
- Large bowl of fruit
  *approximate calories: 325*

## Breakfast #15
■ ■ ■ ■ ■ ■

- Mediterranean Omelet
  *1 t. canola oil or olive oil, 1 egg plus two egg whites, 1 oz. feta cheese, 2 T. sun-dried tomatoes*
- 1 cup fruit
- 1 slice whole-grain toast
  *(Honey Flax Bread, p. 249)*
  *approximate calories: 440*

## Breakfast #16
■ ■ ■ ■ ■ ■

- 1 cup low-fat yogurt
- 1 cup fruit
- 1 slice whole-grain toast
  *(Honey Flax Bread, p. 249)*
- 1 T. jam
  *approximate calories: 325*

## *Breakfast #17*

■ ■ ■ ■ ■ ■

- 1 egg
- 1 English muffin
- 1 t. canola/butter (p. 238)
- Jam or honey
- 1 cup fruit
  *approximate calories: 400*

## *Breakfast #18*

■ ■ ■ ■ ■ ■

- 1½ cups multigrain cereal
- ⅔ cup nonfat milk
- Sugar to taste
- Orange juice
  *approximate calories: 420*

## *Breakfast #19*

■ ■ ■ ■ ■ ■

- Large bowl fruit salad
- ½ cup nonfat yogurt
- Brown sugar to taste
- 1 slice whole-wheat toast
  *approximate calories: 433*

### *Breakfast #20*

▪  ▪  ▪  ▪  ▪

- 1 large slice banana bread
  *(Banana Bread, p. 244)*
- 1 boiled egg
- ½ grapefruit or 1 whole orange
  *approximate calories: 360*

### *Breakfast #21*

▪  ▪  ▪  ▪  ▪

- 2½ ounces whole-grain breakfast cereal
- ⅔ cup nonfat milk
- ½ papaya (or other fruit)
  *approximate calories: 412*

# *21 Lunch Menus— 2,000 Calorie Plan*

### *Lunch #1*

▪  ▪  ▪  ▪  ▪

- Green salad with hard-boiled egg and 1 oz. cheese
  *(Beet and Blue Cheese Salad, p. 252. Add 1 hard-boiled
  egg to recipe.)*
- 1 T. walnut oil, olive oil, or canola oil dressing
  *(Walnut Oil Dressing, p. 259)*
- Whole-grain roll or bread slice *(Honey Flax Bread,
  p. 249)*
  *approximate calories: 450*

## Lunch #2

- 2 cups vegetable soup
  (*Hot and Sour Soup, p. 262*)
- 5 crackers (nonfat or canola-based)
- 1 cup mixed green salad with 2 T. olive oil vinaigrette
  (p. 143)
  *approximate calories: 427*

## Lunch #3

- Chicken salad
  (*Chicken Salad with Vinaigrette, p. 253*)
- Whole-grain roll or bread slice
  (*Honey Flax Bread, p. 249*)
- 1 t. canola/butter (p. 238) or olive oil
  *approximate calories: 450*

## Lunch #4

- Sautéed vegetables
  (*1½ cups Provencal Casserole, p. 273*)
- 1 sliced orange or other fruit
  *approximate calories: 450*

## Lunch #5

■  ■  ■  ■  ■

- Lean beef or vegetable burger 1 patty, 1 multigrain bun, lettuce, tomato, onions, catsup, 1 T. canola mayonnaise
- 12 oz. apple cider, tomato juice, or other juice
  *approximate calories: 425 (veggie burger)*
  *525 (beef patty)*

## Lunch #6

■  ■  ■  ■  ■

- Mixed green salad with 1 oz. cheese, 2 T. olive oil vinaigrette
  *(Chicken Salad with Vinaigrette, p. 253)*
- 1 whole-grain roll
  *approximate calories: 460*

## Lunch #7

■  ■  ■  ■  ■

- 1½ cups tuna and pasta salad
  *(Tuna Pasta Salad, p. 256)*
- ½ cup carrot sticks or raw vegetables or deli salad
  *approximate calories: 540*

## Lunch #8

■  ■  ■  ■  ■

- Turkey sandwich (3 oz. turkey, 2 T. canola oil mayonnaise, 2 slices whole-grain bread, lettuce)
- 1 cup cabbage salad
  *(Fresh Sauerkraut Salad, p. 254)*
  *approximate calories: 532*

## *Lunch #9*

. . . . . .

- Greek salad
  *(1 tomato, $^1/_2$ cucumber, 1 oz. feta cheese, 10 olives, 2 T. Olive Oil Vinaigrette, p. 143)*
- 1 whole-wheat roll or slice of bread
  *approximate calories: 580*

## *Lunch #10*

. . . . . .

- Tuna Salad
  *(Mixed Salad Greens, 2 oz tuna fish, 1 hard-boiled egg, 2 T. salad dressing)*
- 1 bran muffin or roll
  *(Flaxbran Muffin, p. 248)*
  *approximate calories: 425*

## *Lunch #11*

. . . . . .

- Turkey Sandwich
  *3 oz. sliced skinless roasted turkey breast, $1^1/_2$ T. canola oil mayonnaise, lettuce, tomato, 2 slices whole wheat bread (Honey Flax Bread, p. 249) or bagel*
- Small green salad with vinaigrette
  *(Olive Oil Vinaigrette, p. 143)*
  *approximate calories: 550*

## *Lunch #12*

. . . . . .

- Green salad with apple slices, walnuts, and 2 T. olive oil vinaigrette
  (*1 serving Arugula, Walnut and Apple Salad, p. 251*)
- 1 t. canola/butter (p. 238)
- 1 whole-wheat roll
  *approximate calories: 460*

## *Lunch #13*

. . . . . .

- Tuna salad sandwich
  *2 slices whole-wheat bread (Honey Flax Bread, p. 249),
  ½ cup tuna in spring water, 1 T. canola oil mayonnaise,
  green onions, lettuce*
- 1 can V-8 juice or other juice
  *approximate calories: 500*

## *Lunch #14*

. . . . . .

- 1½ cups vegetable soup
  (*Split Pea Soup, p. 263*)
- Green salad with vinaigrette
  (*Olive Oil Vinaigrette, p. 143*)
- 2 bread sticks
  *approximate calories: 610*

## Lunch #15

· · · · · ·

- Open-faced ham sandwich
  *4 oz. trim roasted ham, 1 slice whole-wheat bread
  (Honey Flax Bread, p. 249), 1 T. canola oil mayonnaise,
  tomato, lettuce*
- 1 cup grapes
  *approximate calories: 555*

## Lunch #16

· · · · · ·

- 2 cups bean soup
  *(Bean Soup, p. 260)*
- Green salad with 2 T. olive oil vinaigrette
  *(Olive Oil Vinaigrette, p. 143)*
  *approximate calories: 570*

## Lunch #17

· · · · · ·

- Grilled vegetable sandwich with 1 oz. melted cheese
  with 2 slices whole wheat bread
  *(Grilled Vegetable Sandwich, p. 269)*
- 1 glass nonfat milk
  *approximate calories: 470*

## Lunch #18

• • • • • •

- Chicken salad
  *3 oz. skinless breast meat, 2 T. canola oil mayonnaise,*
  *1 cup lettuce*
- 1 dinner roll
  *(Honey Flax Bread, p. 249)*
- 1 t. canola/butter (p. 238)
  *approximate calories: 430*

## Lunch #19

• • • • • •

- Chicken Fajita
  *4 oz. grilled skinless chicken breast, 2 tortillas, grilled*
  *vegetables in 1 T. canola or olive oil, ¹⁄₂ cup fresh salsa*
  *approximate calories: 550*

## Lunch #20

• • • • • •

- Lean beef or veggie burger
  *(1 beef or veggie patty, 1 multigrain bun, lettuce, tomato,*
  *fresh vegetables, 1 T. canola oil mayonnaise, page 240)*
- Green salad with vinaigrette
  *(Olive Oil Vinaigrette, p. 143)*
  *approximate calories: 475 (veggie burger), 530 (beef patty)*

## Lunch #21

• • • • • •

- Fruit Salad
  *(2 cups fruit, 1 cup lowfat yogurt)*
  *approximate calories: 360*

# 21 Dinner Menus, 2,000 Calorie Plan

## Dinner #1

• • • • • •

- Fatty fish—broiled, simmered in wine or broth, or sautéed in olive oil or canola oil
  (*Trout Simmered in White Wine Sauce, p. 276*)
- ½ baked acorn squash or other squash
- 1 dinner roll
- 1 t. canola/butter (p. 238)
- 1 cup sauerkraut
  (*Fresh Sauerkraut Salad, p. 254*)
  *approximate calories: 620*

## Dinner #2

• • • • • •

- 6 oz. any style chicken, skinless, cooked with olive oil or canola oil
  (*Chicken in Hellfire, p. 281*)
- 1 cup green peas or other vegetables
- Green salad
  *1 cup salad greens and vegetables, 2 T. Olive Oil Vinaigrette (p. 143)*
  *approximate calories: 590*

## Dinner #3

▪ ▪ ▪ ▪ ▪ ▪

- Lean burger
  *(5 oz. lean meat or veggie patty, 1 whole-wheat ham-
  burger bun or roll, 1 T. canola oil mayonnaise, lettuce
  and tomato)*
- ¾ cups cooked carrots marinated in 1 T. olive oil vinaigrette (served cold) *(page 143)*
  *approximate calories: 620*

## Dinner #4

▪ ▪ ▪ ▪ ▪ ▪

- 6 oz. broiled lamb chop
- 1 cup steamed broccoli
  *(Briefly toss in 1 t. olive oil and garlic)*
- 1 whole-wheat roll
  *(Honey Flax Bread, p. 249)*
- Green salad with dressing
  *(2 T. Olive Oil Vinaigrette, p. 143)*
  *approximate calories: 750*

## Dinner #5

▪ ▪ ▪ ▪ ▪

- 6 oz. lean steak
- Bread with canola/butter
- Mixed Green salad
  *(1 cup mixed greens, 2 T. Olive Oil Vinaigrette, page
  143)*
- Brussels sprouts
  *(Brussels sprouts with Walnut Oil and Lemon, p. 267)*
  *approximate calories: 730*

## Dinner #6

▪ ▪ ▪ ▪ ▪

- 5 oz. salmon
  *(Sautéed in 2 t. olive or canola oil)*
- 1 cup yams or sweet potatoes
- ½ cup lima beans
- 1 dinner roll or bread slice
  *(Honey Flax Bread, p. 249)*
  *approximate calories: 640*

## Dinner #7

▪ ▪ ▪ ▪ ▪

- 6 oz. skinless chicken, broiled, sautéed, or poached
  *(Yogurt Chicken, p. 284)*
- ½ cup baked acorn squash or other yellow vegetable
- 1 t. canola margarine
- Green salad
  *(Orange-Walnut Salad, p. 255)*
  *approximate calories: 650*

## Dinner #8

▪ ▪ ▪ ▪ ▪

- 6 oz. skinless roasted chicken breast
  *(Hoisin Chicken or Tofu, p. 282)*
- ¾ cup cooked bulgur, rice. or couscous
- Sauté bulgur with onions and celery in 1 T. canola oil
- Green salad with 2 T. olive oil vinaigrette
  *(Olive Oil Vinaigrette, p. 143)*
  *approximate calories: 710*

## Dinner #9

▪  ▪  ▪  ▪  ▪

- 6 oz. lean pot roast
- 1 large baked potato
- 1 t. canola/butter (p. 238)
- 1 cup baked squash or other yellow vegetable
- Green salad with 2 T. olive oil vinaigrette
  (*Olive Oil Vinaigrette, p. 143*)
  *approximate calories:* 735

## Dinner #10

▪  ▪  ▪  ▪  ▪

- 6 oz. fatty fish, poached, baked, or sautéed
  (*Tuna with Sun-Dried Tomatoes, p. 279*)
- 1 cup steamed broccoli or other vegetable
- 1½ cup bulgur or rice
- 2 t. canola/butter (p. 238)
  *approximate calories:* 720

## Dinner #11

▪  ▪  ▪  ▪  ▪

- Creamed chicken with rice
  (*1½ servings Orange Chicken and Rice, p. 283*)
- 1 cup steamed vegetables
  (*Brussels Sprouts with Lemon, p. 267*)
- 1 dinner roll
- 1 t. canola/butter (p. 238)
  *approximate calories:* 800

## Dinner #12

■ ■ ■ ■ ■ ■

- 6 oz. fatty fish
  (*Tuna Marinated in Dill, p. 278*)
- 1 cup dark green leafy vegetables
  (*Kale with Lemon, p. 271*)
- 2 whole-wheat rolls
  (*Honey Flax Bread, p. 249*)
- 4 T. humus
  (*Humus, p. 270*)
  *approximate calories: 630*

## Dinner #13

■ ■ ■ ■ ■ ■

- 1½ cups bean soup
  (*Bean Soup, p. 260*)
- 1 piece corn bread
  (*Corn Bread, p. 246*)
- 1 t. canola/butter (p. 238)
- Green salad with 2 T. olive oil vinaigrette
  (*Olive Oil Vinaigrette, p. 143*)
  *approximate calories: 720*

## Dinner #14

■ ■ ■ ■ ■ ■

- 2 cups stir fry
  (*Thai Stir Fry, p. 280*)
- 1 cup rice
- Green salad with 2 T. olive oil vinaigrette
  (*Olive Oil Vinaigrette, p. 143*)
  *approximate calories: 760*

## *Dinner #15*

■　■　■　■　■　■

- 2 cups pork stir fry
  *(Pork or Beef Stir Fry, p. 288)*
- 1 cup rice
- Green salad with 2 T. olive oil vinaigrette
  *(Olive Oil Vinaigrette, p. 143)*
  *approximate calories: 760*

## *Dinner #16*

■　■　■　■　■　■

- 1 black bean or beef quesadilla
  *(Black Bean or Beef Quesadillas, p. 264)*
- Black bean salsa
  *(Black Bean Salsa, p. 266)*
- Steamed corn on the cob
  *approximate calories: 650 (black bean); 830 (beef)*

## *Dinner #17*

■　■　■　■　■　■

- 6 oz. salmon with vegetables
  *(Salmon Cilantro with Grilled Vegetables, p. 274)*
- 2 dinner rolls or bread slices
  *(Honey Flax Bread, p. 249)*
- 1 t. canola/butter (p. 238)
  *approximate calories: 638*

## Dinner #18

■ ■ ■ ■ ■ ■

- 2½ cups Pad Thai
  (*Pad Thai, p. 287*)
- 1 cup fresh green beans sautéed in 1 T. olive oil
- Lemon to taste
  *approximate calories: 670*

## Dinner #19

■ ■ ■ ■ ■ ■

- Grilled trout
  (*Trout with Wine and Fine Herbs, p. 276*)
- Swiss chard
  (*Chard with Nuts and Raisins, p. 268*)
- 1 baked potato
- 1 t. canola/butter
  *approximate calories: 730*

## Dinner #20

■ ■ ■ ■ ■ ■

- 6 oz. grilled tuna
- ½ cup baked acorn squash
- ½ cup lima beans
- 1 T. olive oil
- Pepper, garlic to taste
- 1 small dinner roll
  *approximate calories: 710*

## *Dinner #21*

■ ■ ■ ■ ■ ■

- Lamb roast
  (*Lamb, Green Pepper, and Apple Curry, p. 286*)
- 1 whole-wheat roll
  (*Honey Flax Bread, p. 249*)
- 2 t. canola oil mayonnaise or canola/butter (p. 238)
- 6 oz. baked squash
  *approximate calories: 695*

# *50-Calorie Healthy Snacks*

½ cup steamed carrots
1 cup steamed green beans
8 ounces vegetable juice cocktail
½ ounce cheese
6 ounces nonfat milk
½ cup fresh apricots
¾ cup fresh berries
¼ medium cantaloupe
1 small pear
1 cup fresh strawberries
½ grapefruit
1 medium peach
1 medium nectarine
4 walnut halves

# *100-Calorie Healthy Snacks*

1 ounce cheese
1 large apple
1½ ounces dried apples
7 ounces apple juice
½ cup applesauce
1 cup (8 ounces) fresh apricots

¾ cup canned apricots (in juice)
6 ounces apricot nectar
1 small banana
1½ cup fresh blackberries
1¼ cups fresh blueberries
1 cup buttermilk
½, 5-inch diameter cantaloupe
8 ounces carrot juice
1/4 of a 7-inch casaba melon
1 cup fresh cherries
½ cup chocolate milk (1% fat)
⅔ cup lowfat cottage cheese
1 large ear of corn
4 ounces steamed corn kernels
4 ounces of crab meat
2 large fresh figs
⅔ cup canned figs in light syrup
¼ cup dried figs
1 frozen fruit bar (no sugar added)
1 large fruit roll-up
4 ounces fruit sorbet
½ cup fruit compote (see page 291)
1⅔ cups grapes
6 ounces unsweetened grape juice
1 medium grapefruit
9 ounces grapefruit juice
4-inch wedge, honeydew melon
2 medium kiwi fruits
1/3 cup lima beans
3 medium mandarin oranges
1 cup 1% milk
1¼ cup skim milk
1 large nectarine
12 large olives
1 large orange
7 ounces orange juice
⅔ medium papaya
5 ounces papaya nectar

2 medium peaches
1 cup peaches canned in juice
3 ounces dried peaches
5 ounces peach nectar
1 large pear
6 ounces pears canned in juice
3 ounces dried pears
5 ounces steamed green peas
1 small persimmon
3 small or 2 large plums
$\frac{2}{3}$ cup plums canned in juice
1 medium pomegranate
5 dried prunes
3 dried prunes stuffed with walnut halves
3 tablespoons raisins
$1\frac{2}{3}$ cup fresh raspberries
$1\frac{1}{2}$ ounce smoked salmon
2 cups fresh strawberries
8 walnut halves
$\frac{1}{2}$ cup lowfat yogurt

# THIRTEEN

# The Omega Weight-Loss Diet

O NE OUT OF every three adults in this country is overweight. If you're in this category and want to do something about it, read on. This chapter features two weight-loss versions of **The Omega Diet**—a 1,500-calorie diet for gradual weight loss, and a 1,200-calorie diet for more rapid weight loss. The only significant difference between the regular program and these two low-calorie programs is portion size. You will be following the same dietary guidelines, eating the same types and percentages of fat, and reaping all the health benefits of **The Omega Diet**—with the added bonus of losing from one to two pounds a week.

I strongly encourage you to exercise while on **The Omega Weight-Loss Diet**. Exercise is vital to your health whether you are dieting or not, but it is even more important when you're losing weight. First of all, exercise speeds your rate of weight loss. Taking a brisk, hour-long walk is the same as saying "no" to three slices of bread. As you burn calories, you are also firming and toning your muscles, helping to create a taut, sleek body. Just as important, exercise helps preserve your lean body mass. When you diet *without* exercising, you can lose one pound of muscle for every three pounds of fat.[1] It's important to hold on to every muscle fiber you have because your resting metabolic rate (the rate you burn calories while resting) is largely determined by your amount of lean muscle. If you have sixty pounds of muscle, for example, you burn about 1,600 calories to fuel your body while at rest. If you lose five pounds of muscle, you will be burning 150 fewer calories a day.[2] Over a year's time, this could amount to 54,000 extra calories, which could cause you to regain eighteen of those twenty pounds! If you maintain your lean body mass, however, those twenty pounds are far less likely to come back.

---

**WHY EXERCISE?**

1. Double your health benefits.
2. Lose weight faster.
3. Firm and tone your muscles.
4. Preserve your lean muscle mass.
5. Help maintain your weight loss.

---

Proof that exercising helps you lose weight and keep it off comes from a study of overweight men. Some of the men were placed on near-starvation rations—420 calories a day. Others were assigned to a 1,000-calorie diet and were also required to exercise four and a half hours each week. Two months later, the men in the exercise group had lost almost as much weight as the men who had been eating less than half as many calories. But the real benefit of the exercise program was revealed eighteen months later. The men who had *continued* to exercise stayed at their low weight, while the sedentary men regained every pound they had lost.[3]

# How to "Yo!" Instead of "Yo-yo"

Ultimately, there is no "secret" to losing weight and keeping it off. The formula is as old as the hills: Eat fewer calories and exercise more. If you do this faithfully, you will lose a substantial amount of weight. The real challenge, as you well know, is *staying* on a diet and exercise program long enough to get the desired results. The obstacles can seem insurmountable. You're too busy to exercise. Your job requires you to travel much of the time. You have an injury that forces you to jettison your exercise program. Or your life is unusually stressful. And then there's Thanksgiving, Christmas, Easter, Passover, picnics, birthdays, and company dinners. If you also eat for comfort or have decades of self-defeating eating habits to overcome, you need all the help you can get.

There are a number of reasons why **The Omega Weight-Loss Diet** will make it easier for you to succeed at your goals. First, the program is based on sound medical science. If you follow the diet, you *will* lose weight. Sadly, this is not the case for many popular diets. Despite claims to the contrary, you *cannot* lose weight simply by replacing fat with carbohydrates, or combining foods in a particular order, or eating certain foods at specified times of day. *The degree to which you lose weight is the degree to which you burn more calories than you consume.* The eating plan in this book is based on this sound, medically proven principle.

Second, you may find it easier to stay on **The Omega Weight-Loss Diet** than on other diets. If you have tried to lose weight on a low-fat diet, you know how much sacrifice is involved. There is a long list of foods you can't eat, and much of the food you are encouraged to eat is not all that appealing. On **The Omega Weight-Loss Diet**, you will be eating flavorful, *natural* food. It's hard to feel sorry for yourself when you get to eat real cheese, salad dressing, and cooking oils.

Third, **The Omega Weight-Loss Diet** is a drug-free plan, which studies show will make it *easier* for you to maintain your weight loss. Weight-loss drugs trick your brain into thinking you're full, making it easier to cut back on calories. But once you abandon the pharmaceutical crutch—and virtually all diet drugs are to be used for only a limited time—you are at high risk for regaining all the weight because you haven't developed lasting coping skills.

A fourth reason **The Omega Weight-Loss Diet** will help you lose weight successfully is that it is high in fiber and bulk. You will be eating seven or more servings of fruits, vegetables, and legumes every day, food that is low in calories but takes up a lot of room in your gut. Studies show that the bulkier the food and the more fiber people consume, the more satisfied they feel on a low-calorie diet and the more weight they lose.

Finally, **The Omega-Weight Loss Diet** will lessen the temptation to snack between meals. One rarely discussed benefit of eating a moderate amount of fat is that it helps stave off hunger. In a recent French study, healthy male volunteers were given either a low-fat lunch or the same lunch that had been supplemented with butter. They were then put into special rooms that were isolated from all time cues and were told they could request dinner whenever they wanted. The ones who had eaten the higher fat lunch asked for dinner an average of thirty-eight minutes later than the ones who had eaten the low-fat lunch.[4] This half-hour cushion will make it easier to stay away from the refrigerator as mealtime approaches.

## Keeping a Food, Mood, and Exercise Diary

To further enhance your chances for success, I strongly recommend that you keep a journal that records your eating habits, exercise activity, and moods. One of the virtues of keeping such a journal is that you will become more aware of your "unconscious" eating. The vast majority of people, even those without weight or eating problems, eat more food than they realize. They fail to register the size of their portions, the number of times they go back for seconds, and how often they snack. I learned this firsthand while conducting metabolic studies at NIH. In one of my studies, it was important that the volunteers maintain a constant weight. This didn't appear to be a problem, however, because the participants were fit, lean, college-educated women who had had no problem maintaining a healthy weight on their own. To determine how much to feed them, we simply asked them how much they ate on a regular basis and then served them an equivalent amount of food during the course of the study. It didn't work. Invariably, when we fed the women the number of calories they *thought* they'd been eating, they would lose weight. We would have to increase their food intake by at least 15 percent before their weight would stabilize. Even though they had no weight problems or eating disorders, they were in denial about how much food they were putting in their mouths.

Keeping a food diary is one way to remedy this problem. The diary is a simple tool to make you aware of: (1) how much you weigh, (2) how often you eat, (3) how much you eat, and (4) the type of situations and feelings that prompt you to eat. Every time you eat (and this means *nibbling*, too), record the time of day and exactly what you ate. Then, make a brief note describing how you were feeling just prior to eating—happy, sad, angry, anxious, exhilarated, rested, tired, and so on. After a few days review your entries and see if you can identify any emotional or situational triggers that prompted you to eat. Four feelings in particular tend to make people overeat— feeling *h*ungry, *a*ngry, *l*onely, or *t*ired. The initials of these words comprise the word "H.A.L.T.," a memory device used in some 12-Step recovery programs to remind people of the feelings that are most likely to undermine their resolve. If you structure your life so that you avoid these particular feelings as much as possible, you will find it much easier to stay on **The Omega Weight-Loss Diet.**

Another benefit of the journal is that it allows you to keep a record of your physical activity and weight. Every day, write down how long you exercised and what type of exercise you engaged in. Once a week, weigh yourself (preferably at the same time of day and with the same amount of clothing). Record your weight on a graph to give you a visual record.

Surprisingly, when people keep track of their weight in this manner, they are much more likely to maintain their weight loss. In a study published in 1992, seventy-two overweight women were assigned to a weight-loss diet and then divided into two groups. One group was asked to keep a weekly weight chart; the other was not. During the period of active dieting, both groups lost similar amounts of weight. But two years later, the women who continued to chart their weight on a weekly basis had managed to maintain their weight loss, while those who had not kept a chart regained an average of eighteen pounds.[5] Why did such a simple procedure have such a profound effect? The researchers concluded that the weight chart helped people see if and when they were gaining weight, allowing them to make a slight course correction before they had regained too many pounds.

On the next page is a sample page from a food, mood, and exercise diary. As you can see, your comments can be brief. It takes only ten minutes a day to keep an accurate record. Yet, for many, many dieters, this one simple tool has made the difference between success and failure. Is it absolutely essential to go through this drill? No, it isn't. Some people are able to lose weight and keep it off without this tool. But if you match two or more of the descriptions below, a journal will greatly increase your chances for success. (You will find sample blank pages in the resource section, pages 345 to 347.)

---

### SHOULD YOU KEEP A FOOD DIARY?

If you check two or more boxes, keeping a food diary is likely to prove very helpful.

- ❐ I eat between meals.
- ❐ I nibble while I cook.
- ❐ It is difficult for me to lose weight.
- ❐ I've lost and regained weight a number of times.
- ❐ I eat for comfort.
- ❐ I eat quickly.
- ❐ I often eat away from home.
- ❐ I often eat after dinner.
- ❐ There are times of the day or days of the month when I am more vulnerable to overeating.

---

## Removing Eating Triggers

A final strategy that will help you succeed on **The Omega Weight-Loss Diet** is making a conscious effort to eliminate "eating triggers." An eating trigger is something that prompts you to overeat or to eat when you're not hungry. A trigger for many people is simply the sight of tempting food. You might open the refrigerator to get a glass of milk, see a slice of leftover pizza, and devour the pizza while standing up. Shopping while hungry is another common trigger. There you are in the supermarket heading for the paper towels, but you find yourself detouring down the cookie aisle. You are so hungry that you grab a box of cookies and eat six of them on the way home from the store.

| Time | Food | Total Calories | Mood or Situation |
|------|------|----------------|-------------------|
| 7:30 AM | 1 banana<br>1 boiled egg<br>1 piece of flaxseed bread | 310 | Rested, good mood ( The sun was shining.) |
| 1:00 PM | 1 turkey sandwich, 1 green salad plus oil and vinegar dressing | 420 | Pressured to get report out by 5:00. Ordered lunch from the deli. |
| 4:00 | 1 candy bar | 210 | Too rushed to find something healthier |
| 7:00 | 1 skinless chicken breast, bean salad, skim milk, carrots | 460 | Good dinner. Felt less pressured. |
| 9:30 | ½ cup skim milk, fresh strawberries | 70 | Great strawberries! |

| Weight | Daily Exercise | Total Calories | Comments |
|--------|----------------|----------------|----------|
| 164 | Spent 30 minutes on the treadmill (4mph). Walked to the store. 45 minutes total. | 1480 | I'm pleased that I'm continuing to lose one pound a week. Tomorrow I'll bring some fruit to work. |

You probably know many of your eating triggers already. If you take steps to remove them, you will be more successful in holding on to your resolve. Here are some suggestions for you to consider.[6]

### A. Shopping
1. Shop for food after eating.
2. Shop from a written list.
3. Avoid ready-to-eat foods.
4. Pay with cash. Don't carry more cash than you need for essentials.

### B. Advance Planning
1. Plan your snacks for a time of day when you are most likely to be hungry.
2. Plan an activity for a time of day when you are most likely to snack *without* being hungry. (Suggested activities: going for a walk, taking a bath, reading a book, taking a nap.)

3. If possible, plan to cook just after eating a snack or meal.

4. Eat meals and snacks at scheduled times.

5. Develop an emotional support system (diet with a partner or friend; join an on-line diet support group).

6. While on vacation or during the holiday season, plan to maintain your weight, not *lose* weight.

7. Plan in advance how you're going to get back on track once you've strayed away from the plan.

8. Don't order or cook the types of food that tempt you to overeat (pasta, pizza, ribs, ice cream, etc.).

9. Bring your food diary on trips.

10. Plan social events that are centered around sports or exercise, not eating.

### C. Everyday Activities

1. Keep all food hidden behind cupboard doors.

2. Get rid of food that proves too tempting, or store it where it can't be seen.

3. Remove food from inappropriate storage areas (e.g., the TV room, the bedroom).

4. Keep serving dishes off the table (except for the vegetables).

5. Use smaller dishes.

6. Prepare single servings of main dishes.

7. Avoid being the food server.

8. Leave the table immediately after eating.

9. Don't save leftovers.

### D. Holidays, travel, and parties

1. Preorder special meals on airline flights.

2. Rent a motel or hotel room with kitchen facilities so you have an alternative to restaurant fare.

3. Write down in advance what you plan to eat at parties or festive occasions.

4. Eat a small amount of food to ease your hunger before going to a restaurant or party.

5. Volunteer to bring a dish when invited for dinner, and make it something that is on your food plan.

6. Practice polite and creative ways of saying "no."

# *How Many Calories Should You Eat?*

The number of calories you require to lose weight successfully depends on many factors, including your age, body size, metabolic rate, activity level, tolerance for calorie restriction, and desired rate of weight loss. The differences between individuals can be great. If you are a "jittery" person, for example, you might burn as many as 800 calories a day just by jiggling your legs, gesturing, roaming from room to room, and tossing in bed. If so, you can lose weight on a 2,000-calorie diet! On the other hand, if you're placid and slow-moving—which, unfortunately, is often the case for overweight people—you might have to hold the line at 1,200 calories.

In any case, I recommend that you start by following either the 1,200- or 1,500-calorie menu detailed in this chapter and then monitor your progress for two weeks. If you need more food to feel satisfied, or, on the other hand, if you're losing weight too slowly, make the appropriate adjustments. (Don't expect to lose more than two pounds a week, however, unless you are exercising strenuously. This is not a "miracle" diet, just a very reliable, medically sound one.) I recommend that you don't go below 1,200 calories, however, because it's difficult to eat such a low-calorie diet and satisfy all your nutritional needs without the assistance of a dietitian.

Portion size is *critical* on **The Omega Weight-Loss Diet**. To make sure you are eating the right amount of food, you may need to weigh or measure everything you eat. Yes, this is tedious. But given how easy it is to underestimate how much you eat, it may be necessary. It *will* be necessary if you think you are following the program faithfully but not losing weight. Measuring your food more accurately and recording your food intake will get the scales moving.

| What is Your Ideal Weight Range | | |
|---|---|---|
| Height | Men | Women |
| 4′ 9 | | 90–118 |
| 4′ 10 | | 92–121 |
| 4′ 11 | | 95–124 |
| 5′ 0 | | 98–127 |
| 5′ 1 | 105–134 | 101–130 |
| 5′ 2 | 108–137 | 104–134 |
| 5′ 3 | 111–141 | 107–138 |
| 5′ 4 | 114–145 | 110–142 |
| 5′ 5 | 117–149 | 114–146 |
| 5′ 6 | 121–154 | 118–150 |
| 5′ 7 | 125–159 | 122–154 |
| 5′ 8 | 129–163 | 126–159 |
| 5′ 9 | 133–167 | 130–164 |
| 5′ 10 | 137–172 | 134–169 |
| 5′ 11 | 141–177 | |
| 6′ 0 | 145–182 | |
| 6′ 1′ | 149–187 | |
| 6′ 2 | 153–192 | |
| 6′ 3 | 157–197 | |

To use this table, measure your height in feet and inches (minus shoes) and
your weight in pounds (minus clothes.) For women between 18 and 25, sub-
tract 1 pound for each year under 25. (This table is adapted from the 1959
Metropolitan Desirable Weight Table. Although it was created decades ago, it is still
regarded as the best gauge of healthy body weight. Subsequent tables have been based
on *average* weight, not the weight that has been linked with the best health.)

# 21 Breakfast Menus— 1,500 calories

### Breakfast #1
▪ ▪ ▪ ▪ ▪ ▪

- 1 plain bagel
- Tomato slices
- 1 oz. melted mozzarella cheese
- 1 slice honeydew or other melon
  *approximate calories: 360*

### Breakfast #2
▪ ▪ ▪ ▪ ▪ ▪

- 1 bagel toasted
- 1 oz. lox (cold smoked salmon)
- 2 T. low-fat cottage cheese
- Sun-dried tomatoes, sliced red onions (capers)
- 6 oz. orange juice or other juice
  *approximate calories: 430*

### Breakfast #3
▪ ▪ ▪ ▪ ▪ ▪

- 1 cup nonfat yogurt sprinkled with ¼ cup granola
- 1 cup berries
  *approximate calories: 260*

## *Breakfast #4*

■   ■   ■   ■   ■   ■

- 1 slice whole-grain toast
  (*Honey Flax Bread, p. 249*)
- 2 t. jam
- 1 poached or boiled egg
- ½ grapefruit
  *approximate calories: 240*

## *Breakfast #5*

■   ■   ■   ■   ■   ■

- 3 pancakes
  (*Cottage Cheese Pancakes, p. 247*)
- 3 T. maple syrup
- 1 t. canola/butter (p. 238)
  *approximate calories: 440*

## *Breakfast #6*

■   ■   ■   ■   ■   ■

- Smoked Salmon Omelet
  (*2 t. canola oil, 1 egg plus 2 egg whites, 1 oz. smoked
  salmon or lox*)
- 1 slice whole-grain toast or ½ slice flaxseed bread
  (*Honey Flax Bread, p. 249*)
  *approximate calories: 340*

## *Breakfast #7*

■   ■   ■   ■   ■   ■

- 1 English muffin or other toast
  (*Honey Flax Bread, p. 249*)
- 1 oz. Canadian bacon or cheese

- Tomato slices
- 1 cup fruit
  *approximate calories: 310*

## Breakfast #8

■  ■  ■  ■  ■  ■

- ½ cup granola
  *(Canola Granola, p. 245)*
- ½ cup nonfat milk
- ½ grapefruit or other fruit
  *approximate calories: 280*

## Breakfast #9

- 2, 5-inch buttermilk pancakes
  *(Buttermilk Flaxjacks, p. 242)*
- 1 t. canola/butter (p. 238)
- 2 T. maple syrup
- ½ cup sliced strawberries
  *approximate calories: 408*

## Breakfast #10

■  ■  ■  ■  ■  ■

- ¼ cup granola
  *(Canola Granola, p. 245)*
- ½ cup low-fat cottage cheese, yogurt, or nonfat milk
- 1 cup berries
- 6 oz. juice
  *approximate calories: 311*

## *Breakfast #11*

■   ■   ■   ■   ■   ■

- ¼ cup granola
  (*Canola Granola, p. 245*)
- 1 cup low-fat yogurt
- 1 cup fruit
  *approximate calories: 290*

## *Breakfast #12*

■   ■   ■   ■   ■

- ½ cup low-fat yogurt
- ½ cup granola
  (*Canola Granola, p. 245*)
- 1 banana
  *approximate calories: 275*

## *Breakfast #13*

■   ■   ■   ■   ■

- Vegetable Omelet
  (*1 cup fresh vegetables sautéed in 2 t. canola oil, 1 egg
  plus 2 egg whites*)
- 1 slice whole-grain toast
  (*Honey Flax Bread, p. 249*)
- 1 t. canola/butter (p. 238)
  *approximate calories: 330*

## *Breakfast #14*

■   ■   ■   ■   ■

- 1 plain bagel, toasted; or 1 slice any toast
  (*Honey Flax Bread, p. 249*)
- 1 t. canola/butter (p. 238)

- 1 poached egg
- $\frac{1}{2}$ cantaloupe or other melon
  *approximate calories: 285*

## Breakfast #15

■  ■  ■  ■  ■

- Mediterranean Omelet
  *(1 t. canola oil, 1 egg plus two egg whites, 1 oz. feta cheese, 1 T. sun-dried tomatoes)*
- 1 cup fruit
- $\frac{1}{2}$ slice whole-grain toast
  *(Honey Flax Bread, p. 249)*
  *approximate calories: 380*

## Breakfast #16

■  ■  ■  ■  ■

- $\frac{1}{2}$ cup low-fat yogurt
- 1 cup fruit
- 1 slice whole-grain toast
  *(Honey Flax Bread, p. 249)*
- 1 t. canola/butter (p. 238)
  *approximate calories: 250*

## Breakfast #17

■  ■  ■  ■  ■

- 1 poached egg
- 1 English muffin or other toast
  *(Honey Flax Bread, p. 249)*
- 1 t. canola/butter (p. 238)
- 1 T. jam or honey
- $\frac{1}{2}$ cup fruit
  *approximate calories: 321*

## *Breakfast #18*

■ ■ ■ ■ ■ ■

- 1 cup dry cereal
- ⅔ cup nonfat milk
- 1 cup seasonal fruit
*approximate calories: 360*

## *Breakfast #19*

■ ■ ■ ■ ■ ■

- 1 cup cooked cereal
- 1 T. flaxseed
- ⅔ cup nonfat milk
- Sugar or honey to taste
*approximate calories: 310*

## *Breakfast #20*

■ ■ ■ ■ ■ ■

- 1 large slice banana bread
  *(Banana Bread, p. 244)*
- 2 T. low-fat cream cheese
- ½ grapefruit
*approximate calories: 300*

## *Breakfast #21*

■ ■ ■ ■ ■ ■

- 1 cup seven-grain cereal
- 2 t. flaxseed
- ¾ cup nonfat milk
- 1 cup fruit
*approximate calories: 420*

# 1,500-Calorie Menu, 21 Lunches

## Lunch #1
• • • • • •

- Green salad with hard-boiled egg, beans, and 1 T. olive oil or canola dressing
  *(Beet and Blue Cheese Salad,. p. 252. Add 1 hard-boiled egg to recipe.)*
- 1 T. salad dressing
  *(Walnut Oil Dressing, p. 259)*
- Whole-grain roll or bread slice
  *(Honey Flax Bread, p. 249)*
  *approximate calories: 475*

## Lunch #2
• • • • • •

- 2 cups vegetable soup
  *(Hot and Sour Soup, p. 262)*
- 1 oz. low-fat (or canola) crackers or 1 slice bread
  *(Honey Flax Bread, p. 249)*
- 1 t. canola/butter (p. 238)
  *approximate calories: 300*

## Lunch #3
• • • • • •

- Chicken salad
  *(Chicken Salad with Vinaigrette, p. 253.)*
- ½ slice whole-grain bread
  *(Honey Flax Bread, p. 249)*
- 1 t. canola/butter (p. 238)
  *approximate calories: 470*

## *Lunch #4*

. . . . . .

- 1½ cups sautéed vegetables
  *(1½ cups Provençal Casserole, p. 273)*
- 1 sliced orange or other fruit
  *approximate calories: 460*

## *Lunch #5*

. . . . . .

- Lean beef or vegetable burger
  *(1 beef or veggie patty, 1 multigrain bun, lettuce,
  tomato, other fresh vegetables, 1 T. canola oil
  mayonnaise)*
  *approximate calories: 350*

## *Lunch #6*

. . . . . .

- Deli salad with mixed greens, cheese, chicken, carrots,
  tomato, chopped red peppers, 2 T. olive oil vinaigrette
  *(Chicken Salad with Vinaigrette, p. 253)*
  *approximate calories: 385*

## *Lunch #7*

. . . . . .

- 1 cup tuna and pasta salad
  *(Tuna Pasta Salad, p. 256)*
- ½ cup carrot sticks or raw vegetables
  *approximate calories: 370*

## Lunch #8
. . . . . .

- Turkey sandwich
  *(4 oz. turkey, 2 slices whole-grain bread, 1 T. canola oil
  mayonnaise, lettuce, tomatoes)*
- 1 cup low-fat milk
  *approximate calories: 460*

## Lunch #9
. . . . . .

- Greek Salad
  *($^1/_2$ cucumber, 1 tomato, 1 oz. feta cheese, 10 olives, 1$^1/_2$
  T. Olive Oil Vinaigrette, p. 143)*
- 1 whole-wheat roll
- 1 t. canola/butter (p. 238)
  *approximate calories: 510*

## Lunch #10
. . . . . .

- Deli Salad
  *(Greens, 2 oz. tunafish, 1 hard-boiled egg, 2 T. Olive Oil
  Vinaigrette, p. 143)*
- 2 Bread sticks
  *approximate calories: 475*

## *Lunch #11*

■  ■  ■  ■  ■  ■

- Turkey Sandwich
  *4 oz. turkey breast, 1 T. canola oil mayonnaise (p. 240),
  lettuce, tomato, 2 slices whole-wheat bread (Honey Flax
  Bread, p. 249) or bagel*
- 1 cup low-fat milk
  *approximate calories: 475*

## *Lunch #12*

■  ■  ■  ■  ■  ■

- 1 large green salad with vegetables and beans
  *(Arugula, Walnut, and Apple Salad, p. 251;
  omit dressing)*
- 1 T. walnut oil dressing
  *(Walnut Oil Dressing, p. 259)*
- 1 t. canola/butter (p. 238)
- 1 whole-wheat dinner roll
  *(Honey Flax Bread, p. 249)*
  *approximate calories: 450*

## *Lunch #13*

■  ■  ■  ■  ■  ■

- Tuna salad sandwich
  *1 slice whole-wheat bread (Honey Flax Bread, p. 249),
  ¹/₂ cup tuna in spring water, 2 t. canola oil mayonnaise
  (p. 240), green onions, lettuce*
- 6-oz. can V-8 juice or other juice
  *approximate calories: 360*

## *Lunch #14*

■   ■   ■   ■   ■

- 1 cup vegetable soup
  (*Split Pea Soup, p. 263*)
- Green salad with vinaigrette
  (*Olive Oil Vinaigrette, p. 143*)
- 2 bread sticks
  *approximate calories: 450*

## *Lunch #15*

■   ■   ■   ■   ■

- Ham sandwich
  *3 oz. trim roasted ham, 2 slices whole-wheat bread*
  (*Honey Flax Bread, p. 249*), *2 t. canola oil mayonnaise*
  (*p. 240*), *tomato, lettuce*
- 1 cup low-fat milk
  *approximate calories: 450*

## *Lunch #16*

■   ■   ■   ■   ■

- 1½ cups bean soup
  (*Bean Soup, p. 260*)
- Green salad with vinaigrette
  (*Olive Oil Vinaigrette, p. 143*)
  *approximate calories: 475*

## *Lunch #17*

∙  ∙  ∙  ∙  ∙

- Grilled vegetable sandwich
  (*Grilled Vegetable Sandwich, p. 269*)
  *approximate calories: 390*

## *Lunch #18*

∙  ∙  ∙  ∙  ∙

- Chicken salad
  (*4 oz. skinless breast meat, 1¹/₂ cups greens, tomatoes, green pepper*)
- 1¹/₂ T. olive oil vinaigrette
  (*Olive Oil Vinaigrette, p. 143*)
- 1 whole-wheat roll
- 1 t. canola/butter (p. 238)
  *approximate calories: 325*

## *Lunch #19*

∙  ∙  ∙  ∙  ∙

- Chicken Fajita
  (*3 oz. grilled chicken breast, 1 medium flour tortilla, vegetables grilled or sautéed in 1 T. olive oil or canola oil; ¹/₂ cup fresh salsa*)
  (*Black Bean Salsa, p. 266*)
  *approximate calories: 403*

### Lunch #20

. . . . . .

- Lean Beef or Vegetable burger
  (*1 meat or veggie patty, 1 multigrain bun, lettuce,
  tomato, fresh vegetables, 2 t. canola oil mayonnaise,
  p. 240*)
- 1 baked potato
  *approximate calories: 411*

### Lunch #21

. . . . . .

- yogurt and fruit salad
  (*2 cups fruit, 1 cup low-fat yogurt*)
  *Approximate calories: 270*

# 1,500-Calorie Menu, 21 Dinners

### Dinner #1

. . . . . .

- 4 oz. fatty fish—broiled, simmered in wine or broth or
  sautéed in olive oil or canola oil
  (*Trout Simmered in White Wine, p. 276*)
- ½ baked acorn squash or other yellow vegetable
- 1 cup canned or fresh sauerkraut
  (*Fresh Sauerkraut Salad, p. 254*)
  *approximate calories: 506*

## Dinner #2

∙ ∙ ∙ ∙ ∙ ∙

- 6 oz. chicken, skinless, cooked with olive oil or canola oil
  *(Chicken in Hellfire, p. 281)*
- ¾ cup green peas or other vegetables
- Green salad
  *(1 cup salad greens and vegetables, 1 T. Olive Oil Vinaigrette, p. 143)*
- 1 whole-wheat dinner roll
  *approximate calories: 440*

## Dinner #3

∙ ∙ ∙ ∙ ∙ ∙

- Lean burger
  *(4 oz. lean meat or vegie patty, 1 whole-wheat hamburger bun or roll, 1 T. canola oil mayonnaise, catsup, lettuce, and tomato)*
- ¾ cups cooked carrots marinated in 1 T. olive oil vinaigrette (served cold)
  *(Olive Oil Vinaigrette, p. 143)*
  *approximate calories: 575*

## Dinner #4

∙ ∙ ∙ ∙ ∙ ∙

- 6 oz. broiled lamb chop
- 1 cup steamed broccoli
- Briefly sauté in 1 T. olive oil and garlic
- 1 whole-wheat roll
  *(Honey Flax Bread, p. 249)*
- 1 t. canola/butter (p. 238)
  *approximate calories: 570*

## *Dinner #5*

∎ ∎ ∎ ∎ ∎

- 5 ounces lean steak
- 1 slice whole-wheat bread
- 1 t. canola/butter (p. 238)
- Mixed greens salad with 1 T. olive oil vinaigrette
  (*Olive Oil Vinaigrette, p. 143*)
  *approximate calories: 630*

## *Dinner #6*

∎ ∎ ∎ ∎ ∎

- 4 oz. salmon
- Sautéed in 2 t. canola oil or olive oil, garlic
- ¾ cup yams, sweet potatoes, or squash
- ½ cup lima beans or other vegetables
  *approximate calories: 505*

## *Dinner #7*

∎ ∎ ∎ ∎ ∎

- 5 oz. skinless chicken, broiled, sautéed, or poached
  (*Yogurt Chicken, p. 284*)
- ½ cup baked acorn squash or other yellow vegetable
- Green salad
  (*Orange Walnut Salad, p. 255*)
  *approximate calories: 650*

## Dinner #8

• • • • • •

- 3 oz. skinless roasted chicken breast
- ¾ cup cooked bulgur or rice or couscous
  *Sauté bulgur with onions and celery in 1 T. canola oil.*
- Green salad with 2 t. olive oil vinaigrette
  *(Olive Oil Vinaigrette, p. 143)*
  *approximate calories: 575*

## Dinner #9

• • • • • •

- 4 oz. lean roast beef
- 1 baked potato
- 1 t. canola/butter (p. 238)
- 1 cup baked squash or other yellow vegetable
  *approximate calories: 478*

## Dinner #10

• • • • • •

- 4 oz. fatty fish, poached, baked or sautéed
  *(Tuna with Sun-Dried Tomatoes, p. 279)*
- 1 cup steamed broccoli or other vegetable
- ¾ cup cooked bulgur or rice
- 1 t. canola/butter (p. 238)
  *approximate calories: 538*

## Dinner #11

• • • • • •

- 6 oz. skinless chicken with rice
  *(Orange Chicken and Rice, p. 283)*

- 1 cup brussels sprouts
  (*Brussels Sprouts with Walnut Oil and Lemon, p. 267*)
- 1 whole-grain dinner roll
- 1 t. canola/butter (*p. 238*)
  *approximate calories: 573*

### Dinner #12

∎　∎　∎　∎　∎　∎

- 5 oz. any fatty fish
  (*Tuna Marinated in Dill, p. 278*)
- 1 serving kale, spinach or mustard greens
  (*Kale with Lemon, p. 271*)
- 1 whole-wheat roll
  (*Honey Flax Bread, p. 249*)
- 2 T. humus
  (*Humus, p. 270*)
  *approximate calories: 585*

### Dinner #13

∎　∎　∎　∎　∎　∎

- 1½ cups bean soup
  (*Bean Soup, p. 260*)
- 1 piece corn bread
  (*Corn Bread, p. 246*)
- 1 t. canola/butter (p. 238)
  *approximate calories: 531*

## Dinner #14

■ ■ ■ ■ ■ ■

- 1½ cups stir fry
  (*Thai Stir Fry, p. 280*)
- ¾ cup rice
- Green salad with vinaigrette
  (*Olive Oil Vinaigrette, p. 143*)
  *approximate calories: 560*

## Dinner #15

■ ■ ■ ■ ■ ■

- 1½ cup pork stir fry
  (*Pork or Beef Stir Fry, p. 288*)
- ¾ cup rice or bulgur
- Green salad with 1 T. vinaigrette
  (*Olive Oil Vinaigrette, p. 143*)
  *approximate calories: 628*

## Dinner #16

■ ■ ■ ■ ■ ■

- 1 black bean quesadilla
  (*Black Bean or Beef Quesadillas, p. 264*)
- ½ cup black bean salsa
  (*Black Bean Salsa, p. 266*)
- ½ corn on the cob
  *approximate calories: 550*

## Dinner #17

■ ■ ■ ■ ■ ■

- 5 oz. salmon with vegetables
  (*Salmon Cilantro with Grilled Vegetables, p. 274*)

- 1 dinner roll or bread slice
  (*Honey Flax Bread, p. 249*)
- 1 t. canola/butter (p. 238)
  *approximate calories: 538*

## *Dinner #18*

■ ■ ■ ■ ■

- 1½ cups Pad Thai
  (*Pad Thai, p. 287*)
- 1 cup fresh green beans sautéed in 2 t. olive oil
- Lemon to taste
  *approximate calories: 525*

## *Dinner #19*

■ ■ ■ ■ ■

- 5 oz. grilled trout
  (*Trout with Wine and Fine Herbs, p. 277*)
- 1 cup Swiss chard
  (*Chard with Nuts and Raisins, p. 268*)
- ¾ cup brown rice
- 1 t. canola/butter (p. 238)
  *approximate calories: 625*

## *Dinner #20*

■ ■ ■ ■ ■

- 5 oz. grilled tuna
- ½ baked acorn squash
- 1 cup steamed broccoli
- 1 T. olive oil
- Pepper, garlic to taste
  *approximate calories: 495*

### Dinner #21

. . . . . .

- Lamb curry
  (*Lamb, Green Pepper, and Apple Curry, p. 286*)
- 1 small dinner roll
- 2 t. canola/butter (p. 238)
- 4 oz. baked squash
  *approximate calories: 540*

See Healthy Snack List on page 232

# 1,200-Calorie Menu, 21 Breakfasts

### Breakfast #1

. . . . . .

- ½ plain bagel
- Tomato slices
- ½ oz. melted, mozzarella cheese
- 1 cup honeydew or other melon
  *approximate calories: 214*

### Breakfast #2

. . . . . .

- ½ bagel, toasted
- 1 oz. lox (cold smoked salmon)
- 2 T. low-fat cottage cheese or 1 oz. low-fat cream cheese
- 4 oz. orange juice
  *approximate calories: 310*

## *Breakfast #3*

. . . . . .

- ¾ cup nonfat yogurt sprinkled with 2 T. granola
- 1 cup fresh berries
  *approximate calories: 230*

## *Breakfast #4*

. . . . . .

- 1 slice whole-grain toast
  *(Honey Flax Bread, p. 249)*
- 2 t. jam
- 1 poached or boiled egg
- ½ grapefruit or 1 orange
  *approximate calories: 240*

## *Breakfast #5*

. . . . . .

- 2 pancakes
  *(Cottage Cheese Pancakes, p. 247)*
- 2 T. maple syrup
- ½ t. canola/butter (p. 238)
  *approximate calories: 295*

## *Breakfast #6*

. . . . . .

- Smoked Salmon Omelet
  *2 t. canola oil, 1 egg plus 2 egg whites, 1 oz. smoked salmon or lox*
- ½ slice whole-grain toast or flaxseed bread
  *(Honey Flax Bread, p. 249)*
  *approximate calories: 290*

## *Breakfast #7*

. . . . . .

- 1 English muffin or other toast
- 1 oz. Canadian bacon
- Tomato slices
- ¾ cup fresh fruit
  *approximate calories: 300*

## *Breakfast #8*

. . . . . .

- 1 cup dry cereal
  *(1/2 cup Canola Granola, p. 245)*
- ½ cup nonfat milk
- ½ grapefruit or other fruit
  *approximate calories: 275*

## *Breakfast #9*

. . . . . .

- 2, 5-inch buttermilk pancakes
  *(Buttermilk Flaxjacks, p. 242)*
- 1 T. maple syrup
- ½ cup sliced strawberries
  *approximate calories: 350*

## *Breakfast #10*

. . . . . .

- ¼ cup canola granola
  *(Canola Granola, p. 245)*
- ½ cup nonfat yogurt
- ½ banana
  *approximate calories: 240*

## *Breakfast #11*

- ¼ cup canola granola
  *(Canola Granola, p. 245)*
- ¾ cup nonfat yogurt
- 1 cup fruit
  *approximate calories: 260*

## *Breakfast #12*

- 1 cup plain nonfat yogurt
- 2 T. granola
  *(Canola Granola, p. 245)*
- 1 cup fruit
  *approximate calories: 250*

## *Breakfast #13*

- Vegetable Omelet
  *(1 cup fresh vegetables sautéed in 1 t. canola oil, 1 egg
  plus 2 egg whites)*
- 1 slice whole-grain toast
  *(Honey Flax Bread, p. 249)*
- 1 t. canola/butter (p. 238)
  *approximate calories: 295*

## Breakfast #14

• ¹⁄₂ plain bagel, toasted, or 1 slice any toast
  (*Honey Flax Bread, p. 249*)
• ¹⁄₂ cup nonfat yogurt
• ¹⁄₂ cantaloupe or other melon
  *approximate calories: 310*

## Breakfast #15

• Mediterranean Omelet
  *1 t. canola oil, 1 egg plus 2 egg whites, ¹⁄₂ oz. feta
  cheese, 1 T. sun-dried tomatoes*
• ¹⁄₂ slice whole-grain toast
  (*Honey Flax Bread, p. 249*)
• ¹⁄₂ grapefruit
  *approximate calories: 300*

## Breakfast #16

• ³⁄₄ cup nonfat yogurt
• ¹⁄₂ cup fresh fruit
• ¹⁄₂ slice whole-grain toast
  (*Honey Flax Bread, p. 249*)
• 1 T. jam
  *approximate calories: 340*

## Breakfast #17

• 1 English muffin or other toast
  (*Honey Flax Bread, p. 249*)

- 1 poached egg
- 1 t. canola/butter (p. 238)
- Sliced tomato
  *approximate calories: 310*


## Breakfast #18

■  ■  ■  ■  ■  ■

- 1 cup dry cereal
- ¾ cup seasonal fruit
- ⅔ cup nonfat milk
  *approximate calories: 300*


## Breakfast #19

■  ■  ■  ■  ■  ■

- 1 cup cooked cereal
- Sugar or honey to taste
- ½ cup nonfat milk
- ½ cup fresh fruit
  *approximate calories: 270*


## Breakfast #20

■  ■  ■  ■  ■  ■

- 1 medium slice banana bread
  (*Banana Bread, p. 244*)
- 2 T. low-fat cream cheese
- ½ grapefruit
  *approximate calories: 275*

*Breakfast #21*
■  ■  ■  ■  ■

- 1 cup 7-grain cereal
- 1 t. flaxseed
- ²/₃ cup nonfat milk
- ³/₄ cup fresh fruit
  *approximate calories: 360*

# 1,200-Calorie Menu, 21 Lunches

## *Lunch #1*
■  ■  ■  ■  ■

- Green salad with hard-boiled egg
  *(Beet and Blue Cheese Salad, p. 252)*
- 2 t. walnut oil, olive oil, or canola oil dressing
  *(Walnut Oil Dressing, p. 259)*
- Whole-grain roll or bread slice
  *(Honey Flax Bread, p. 249)*
  *approximate calories: 265*

## *Lunch #2*
■  ■  ■  ■  ■

- 1½ cups vegetable soup
  *(Hot and Sour Soup, p. 262)*
- Raw vegetables
- ³/₄ cup nonfat milk
  *approximate calories: 270*

## Lunch #3

▪ ▪ ▪ ▪ ▪

- Chicken salad
  (*Chicken Salad with Vinaigrette, p. 253*)
- ½ slice whole-grain bread
  *approximate calories: 430*

## Lunch #4

▪ ▪ ▪ ▪ ▪

- 1 cup sautéed vegetables
  (*1 cup Provençal Casserole, p. 273*)
- 1 sliced orange
  *approximate calories: 375*

## Lunch #5

▪ ▪ ▪ ▪ ▪

- Lean beef or vegetable burger
  (*1 beef or veggie patty, ½ multigrain bun, lettuce, tomato, 1 T. canola oil mayonnaise, p. 240*)
- 6 oz. vegetable juice
  *approximate calories: 290*

## Lunch #6

▪ ▪ ▪ ▪ ▪

- Deli salad with mixed greens, cheese, chicken, mushrooms, chopped red peppers, 1 T. olive oil vinaigrette
  (*Olive Oil Vinaigrette, p. 143*)
  *approximate calories: 310*

## Lunch #7

. . . . . .

- 1 cup tuna and pasta salad
  (*Tuna Pasta Salad, p. 256*)
- ½ cup carrot sticks or raw vegetables
  *approximate calories: 370*

## Lunch #8

. . . . . .

- Turkey sandwich
  (*3 ounces turkey breast, 2 slices whole-grain bread, 2 T. canola oil mayonnaise, lettuce, tomatoes.*)
- ¾ cup nonfat milk
  *approximate calories: 390*

## Lunch #9

. . . . . .

- Greek Salad
  (*½ cucumber, 1 tomato, 1 oz. feta cheese, 8 olives, 1½ T. Olive Oil Vinaigrette, p. 143*)
- 1 whole-wheat roll
  *approximate calories: 420*

## Lunch #10

. . . . . .

- Deli Salad
  (*Greens, 2 oz. tuna fish, 2 T. olive oil vinaigrette*)
- 1 T. olive oil dressing
  (*Olive Oil Vinaigrette, p.143*)
  *approximate calories: 258*

## *Lunch #11*

■  ■  ■  ■  ■  ■

- Turkey Sandwich
  *(3 oz. roasted turkey breast, 2 t. canola oil mayonnaise,
  lettuce, tomato, 1 slice whole-wheat bread or bagel)*
- 1 cup nonfat milk
  *approximate calories: 380*

## *Lunch #12*

■  ■  ■  ■  ■  ■

- 1 green salad with 1 T. walnut dressing, (p. 259)
  *(Arugula, Walnut, and Apple Salad, p. 251)*
- 1 t. canola/butter (p. 238)
- 1 whole-wheat dinner roll
  *approximate calories: 425*

## *Lunch #13*

■  ■  ■  ■  ■  ■

- Tuna salad sandwich
  *1 slice whole-wheat bread (Honey Flax Bread, p. 249),
  ¼ cup tuna in spring water, 1 T. canola oil mayonnaise,
  green onions, lettuce*
- 1 can vegetable juice
  *approximate calories: 280*

## *Lunch #14*

▪ ▪ ▪ ▪ ▪

- 1 cup vegetable soup
  *(Split Pea Soup, p. 263)*
- Green salad with vinaigrette
  *(Olive Oil Vinaigrette, p. 143)*
  *approximate calories: 350*

## *Lunch #15*

▪ ▪ ▪ ▪ ▪

- Ham sandwich
  *3 oz. lean ham, 1 slice whole-wheat bread (Honey Flax Bread, p. 249), 1 t. canola oil mayonnaise, tomato, let-tuce*
- ³⁄₄ cup nonfat milk
  *approximate calories: 375*

## *Lunch #16*

▪ ▪ ▪ ▪ ▪

- 1 cup bean soup
  *(Bean Soup, p. 260)*
- Green salad with vinaigrette
  *(Olive Oil Vinaigrette, p.143)*
  *approximate calories: 370*

## *Lunch #17*

▪ ▪ ▪ ▪ ▪

- Grilled Vegetable Sandwich
  *(Grilled Vegetable Sandwich, p. 269.)*
  *approximate calories: 390*

## Lunch #18
• • • • • •

- Chicken salad
  *3 oz. skinless breast meat, 1 T. canola oil mayonnaise,
  1 cup lettuce, green onions, red peppers*
- Dinner roll
- 1 t. canola/butter (p. 238)
  *approximate calories: 320*

## Lunch #19
• • • • • •

- Chicken Fajita
  *2 oz. grilled skinless chicken breast meat, 1 tortilla,
  grilled vegetables in 1 T. canola or olive oil, ½ cup fresh
  salsa*
  *approximate calories: 325*

## Lunch #20
• • • • • •

- Lean beef or vegetable burger
  *1 meat or veggie patty, 1 multigrain bun, lettuce,
  tomato, fresh vegetables, 2 t. canola oil mayonnaise
  (p. 240)*
- ½ baked potato
  *approximate calories: 380*

## Lunch #21
• • • • • •

- Fruit salad
  *(2 cups fruit, ½ cup low-fat yogurt)*
  *approximate calories: 195*

# 1,200-Calorie Menu, 21 Dinners

### Dinner #1
▪ ▪ ▪ ▪ ▪

- 4 oz. fatty fish—broiled, simmered in wine or broth or sautéed in olive oil or canola oil
  (*Trout Simmered in White Wine Sauce, p. 276*)
- ½ cup baked acorn squash or other yellow vegetable
- ½ cup canned or fresh sauerkraut
  (*Fresh Sauerkraut Salad, p. 254*)
  *approximate calories: 470*

### Dinner #2
▪ ▪ ▪ ▪ ▪

- 4 oz. chicken, skinless, sautéed in olive oil or canola oil
  (*Chicken in Hellfire, p. 281*)
- ½ cup green peas or other vegetables
- Green salad
  (*1 cup salad greens and vegetables, 1 T. Olive Oil Vinaigrette, p. 143*)
  *approximate calories: 376*

### Dinner #3
▪ ▪ ▪ ▪ ▪

- Lean burger
  (*4 oz. lean meat or vegie patty, ½ whole-wheat hamburger bun or roll, 1 T. canola oil mayonnaise, catsup, lettuce, and tomato*)
- ¾ cups cooked carrots marinated in 1 T. olive oil vinaigrette (served cold)
  (*Olive Oil Vinaigrette, p.143*)
  *approximate calories: 510*

## *Dinner #4*

■  ■  ■  ■  ■

- 5 oz. broiled lamb chop
- 1 cup steamed broccoli
- Briefly sauté in 1 t. olive oil and garlic
- ½ dinner roll
- Carrot sticks
  *approximate calories: 350*

## *Dinner #5*

■  ■  ■  ■  ■

- 5 ounces lean steak
- Large green salad
  1 cup greens, 1 T. olive oil vinaigrette, 1 oz. roasted chicken breast
  *(Olive Oil Vinaigrette, p. 143)*
  *approximate calories: 475*

## *Dinner #6*

■  ■  ■  ■  ■

- 4 oz. salmon with lemon and garlic
- Sautéed in 2 t. canola oil or olive oil
- ½ cup yams
- ½ cup green beans
  *approximate calories: 407*

## *Dinner #7*

. . . . . .

- 5 oz. skinless chicken, broiled, sautéed, or poached
  (*Yogurt Chicken, p. 284*)
- ¼ cup baked acorn squash or other yellow vegetable
- Green salad
  (*Orange-Almond Salad, p. 255*)
  *approximate calories: 420*

## *Dinner #8*

. . . . . .

- 3 oz. skinless roasted chicken breast
- ½ cup cooked bulgur or rice or couscous
- Green salad with 2 t. olive oil vinaigrette
  (*Olive Oil Vinaigrette, p. 143*)
  *approximate calories: 500*

## *Dinner #9*

. . . . . .

- 4 oz. lean roast beef
- ½ baked potato
- 2 t. canola/butter (p. 238)
- ½ cup baked squash or other yellow vegetable
  *approximate calories: 425*

## Dinner #10

• • • • •

- 4 oz. fatty fish, poached, baked, or sautéed
  *(Tuna with Sun-Dried Tomatoes, p. 279)*
- 1 cup steamed broccoli or other vegetable
- ¾ cup bulgur or rice
- 1 t. canola/butter (p. 238)
  *approximate calories: 463*

## Dinner #11

• • • • •

- 4 oz. chicken with rice
  *(Orange Chicken and Rice, p. 283)*
- 1 cup brussels sprouts
  *(Brussels Sprouts with Walnut Oil and Lemon, p. 267)*
  *approximate calories: 475*

## Dinner #12

• • • • •

- 4 oz. any fatty fish
  *(Tuna Marinated in Dill, p. 278)*
- 1 serving kale, spinach, or mustard greens
  *(Kale with Lemon, p. 271)*
- 1 whole-wheat roll
  *(Honey Flax Bread, p. 249)*
- 1 T. humus
  *(Humus, p. 270)*
  *approximate calories: 480*

### Dinner #13

·  ·  ·  ·  ·

- 1 cup bean soup
  (*Bean Soup, p. 260*)
- 1 piece corn bread
  (*Corn Bread, p. 246*)
- 1 t. canola/butter (p. 238)
  *approximate calories: 472*

### Dinner #14

·  ·  ·  ·  ·

- 1½ cups stir fry
  (*Thai Stir Fry, p. 280*)
- ½ cup rice
- Green salad with vinaigrette
  *approximate calories: 530*

### Dinner #15

·  ·  ·  ·  ·

- 1½ cups pork stir fry
  (*Pork or Beef Stir Fry, p. 288*)
- ½ cup rice or bulgur
  *approximate calories: 500*

### Dinner #16

·  ·  ·  ·  ·

- 1 black bean quesadilla
  (*Black Bean or Beef Quesadillas, p. 264*)
- ½ cup salsa
  (*Black Bean Salsa, p. 266*)
  *approximate calories: 350*

## Dinner #17

▪ ▪ ▪ ▪ ▪ ▪

- 5 oz. salmon with vegetables
  (*Salmon Cilantro with Grilled Vegetables, p. 274*)
- 1 multigrain bun
- 1 t. canola oil mayonnaise
  *approximate calories: 540*

## Dinner #18

▪ ▪ ▪ ▪ ▪ ▪

- 1½ cups Pad Thai
  (*Pad Thai, p. 287*)
- 1 cup fresh green beans sautéed in 2 t. olive oil
- Lemon to taste
  *approximate calories: 580*

## Dinner #19

▪ ▪ ▪ ▪ ▪ ▪

- 5 oz. grilled trout
  (*Trout with Wine and Fine Herbs, p. 277*)
- Swiss chard
  (*Chard with Nuts and Raisins, p. 268*)
  *approximate calories: 491*

## Dinner #20

▪ ▪ ▪ ▪ ▪ ▪

- 6 oz. grilled tuna
- ½ cup baked acorn squash
- ¾ cup steamed spinach
- 1 small dinner roll
  *approximate calories: 510*

## Dinner #21

■　■　■　■　■　■

- Lamb roast
  (*Lamb, Green Pepper, and Apple Curry, p. 286*)
- 1 cup cooked carrots
- 1 t. olive oil plus lemon
  *approximate calories: 610*

# 50-Calorie Healthy Snacks

½ cup steamed carrots
1 cup steamed green beans
8 ounces vegetable juice cocktail
½ ounce cheese
6 ounces nonfat milk
½ cup fresh apricots
¾ cup fresh berries
¼ medium cantaloupe
1 small pear
1 cup fresh strawberries
½ grapefruit
1 medium peach
1 medium nectarine
4 walnut halves

# 100-Calorie Healthy Snacks

1 ounce cheese
1 large apple
1½ ounces dried apples
7 ounces apple juice
½ cup applesauce
1 cup (8 ounces) fresh apricots
¾ cup canned apricots (in juice)
6 ounces apricot nectar

1 small banana
1½ cups fresh blackberries
1¼ cups fresh blueberries
1 cup buttermilk
½, 5-inch-diameter cantaloupe
8 ounces carrot juice
¼ of a 7-inch casaba melon
1 cup fresh cherries
½ cup chocolate milk (1% fat)
⅔ cup lowfat cottage cheese
1 large ear of corn
4 ounces steamed corn kernels
4 ounces of crab meat
2 large fresh figs
⅔ cup canned figs in light syrup
¼ cup dried figs
1 frozen fruit bar (no sugar added)
1 large fruit roll-up
4 ounces fruit sorbet
½ cup fruit compote (see page 291)
1⅔ cups grapes
6 ounces unsweetened grape juice
1 medium grapefruit
9 ounces grapefruit juice
4-inch wedge, honeydew melon
2 medium kiwifruits
1/3 cup lima beans
3 medium mandarin oranges
1 cup 1% milk
1¼ cup nonfat milk
1 large nectarine
12 large olives
1 large orange
7 ounces orange juice
⅔ medium papaya
5 ounces papaya nectar
2 medium peaches
1 cup peaches canned in juice

3 ounces dried peaches
5 ounces peach nectar
1 large pear
6 ounces pears canned in juice
3 ounces dried pears
5 ounces steamed green peas
1 small persimmon
3 small or 2 large plums
⅔ cup plums canned in juice
1 medium pomegranate
5 dried prunes
3 dried prunes stuffed with walnut halves
3 tablespoons raisins
1⅔ cups fresh raspberries
1½ ounces smoked salmon
2 cups fresh strawberries
8 walnut halves
½ cup lowfat yogurt

# FOURTEEN

# In the Omega Kitchen

THIS CHAPTER CONTAINS fifty recipes that illustrate The Seven Dietary Guidelines of **The Omega Diet**. Scan through them and you will see a number of common denominators. First of all, olive oil and canola oil are the primary oils, with butter and walnut oil making an occasional appearance. Flaxseeds, flaxseed meal (or flaxmeal), walnuts, and Brazil nuts—rich sources of LNA—are added to many of the baked goods. All of the recipes are relatively low in saturated fat and omega-6 oils, and they contain no partially hydrogenated oils. The most common sources of protein are lean meat, chicken, fish, cheese, and legumes. The overall ratio of omega-6 to omega-3 is kept below 4 to 1, and omega-3 fatty acids are found in all the meals, just as in the traditional diet of Crete and in the Lyon Diet Heart Study.[1]

Most of the recipes are also relatively low in calories to accommodate those people on one of the **Omega Weight-Loss Diets**. If you are not concerned about calories, eat larger portions or choose the high-calorie options, such as adding walnuts or more oil. Some recipes give you a choice between using either whole eggs, egg whites, or a combination of the two. If you have high cholesterol (or a family history of high cholesterol), use omega-3-enriched eggs, egg whites, or a combination of yolks and whites.

Each recipe concludes with a nutritional breakdown. In addition to the usual categories—total fat, saturated fat, calories, carbohydrates, protein, and sodium—you will find information about fatty acids, specifically the omega-6 fatty acid linoleic acid (LA) and three omega-3 fatty acids: eicosapentaenoic acid (EPA), docosahexaenoic acid (DHA), and alpha-linolenic acid (LNA). The last column in the nutritional summary shows the overall ratio of omega-6 to omega-3 fatty acids.[2]

We've made a special effort to keep the recipes simple. Most involve fifteen minutes or less of actual preparation time. To further simplify your life, we've compiled detailed shopping lists for all the recipes, which you will find at the end of the next chapter. Take the book to the store with you, and you can plan your menus as you shop.

If you rarely cook, take heart. The next chapter gives you advice on how to order the healthiest meals at fast-food outlets and restaurants, and how to bring home "Omega-friendly" convenience food from the grocery store.

## Make Your Own Recipes "Omega-Friendly"

The recipes in this chapter can serve as a model for modifying your own recipes. Consider the recipe for "Jo's Brownies" on page 292. The original recipe was a standard, one-bowl brownie recipe. We reduced the sugar by a quarter of a cup, eliminating some empty calories. Then we cut the overall fat from eight tablespoons to five and replaced the butter with a mixture of butter and canola oil, thereby lowering the saturated fat content and adding omega-3 fatty acids. The changes were minor enough to retain the rich, chocolate flavor of the brownies. There's no point in altering a dessert recipe to the point that it is no longer appealing. Nonetheless, these alterations shaved 50 calories off each brownie, eliminated 49 milligrams of cholesterol, dropped the saturated fat content from 7 grams to 2, and just as important, added lots of omega-3 fatty acids.

You can apply similar exchange principles to other recipes. They are fairly simple:

- If a recipe calls for eggs, use omega-3-enriched eggs or substitute two egg whites for one or more of the yolks.
- If a recipe calls for sugar, try using slightly less.
- If a recipe specifies vegetable oil, use either canola oil, olive oil, or a combination of the two.

- If a recipe requires a solid fat such as shortening, butter, or margarine, lower the total amount of fat if possible and then substitute a butter/canola or butter/olive oil blend.
- For every cup of flour, substitute 2 tablespoons of flaxmeal for 2 of the tablespoons of flour.

Some recipes are fussy and won't tolerate these changes, but most will. You'll need to experiment.

## Baking Tips for Using Flaxmeal and Flaxseeds

As indicated above, one way to add more omega-3 fatty acids to your diet is to use flaxmeal in much of your baking. This nutritious ingredient does more than add healthy fiber and essential fatty acids; it also improves the volume and texture of breads, muffins, and cookies, at the same time that it extends their shelf life. (Flaxmeal has excellent water-binding properties, which makes baked goods taste fresher longer.)

For optimal results, heed the following advice:

- You can replace from 10 to 15 percent of the amount of flour in a recipe with flaxmeal and get excellent results. That means that for each 1 cup of flour, you can replace as much as 2 tablespoons of the flour with flaxmeal.
- Flaxmeal is high in fat (healthy fat), so when adding it to a recipe, you can reduce some of the other fat if you wish. As a general rule, you can substitute three parts flaxmeal for one part oil. If you add three tablespoons of flaxmeal to a recipe, for example, you can eliminate one tablespoon of the oil.
- Flaxmeal makes baked goods brown faster, so reduce the heat 25 degrees or cook for a shorter period of time. (In a bread machine, use the "light" crust setting.)
- For optimum results when adding flaxmeal to yeast bread, increase the amount of yeast by 25 percent and add slightly more water.
- Flaxmeal does not contain gluten (the protein in flour that creates the internal structure that allows bread to rise). When adding a significant amount of flaxmeal to yeast bread, you will

get better results if you also add gluten. Add one tablespoon for each one-half cup of flax.

- If using whole flaxseeds, soak them in warm water for ten minutes before adding them to your baked goods.

People who do not eat eggs can substitute flaxmeal for eggs in many recipes because the ground flaxseeds have a natural gum that thickens batter in much the same way as eggs. To replace one egg, mix together one tablespoon of flaxmeal and three tablespoons of water. Let sit for one to two minutes and then add the combined mixture to the recipe as you would an egg.

The only recipes where the ratio of omega-6 to omega-3 is higher than 4 to 1 are those few recipes that rely on olive oil exclusively and are not based on fish. When these dishes are combined with other dishes with a lower ratio, the overall daily intake is within the desired guidelines.

---

A few additional comments about the fatty acid calculations: First, in most instances, the omega-6 to omega-3 ratio noted in tables is the ratio of LA to LNA, and the source is predominately oils. Second, in recipes containing fish, we include amounts of EPA and DHA because this is the predominant source of omega-3 fatty acids in the fish. Although eggs and some other animal products also contain EPA and DHA, we do not list the amount because either the amount is negligible, we do not have good data, or there is too much variety between products. (For example, eggs from hens raised in a natural environment contain far more EPA and DHA than eggs from ordinary hens.)[1] Third, in the meat dishes, no information is given for the AA content (although all meat contains AA) because there is inadequate data about the AA content in the food supply.

---

# The Basics

## CANOLA/BUTTER OR OLIVE/BUTTER

Consider making canola/butter and olive/butter your daily spreads. They have about half the amount of saturated fat as regular butter, and, unlike margarine, they have negligible amounts of trans-fatty acids. Either one of these butter mixtures is the perfect consistency for spreading on bread right from the refrigerator. (If left at room temperature for an hour or more, they'll become almost liquid.)

The two spreads are quite different. Canola/butter tastes much like butter, while olive/butter retains the flavor of the olive oil. They also have different nutritional content. Canola/butter gives you mono-unsaturated fatty acids and omega-3 fatty acids, while olive/butter provides monounsaturated fatty acids and a substance called "squa-lene," which, by itself, can lower cholesterol. Try them both and see which you like best. Some people like canola/butter on their breakfast toast but olive/butter on their dinner rolls.

You can buy canola/butter premixed in some health food stores. The only difference between the store-bought variety and the kind you make at home is that the commercial product has an added sta-bilizer to keep the oil and butter from separating.

MAKES: *1 cup*
TIME: *5 minutes*

### Canola/butter
$\frac{1}{2}$ cup butter (1 cube) brought to room temperature
$\frac{1}{2}$ cup canola oil

### Olive/butter
$\frac{1}{2}$ cup butter (1 cube) brought to room temperature
$\frac{1}{2}$ cup olive oil

Place butter and oil into a blender or food processor. Blend until thoroughly combined. (The spread will be the consistency of yogurt or thick cream.) Spoon into a cup, bowl, or mold; cover and place in refrigerator to firm.

For variety add: herbs of your choice, grated citrus fruit rind, or garlic (fresh, not powdered).

## NUTRITIONAL VALUE PER TEASPOON:

### Canola/Butter

| Calories | Protein | Carbs | Sodium | Total Fat | Sat. Fat | Chol. |
|----------|---------|-------|--------|-----------|----------|-------|
| 37 | <1 gms. | 0 gms. | 20 mgs. | 4 gms. | 1 gms. | 5 mgs. |

| LA | LNA | EPA | DHA | Omega-6/Omega-3 |
|----|-----|-----|-----|-----------------|
| 0.4 gms. | 0.2 gms. | 0 gms. | 0 gms. | 2 |

### Olive/Butter

| Calories | Protein | Carbs | Sodium | Total Fat | Sat. Fat | Chol. |
|----------|---------|-------|--------|-----------|----------|-------|
| 37 | <1 gms. | 0 gms. | 20 mgs. | 4 gms. | 1 gms. | 5 mgs. |

| LA | LNA | EPA | DHA | Omega-6/Omega-3 |
|----|-----|-----|-----|-----------------|
| 0.2 gms. | 0.3 gms. | 0 gms. | 0 gms. | 6.6 |

# CANOLA OIL MAYONNAISE

Can't find canola oil mayonnaise at your grocery store? Make your own. It's easier than you think. If you like to experiment, you can add a number of different flavorings, including prepared mustard, garlic, orange, tarragon, or vinegar. You can also use olive oil instead of canola oil for an entirely different flavor.

Purists recommend making mayonnaise with a wire whisk, but you can make a fine mayonnaise using an egg beater, mixer, blender, or food processor. The directions below are for a food processor or blender.

MAKES: *About 1³/₄ cups*
TIME: *10 minutes*

1 egg
¹/₂ t. salt
1¹/₂ t. dried mustard
¹/₈ t. cayenne
¹/₂ t. sugar
1¹/₄ cups canola oil (divided)
4 T. lemon juice (fresh, not bottled)

Allow the oil and egg to come to room temperature. (You can speed matters by placing the egg and measuring cup filled with oil in hot water for ten minutes.) Place ¼ cup of the oil plus the egg, salt, mustard, cayenne, and sugar into the food processor or blender. Blend until thoroughly combined. With the food processor, beater, or blender running, add an additional ½ cup of oil in a *very* thin stream (about the diameter of a thin strand of yarn). When the ½ cup of oil has been added, add the lemon juice and blend briefly until combined. Add the final ½ cup of oil, once again in a fine stream. Refrigerate.

For variety add: 2 cloves of crushed garlic, 1 teaspoon of dried tarragon or dill, or more cayenne. You can also substitute vinegar for the lemon juice. For a wonderful fish sauce, use orange juice rather than lemon juice and add 1 teaspoon paprika for more color. To make low-fat mayonnaise, blend fifty-fifty with low-fat yogurt.

**NUTRITIONAL VALUE PER TABLESPOON:**

| Calories | Protein | Carbs | Sodium | Total Fat | Sat. Fat | Chol. |
|---|---|---|---|---|---|---|
| 91 | .24 gms. | .28 gms. | 46 mgs. | 9.9 gms. | .71 gms. | 7.57 mgs. |

| LA | LNA | EPA | DHA | Omega-6/Omega-3 | |
|---|---|---|---|---|---|
| 1.7 gms. | 0.9 gms. | NA* | NA | 1.9 | |

* NA = information not available

# FLAXMEAL

Flaxmeal, or flaxseed meal, is a standard ingredient in the Omega kitchen. When flaxseeds are ground to a wheat-germ-like texture, they can be added in small amounts to virtually everything you bake without making a noticeable alteration in flavor or texture. Consider it your secret ingredient for restoring omega-3 fatty acids to the food chain. A must for people who do not eat fish.

You can buy flaxmeal at some natural foods stores, or you can order it from a mail-order catalogue. (See p. 360 for mail-order information.) To make your own flaxmeal, you will need a coffee grinder or similar apparatus. (You can't grind the flaxseeds in a food processor or blender because they will bounce around.) If you don't have a coffee grinder or food mill, consider buying one. The nutritional payoff of having a fresh supply of flaxmeal will more than justify the cost.

MAKES: *1³/₄ cups*
TIME: *5 minutes*

1 cup whole flaxseeds

Pour flaxseeds into a grinder and process on a fine setting. (Use the espresso setting on a coffee grinder.) Store in a covered jar in the refrigerator or freezer. Use within a few weeks. (If you use the coffee grinder for both coffee beans and flaxseeds, clean carefully between use.)

### Variation: Toasted Flaxmeal

You can toast flaxmeal and flavor it with honey, brown sugar, or maple syrup, creating a nutritious topping to sprinkle on cereal, fruit, cottage cheese, yogurt, pies, crumb cakes, and pastries. It tastes a bit like toasted wheat germ, only better. Even Mikey will like it.

**NUTRITIONAL VALUE PER RECIPE (1 CUP FLAXSEEDS):**

| Calories | Protein | Carbs | Sodium | Total Fat | Sat. Fat | Chol. |
|---|---|---|---|---|---|---|
| 675 | 31.5 gms. | .375 gms. | TR mgs. | 63 gms. | 6 gms. | 0 mgs. |

| LA | LNA | EPA | DHA | Omega-6/Omega-3 |
|---|---|---|---|---|
| 11 gms. | 36 gms. | 0 gms. | 0 gms. | 0.3 |

# Breads and Grains

## BUTTERMILK FLAXJACKS

These light and flavorful pancakes are rich with omega-3 fatty acids. Serve with canola/butter and top with maple syrup, berries, yogurt, applesauce, cottage cheese, jam, or powdered sugar and lemon juice. Yumm.

If you have a favorite pancake recipe already, you can increase the omega-3 content by adding 3–4 tablespoons of flaxmeal. Add more milk if necessary. Or buy a whole-grain pancake mix from the health food section of your local store and enrich with flaxmeal.

MAKES: *7–8, 5-inch pancakes*
TIME: *10 minutes of prep, 10 minutes to cook*

1 egg
1 T. canola oil
1½ cups buttermilk (or 1 cup milk plus ½ cup plain yogurt)
3 T. ground flaxseeds (flaxmeal)
1¼ cups white, whole-wheat, or whole-wheat pastry flour
1 t. baking soda
1/8 t. salt
1–2 T. sugar

*Variations:*
Add grated orange or lemon peel, berries, sliced bananas or nuts.

Heat a griddle or skillet to approximately 325 degrees.

Beat egg, milk, and oil in a small bowl. Add the dry ingredients to a larger mixing bowl and stir until combined. Add the liquid ingredients to the dry ingredients and stir until combined. Cook on the griddle until golden brown. (Do not undercook.)

Note: For even lighter pancakes, separate the egg and beat white separately. Fold the beaten egg white into the batter after the liquid and dry ingredients have been combined.

## NUTRITIONAL VALUE PER 5" FLAXJACK:

| Calories | Protein | Carbs | Sodium | Total Fat | Sat. Fat | Chol. |
|---|---|---|---|---|---|---|
| 122 | 5 gms. | 16 gms. | 184 mgs. | 4 gms. | .59 gms. | 32 mgs. |

| LA | | LNA | | EPA | DHA | Omega-6/Omega-3 | |
|---|---|---|---|---|---|---|---|
| .06 gms. | | .07 gms. | | NA | NA | 0.86 | |

# BANANA BREAD

MAKES *1 loaf, 10 slices*
TIME: *20 minutes of preparation, 45 minutes to bake*

$1/3$ cup canola oil
2 large eggs or 1 egg and 2 whites
$1/4$ cup low-fat sour cream or yogurt
1 cup mashed ripe banana
1 t. vanilla
$1 1/2$ cups white flour or whole-wheat pastry flour
$2/3$ cup sugar
$1 1/2$ t. baking powder
$1/2$ t. baking soda
$1/4$ t. salt
$1/2$ cup chopped walnuts
4 T. flaxmeal (ground flaxseed)

If making in a bread machine, select for quick bread and follow the directions for your individual machine. (You may be instructed to add the bananas and nuts mid-cycle.)

By hand: Preheat oven to 325 degrees. Lightly oil a standard bread pan. Beat the oil, eggs, sour cream, banana, and vanilla in a mixer or by hand until creamy. Mix the dry ingredients in a separate bowl. Add dry ingredients to liquid ingredients and stir until combined. Add walnuts and flaxmeal and stir a couple of strokes just to combine. Spoon into bread pan and bake for 45 minutes or until done.

Remove from pan and cool.

NOTE: Banana bread is high in calories. On the 1,200-calorie version of **The Omega Weight-Loss Diet,** for example, you may be allotted only half a slice. To lower the calories, leave out the walnuts. (Walnuts, however, are a good source of linolenic acid. A better choice would be to keep the walnuts and go for a 45-minute walk.)

## NUTRITIONAL VALUE PER GENEROUS SLICE ($^1/_{10}$ OF LOAF):

| Calories | Protein | Carbs | Sodium | Total Fat | Sat. Fat | Chol. |
|---|---|---|---|---|---|---|
| 260 | 4.9 gms. | 32.6 gms. | 163 mgs. | 13 gms. | 2.4 gms. | 42.6 mgs. |

| LA | LNA | EPA | DHA | Omega-6/Omega-3 | |
|---|---|---|---|---|---|
| 3.4 gms. | 1.4 gms. | NA | NA | 2.4 | |

# CANOLA GRANOLA

Nutritionally speaking, this granola wins hands down over regular granola. Store-bought granola has less fruit, more sugar, a high ratio of omega-6 to omega-3 fatty acids, and often a significant amount of partially hydrogenated oil as well.

Make up a big batch of canola granola on the weekend and it will last you all week. If you have young children (or grandchildren), they'll want to help out. For variety, you can add shredded coconut, sunflower seeds, Cheerios, or pumpkin seeds. Given time, many people create their own "house" granola. (This particular recipe tastes like a cross between granola and muesli.)

MAKES: *7 cups*
TIME: *10 minutes of prep, plus up to 30 minutes baking time*

> 6 cups raw oats, quick-cooking or regular
> $^1/_3$ cup ground flaxseed or chopped walnuts
> 2–3 T. canola oil
> 2–4 T. of honey or brown sugar (or to taste)
> 1 cup dried fruit such as raisins, blueberries, cranberries, or papaya
> 1$^1/_2$ cups dried apples, chopped into $^1/_4$-inch pieces (Chop apples in a blender or food processor or by hand. Coat the knife or blade with cooking oil to keep apples from sticking.)

Preheat oven to 350. Mix all the ingredients except the dried fruit in a large bowl. Spread evenly in a shallow baking pan and bake for 15 minutes. Remove from the oven and stir so the granola will cook uniformly. Continue to bake until golden (10–15 additional minutes. Watch carefully. Stir if necessary). Remove from oven and mix in dried fruit. Cool and then store in a covered container.

**NUTRITIONAL VALUE PER ½ CUP:**

| Calories | Protein | Carbs | Sodium | Total Fat | Sat. Fat | Chol. |
|---|---|---|---|---|---|---|
| 191 | 5 gms. | 34.4 gms. | 193 mgs. | 5 gms. | <1 gms. | 0 mgs. |

| LA | LNA | EPA | DHA | Omega-6/Omega-3 |
|---|---|---|---|---|
| 1.7 gms. | 0.64 gms. | 0 gms. | 0 gms. | 2.6 |

# CORN BREAD

MAKES: *8 servings*
TIME: *10 minutes of prep, 20 minutes to bake*

1 egg or 2 egg whites
2 T. canola oil
1 cup nonfat milk
1 cup flour
1 cup cornmeal
2½ t. baking powder
3–4 T. sugar
½ t. salt
¼ cup flaxmeal (ground flaxseed)

Heat oven to 325 degrees. Mix egg, oil, and milk and beat well. Mix the dry ingredients and add to the egg mixture. Stir until just blended. Pour batter into a lightly oiled bread pan and cook for 25 minutes or until corn bread springs back when touched in the center.

**NUTRITIONAL VALUE PER ⅛ OF TOTAL RECIPE:**

| Calories | Protein | Carbs | Sodium | Total Fat | Sat. Fat | Chol. |
|---|---|---|---|---|---|---|
| 204 | 6 gms. | 33 gms. | 267 mgs. | 6 gms. | <1 gms. | 27 mgs. |

| LA | LNA | EPA | DHA | Omega-6/Omega-3 |
|---|---|---|---|---|
| 1.4 gms. | 0.9 gms. | NA | NA | 1.5 |

# COTTAGE CHEESE PANCAKES

These pancakes are tender with a cornmeal crunch. They're simple to make and provide a welcome change from ordinary pancakes. They're also healthier. Pancakes from a standard pancake mix contain twice as much sodium, twice as much saturated fat, no omega-3 fatty acids, and only one third as much protein.

MAKES: *7–8 medium-sized pancakes*
*(⅓ cup batter per pancake)*
TIME: *5–10 minutes of prep*

2 eggs or 1 egg and 2 egg whites
⅔ cup low-fat cottage cheese
2 T. white or whole-wheat flour
½ cup cornmeal (preferably whole-grain)
1 t. baking powder
1 T. sugar
⅓ cup nonfat milk
2 T. flaxmeal
(½ t. grated orange or lemon peel)

Place all ingredients in a blender or food processor and blend for 5–10 seconds. Bake on a 350-degree griddle or a medium-hot skillet lightly greased with canola oil.

**NUTRITIONAL VALUE PER PANCAKE (MADE WITH 1 EGG AND 2 EGG WHITES. DOES NOT INCLUDE BUTTER OR SYRUP):**

| Calories | Protein | Carbs | Sodium | Total Fat | Sat. Fat | Chol. |
|----------|---------|--------|---------|-----------|----------|-------|
| 83 | 5 gms. | 12 gms. | 161 mgs. | 2 gms. | 0.7 gms. | 54 mgs. |

| LA | LNA | EPA | DHA | Omega-6/Omega-3 |
|----|-----|-----|-----|-----------------|
| 0.5 gms. | 0.3 gms. | NA | NA | 1.7 |

# FLAXBRAN MUFFINS

Make a full batch of these muffins even if you have a small household. Store the extra ones in the freezer. Muffins make great snacks or additions to any meal. They're also ideal for taking to work. If you don't have time to make these muffins from scratch, buy a bran muffin mix (preferably one that does not contain partially hydrogenated oil) and add ½ cup ground flaxseed and ¼ cup milk. Use canola oil for the oil.

MAKES: *10, 2½-inch muffins*
TIME: *10 minutes of prep, approximately 20 minutes to bake*

> 1½ cups all-purpose white flour or whole-wheat
>    pastry flour
> ½ cup wheat bran
> ½ cup flaxmeal
> ½ cup white or brown sugar
> ¼ t. salt
> 2½ t. baking powder
> (⅔ cup raisins or other dried fruit)
> (grated orange rind)
> 1 cup low-fat milk or buttermilk
> 1 egg
> 2 T. molasses
> 2 T. canola oil

Preheat oven to 350. Grease muffin tins with canola oil. Mix dry ingredients thoroughly (including optional dried fruit). In a separate bowl, beat together milk, egg, molasses, and canola oil. Add liquid ingredients to dry ingredients, and stir with a few deft strokes. (The more you stir the muffin batter, the tougher the muffins will be. Muffins contain the ideal ratio of flour to water to develop gluten.) Spoon into muffin tins and bake 18–20 minutes or until done.

**NUTRITIONAL VALUE PER AVERAGE-SIZED MUFFIN ($^{1}/_{10}$ OF RECIPE):**

| Calories | Protein | Carbs | Sodium | Total Fat | Sat. Fat | Chol. |
|---|---|---|---|---|---|---|
| 223 | 4.8 gms. | 36 gms. | 157 mgs. | 7.5 gms. | 1.4 gms. | 23 mgs. |

| LA | LNA | EPA | DHA | Omega-6/Omega-3 | |
|---|---|---|---|---|---|
| 0.63 gms. | 1.09 gms. | NA | NA | 0.58 | |

# HONEY FLAX BREAD

There are a number of reasons why honey flax bread should be your daily bread. First, it tastes great. Second, it is made primarily from whole-wheat flour, which contains more nutrients and fiber than white flour. Third, it's rich in flaxmeal, so it has a ratio of omega-6 to omega-3 fatty acids of less than one—in harmony with the balance of fatty acids found in the evolutionary diet. Flaxmeal also gives you a cancer-fighting substance called "lignan" plus ample amounts of soluble and insoluble fiber. Have a piece of toast for breakfast, and you will stay satisfied from breakfast until lunch.

Pressed for time? You can make flaxmeal bread from a prepared whole-wheat bread mix. (We recommend Bob's Red Mill 100% Whole Wheat Bread Mix. See mail-order information on page 360.) Simply add ½ cup of flaxmeal and one tablespoon of water to the regular recipe. A few natural food stores carry flaxseed bread.

MAKES *1 large loaf, 14 slices*
TIME: *5 minutes of preparation if using a bread machine;
30-plus minutes if making the bread by hand or using a
heavy-duty mixer. The bread takes several hours to rise
and 30 or more minutes to bake.*

> 1½ cups warm water (add slightly more if
>   needed)
> 1 cup white flour (ideally bread flour)
> 3 cups whole-wheat bread or all-purpose flour
> ½ cup ground flaxseeds (flaxmeal)
> 1 T. canola oil
> 3 T. honey or sugar
> 1 t. salt
> 1 T. plus 1 t. yeast

**BREAD MACHINE.** Select for whole-wheat bread and light crust. (The flaxmeal makes the bread brown more quickly.) Combine the ingredients in the order given and begin the mixing process. After a few minutes of kneading, check to make sure that the dough has formed a smooth, round ball. If not, add a small amount of water or flour as needed.

**BY HAND OR HEAVY-DUTY MIXER.** Place water and yeast in a large mixing bowl. Let rest for several minutes. Add the white flour and 1 cup of the whole-wheat flour. Beat into a sponge. (Use the dough hook on the mixer.) Add the remaining flour along with the flaxseed meal, oil, honey, and salt. Knead thoroughly, either by hand or mixer.

Let rise in a warm place until double in bulk. Punch down, shape into a loaf, and place into a greased bread pan. Let rise again and bake in a preheated 375-degree oven for 30 minutes or until done.

**NUTRITIONAL VALUE PER SLICE:**

| Calories | Protein | Carbs | Sodium | Total Fat | Sat. Fat | Chol. |
|---|---|---|---|---|---|---|
| 173 | 5 gms. | 32 gms. | 165 mgs. | 3 gms. | <1 gms. | 0 mgs. |

| LA | LNA | EPA | DHA | Omega-6/Omega-3 | |
|---|---|---|---|---|---|
| 0.7 gms. | 0.8 gms. | 0 gms. | 0 gms. | 0.87 | |

# Salads and Salad Dressings
## ARUGULA, WALNUT, AND APPLE SALAD

MAKES: *4 servings*
TIME: *20 minutes*

**Dressing:**
5 T. walnut oil
2 T. olive oil
3 T. balsamic vinegar (or wine vinegar)
salt and pepper to taste

**Salad:**
2 apples, peeled and cored
1 bunch arugula (preferably from young plants)
⅓ cup chopped walnuts
(2 ounces goat or feta cheese, crumbled)

Combine dressing ingredients. Wash the arugula, removing woody stems. Slice the apples into thin slices. Arrange apple slices over a bed of arugula, and top with cheese, walnuts, and dressing.

As you can see, some salads can be quite high in calories.

**NUTRITIONAL VALUE OF 1 SALAD (¼ OF RECIPE):**

**With Cheese**

| Calories | Protein | Carbs | Sodium | Total Fat | Sat. Fat | Chol. |
|---|---|---|---|---|---|---|
| 357 | 5 gms. | 12 gms. | 159 mgs. | 33 gms. | 6 gms. | 11 mgs. |

| LA | LNA | EPA | DHA | Omega-6/Omega-3 | |
|---|---|---|---|---|---|
| 12 gms. | 3 gms. | 0 gms. | 0 gms. | 4 | |

**Without Cheese**

| Calories | Protein | Carbs | Sodium | Total Fat | Sat. Fat | Chol. |
|---|---|---|---|---|---|---|
| 305 | 2 gms. | 12 gms. | 5 mgs. | 29 gms. | 3 gms. | 0 mgs. |

| LA | LNA | EPA | DHA | Omega-6/Omega-3 | |
|---|---|---|---|---|---|
| 10 gms. | 2.7 gms. | 0 gms. | 0 gms. | 3.7 | |

# BEET AND BLUE CHEESE SALAD

This is a beautiful and delicious salad that you'll be proud to serve to company.

MAKES: *2 servings*
TIME: *10 minutes*

1 cup canned sliced beets (or fresh-cooked
   beets)
1 ounce blue or Stilton cheese (Stilton is a mild,
   creamy blue cheese)
2 T. chopped walnuts
Bed of arugula or other lettuce, about 1 cup
   packed

Drain beets and arrange on a bed of arugula. Top with crumbled blue cheese, walnuts, and serve with Walnut Oil Dressing *(p. 259)* or other mild dressing

**NUTRITIONAL VALUE PER ½ RECIPE:**

| Calories | Protein | Carbs | Sodium | Total Fat | Sat. Fat | Chol. |
|---|---|---|---|---|---|---|
| 105 | 5.2 gms. | 7.6 gms. | 439 mgs. | 6.5 gms. | 2.8 gms. | 10.5 mgs. |

| LA | LNA | EPA | DHA | Omega-6/Omega-3 | |
|---|---|---|---|---|---|
| 2.5 gms. | 0.5 gms. | 0 gms. | 0 gms. | 5 | |

# CHICKEN SALAD WITH VINAIGRETTE

You can now buy roast chicken that is free from artificial and added ingredients. There is a world of difference between regular deli meat and this unadulterated deli meat. It costs more, but once you taste the difference, you may feel the added cost is justified.

MAKES: *2 servings*
TIME: *10 minutes, plus cooking time for chicken*

6 ounces roasted skinless chicken breast (or deli meat), cubed or cut into shreds
2 cups mixed salad greens
1 carrot, chopped
1 fresh tomato, chopped
$1/2$ green or red pepper, chopped

Prepare salad. Toss with 2 tablespoons olive oil vinaigrette.

## NUTRITIONAL VALUE FOR $1/2$ OF RECIPE:

| Calories | Protein | Carbs | Sodium | Total Fat | Sat. Fat | Chol. |
|---|---|---|---|---|---|---|
| 197 | 21 gms. | 12 gms. | 109 mgs. | 3.4 gms. | 1 gms. | 72 mgs. |

| LA | LNA | EPA | DHA | Omega-6/Omega-3 | |
|---|---|---|---|---|---|
| .9 gms. | .04 gms. | 0 gms. | 0 gms. | 22 | |

NOTE: Use canola oil or a combination of canola oil and olive oil to lower the omega-6 to omega-3 ratio.

# FRESH SAUERKRAUT SALAD

This crisp, refreshing salad goes well with meat dishes, especially pork chops, fish, and barbecued ribs. If you use green cabbage, use the red onion. If you use red cabbage, use the white onion. (The combination of cabbage and onion is a potent cancer-fighting duo.)

MAKES: *7 cups*

TIME: *15 minutes of prep, 12+ hours to marinate*

½ red or green cabbage
1 medium onion (red or white)
⅓ cup sugar
½ t. dried dillweed or 2 T. chopped fresh dill-
    weed
½ cup vinegar
½ t. salt or to taste
2 T. canola oil
1 t. prepared mustard

Slice cabbage and onion into thin slices. Layer in the bottom of a bowl or pan. Mix remaining ingredients in a saucepan, bring to a boil, and pour over the cabbage while still hot. Marinate in refrigerator for 12 hours or more. Stir occasionally.

**NUTRITIONAL VALUE PER CUP:**

| Calories | Protein | Carbs | Sodium | Total Fat | Sat. Fat | Chol. |
|----------|---------|-------|--------|-----------|----------|-------|
| 80 | 1 gms. | 16 gms. | 178 mgs. | 4 gms. | <1 gms. | 0 mgs. |

| LA | LNA | EPA | DHA | Omega-6/Omega-3 |
|----|-----|-----|-----|-----------------|
| 0.6 gms. | 0.4 gms. | 0 gms. | 0 gms. | 1.5 |

# ORANGE WALNUT SALAD

One overlooked way to add more fruit to your diet is to add it to a "vegetable" salad. This particular salad uses orange slices, but try it with sliced apples, pears—or even kiwifruit!

MAKES: *6 servings*
TIME: *15 minutes*

6 cups mixed salad greens, washed and dried
2 medium oranges, peeled and thinly sliced (or 1
    small can mandarin oranges)
1/3 cup walnuts, coarsely chopped
1 cup celery, chopped
5 stalks of green onions, chopped
(2 ounces blue cheese or goat cheese)

Tear lettuce and place in salad bowl. Add remaining ingredients. For a salad dressing, consider using the Walnut Oil Dressing *(p. 259)* or Citrus Vinaigrette *(p.258)*.

## NUTRITIONAL VALUE PER ⅙ OF RECIPE (DOES NOT INCLUDE CHEESE):

| Calories | Protein | Carbs | Sodium | Total Fat | Sat. Fat | Chol. |
|---|---|---|---|---|---|---|
| 98.5 | 5 gms. | 10 gms. | 70 mgs. | 4 gms. | <1 gms. | 0 mgs. |

| LA | LNA | EPA | DHA | Omega-6/Omega-3 | |
|---|---|---|---|---|---|
| 2 gms. | 0.4 gms. | 0 gms. | 0 gms. | 5 | |

# TUNA PASTA SALAD

MAKES: *4¹/₂ cups*
TIME: *30 minutes*

2 cups colorful pasta shells
1 can tuna (drained) or 1 cup fresh-cooked tuna
1 red pepper, chopped
3 T. canola oil mayonnaise
1 T. lime juice
¹/₂ cup chopped green onion

Cook the pasta in boiling water until just tender. Mix the tuna, pepper, mayonnaise, lime juice, and green onion. Toss with pasta. Serve warm or cold.

**NUTRITIONAL VALUE PER CUP:**

| Calories | Protein | Carbs | Sodium | Total Fat | Sat. Fat | Chol. |
|---|---|---|---|---|---|---|
| 205 | 11 gms. | 34 gms. | 120 mgs. | 3 gms. | 0.5 gms. | 10.3 mgs. |

| LA | LNA | EPA | DHA | Omega-6/Omega-3 |
|---|---|---|---|---|
| 1 gms. | 0.6 gms. | 0.13 gms. | 0.44 gms. | 0.85 |

# BUTTERMILK SALAD DRESSING

There's no point in buying salad dressing when you can make a healthier, better tasting dressing in a matter of minutes. This buttermilk salad dressing will store in your refrigerator for at least a week.

MAKES: *³/₄ cup*
TIME: *5 minutes*

¹/₂ cup canola or olive oil mayonnaise
¹/₄ cup buttermilk
Dried dill, to taste

        Garlic, to taste (minced or pressed through a
            garlic press)
        Salt and pepper, to taste

Combine all ingredients. Keep in the refrigerator.

*Variations:*
Eliminate the dill and add 2 tablespoons of blue cheese. Use tarragon instead of dill. For a thousand island–type dressing, eliminate dill and add 3 tablespoons of catsup. (Garlic is optional.) Eliminate the dill and add 3 tablespoons of finely grated Parmesan cheese. Eliminate the dill and add 2 teaspoons of mustard and 1 teaspoon of warm honey.

## NUTRITIONAL VALUE PER TABLESPOON:

| Calories | Protein | Carbs | Sodium | Total Fat | Sat. Fat | Chol. |
|----------|---------|----------|---------|-----------|----------|----------|
| 15.4 | 0.2 gms. | 1.5 gms. | 35 mgs. | 1.4 gms. | <1 gms. | 1.5 mgs. |

| LA | LNA | EPA | DHA | Omega-6/Omega-3 | |
|----------|----------|---------|---------|-----------------|---|
| 1 gms. | .5 gms. | 0 gms. | 0 gms. | 2 | |

# CITRUS VINAIGRETTE

MAKES: *4 servings*
TIME: *10 minutes*

¼ cup olive oil or canola oil
5 T. orange juice (fresh or made from concen-
    trate)
2 T. rice wine or other vinegar
1 t. prepared Dijon mustard
1 t. dried or 1 T. fresh tarragon
½ t. paprika
1 clove garlic, minced or pressed through a
    garlic press
¼ t. salt
Pepper to taste

Combine all ingredients with a whisk or in a blender. Try on a green salad garnished with orange slices and walnuts.

## NUTRITIONAL VALUE PER ¼ TOTAL RECIPE (APPROXIMATELY 2½ TABLESPOONS):

| Calories | Protein | Carbs | Sodium | Total Fat | Sat. Fat | Chol. |
|----------|---------|-------|--------|-----------|----------|-------|
| 132 | <1 gms. | 3 gms. | 146 mgs. | 13.7 gms. | 1.9 gms. | 0 mgs. |

| LA | LNA | EPA | DHA | Omega-6/Omega-3 | |
|----|-----|-----|-----|-----------------|--|
| 1.25 gms. | 0.07 gms. | 0 gms. | 0 gms. | 16 | |

°Use canola oil or a combination of canola oil and olive oil to lower the omega-6 to omega-3 ratio.

# WALNUT OIL DRESSING

Walnut oil is available in health food stores (or the health food section of your supermarket) and specialty stores. It has a delicate, slightly nutty flavor that is wonderful for salad dressing or for sprinkling on steamed vegetables. Like canola oil, walnut oil is rich in omega-3 fatty acids.

MAKES: $1/2$ cup
TIME: 5 minutes

$1/3$ cup walnut oil
2 T. rice wine or other vinegar
$1/2$ t. dried tarragon or 1 T. fresh
$1/2$ t. prepared mustard
Salt and pepper to taste

Blend all ingredients. Store extra dressing in the refrigerator.

**NUTRITIONAL VALUE PER TABLESPOON:**

| Calories | Protein | Carbs | Sodium | Total Fat | Sat. Fat | Chol. |
|---|---|---|---|---|---|---|
| 83 | 0 gms. | 0 gms. | 4.3 mgs. | 9 gms. | <1 gms. | 0 mgs. |

| LA | LNA | EPA | DHA | Omega-6/Omega-3 |
|---|---|---|---|---|
| 4.6 gms. | 1.3 gms. | 0 gms. | 0 gms. | 3.5 |

# Soups

## BEAN SOUP

MAKES: *10 cups*

TIME: *20 minutes to prepare, 3+ hours to cook*

1 pound mixed beans, soaked overnight, rinsed
   and drained (or use canned beans)
6 cups beef or vegetable broth
2 carrots, peeled and chopped
1 medium onion, chopped
1 T. olive oil
1 large can (28 ounces) whole tomatoes
2 cloves garlic, minced or pressed through a
   garlic press
½ t. thyme
½ bay leaf
¼ t. hot red pepper flakes
Salt and pepper to taste

Dice carrots and onions and sauté in the olive oil in a soup pot on medium high until slightly brown and caramelized (about ten minutes). Add beans, tomatoes, broth, and seasonings. Simmer for three hours or more. (Two hours if using canned beans.)

**NUTRITIONAL VALUE PER CUP:**

| Calories | Protein | Carbs | Sodium | Total Fat | Sat. Fat | Chol. |
|---|---|---|---|---|---|---|
| 100 | 6.2 gms. | 15 gms. | 607 mgs. | 2 gms. | <1 gms. | 0.4 mgs. |
| LA | | LNA | EPA | DHA | Omega-6/Omega-3 | |
| 0.3 gms. | | 0.34 gms. | 0 gms. | 0 gms. | 0.9 | |

# BEET AND CABBAGE SOUP

MAKES: *8 cups*
TIME: *15 minutes of prep, 30–45 minutes to cook*

2 T. canola oil or olive oil
$\frac{1}{2}$ red onion
$\frac{2}{3}$ of a small head of cabbage, chopped (about 5
    cups)
$\frac{1}{2}$ t. freshly ground pepper
$\frac{1}{2}$ t. dry mustard
1 T. chopped fresh dill or 1 t. dried dillweed
3 cans beef broth or $5\frac{1}{2}$ cups homemade beef
    stock (use low-salt beef broth if you are con-
    cerned about sodium intake)
2, $14\frac{1}{2}$-oz. cans diced beets and their juice (or
    use fresh-cooked)
1 T. Worcestershire sauce
Low-fat plain yogurt to garnish

Sauté red onion in the oil until soft. Add remaining ingredients to
soup pot and simmer for 45 minutes. Serve with a few tablespoons
of yogurt in each soup bowl. If desired, sprinkle with dill.

**NUTRITIONAL VALUE PER CUP:**

| Calories | Protein | Carbs | Sodium | Total Fat | Sat. Fat | Chol. |
|----------|---------|-------|--------|-----------|----------|-------|
| 78 | 4.5 gms. | 10 gms. | 882 mgs. | 4 gms. | <1 gms. | 0.4 mgs. |
| LA | LNA | EPA | DHA | | Omega-6/Omega-3 | |
| 0.6 gms. | 0.3 gms. | 0 gms. | 0 gms. | | 2 | |

# HOT AND SOUR SOUP

Tofu (soy bean curd) is a good source of LNA. It also contains genistein, a cancer-fighting phytochemical. This soup is delicious and very low in calories.

MAKES: *8 cups*
TIME: *40 minutes*

3, 14½-ounce cans beef broth (or six cups
   homemade stock)
10 fresh or dried shiitake mushrooms, coarsely
   chopped (if using dried mushrooms, soak them
   in warm water for 10 minutes before adding)
½ cup bamboo shoots, sliced
½ cup water chestnuts, sliced
1 t. fresh ginger, minced
4 oz. firm tofu cut into small squares
1 T. soy sauce
2 T. rice wine vinegar
2 ounce bean thread noodles
½ pound rinsed and coarsely chopped spinach
   or mustard greens
½ t. chili oil (or to taste)
1 t. sesame oil

Bring broth to boil in a large saucepan. Add mushrooms, bamboo shoots, water chestnuts, and ginger. Simmer 10 minutes. Add tofu, soy, rice wine vinegar, noodles, and greens. Bring to serving temperature. Remove from heat and stir in the oils.

## NUTRITIONAL VALUE PER 2 CUPS:

| Calories | Protein | Carbs | Sodium | Total Fat | Sat. Fat | Chol. |
|---|---|---|---|---|---|---|
| 107 | 11 gms. | 16 gms. | 1551 mgs. | 8 gms. | 1.2 gms. | 0.9 mgs. |

| LA | LNA | EPA | DHA | Omega-6/Omega-3 |
|---|---|---|---|---|
| 0.1 gms. | 0.2 gms. | 0 gms. | 0 gms. | 0.5 |

# SPLIT PEA SOUP

Instead of soaking the peas overnight, you can boil them for 2 minutes in 6 cups of water and then soak for 2 hours. For some reason, split pea soup is notorious for sticking to the bottom of the pot and scorching. You'll need to hover during the last hour of cooking.

MAKES: *5¹/₂ cups*
TIME: *10–15 minutes of preparation.*
*Soak overnight; cook for 2 or more hours.*

2 cups split peas, soaked overnight and drained
2 T. canola or olive oil
2 medium carrots, diced
1 medium onion, diced
¹/₂ t. salt or to taste
Pepper to taste
¹/₄ t. dried thyme
1 T. Worcestershire sauce
1–2 cloves garlic, minced or pressed through a
    garlic press
1 quart chicken broth
(²/₃ cup evaporated skim milk)
(1 cup smoked salmon, flaked into ¹/₂-inch
    pieces)

Sauté the onions and carrots in the oil until the onions are caramelized. Combine all ingredients except for the milk and salmon in a soup pot, cover, and simmer on low for two or more hours. For a creamy texture, press through a sieve or food mill. (A blender will make the soup too frothy.) The optional milk and smoked salmon can be added ten minutes before serving.

**NUTRITIONAL VALUE PER CUP:**

| Calories | Protein | Carbs | Sodium | Total Fat | Sat. Fat | Chol. |
|----------|---------|-------|--------|-----------|----------|-------|
| 248 | 20 gms. | 24 gms. | 1156 mgs. | 8.2 gms. | 1.4 gms. | 11.4 mgs. |

| LA | | LNA | | EPA | DHA | Omega-6/Omega-3 | |
|----|--|-----|--|-----|-----|-----------------|--|
| 0.6 gms. | | 0.6 gms. | | NA | NA | 1 | |

# Vegetables and Vegetable Entrées

## BLACK BEAN OR BEEF QUESADILLAS

You can add many different kinds of vegetables to these quesadillas, including green and red peppers, mushrooms, or celery. This is a good excuse to clean out the vegetable drawer.

If you're going to use beef and you're short of time, use deli meat (preferably nitrate-free).

This recipe introduces a novel way to "fry" tortillas. You're going to brush or spritz them with a slight amount of water; place then in a heated, lightly oiled pan; and cook until brown. You will get a crisp, but not greasy, quesadilla.

*Makes: 4 servings*
*Time: 20 minutes*

1½ T. canola or olive oil
1 small onion, chopped
1 carrot, thinly sliced or grated
½ cup chopped or grated purple or green cabbage
2 cups chopped spinach leaves (rinse first and
 remove stems)
3 T. fresh cilantro or parsley
1 15-ounce can black beans (canned or home-
 cooked)

(½ pound of lean beef, cut into strips)
Salt to taste
½ t. cumin
½ t. chili powder
4 tortillas (whole wheat or white)
4 T. grated cheese (such as jack, feta, moz-
    zarella, or Parmesan)
Optional toppings: yogurt, salsa, and/or avocados

Sauté onion, carrot, (beef), and purple cabbage in oil for 3–5 minutes. Add spinach, cilantro, or parsley, beans or beef, and seasonings. Cook until the spinach is wilted. Keep warm. Heat 1 teaspoon of canola oil in a frying pan over medium high. (Don't let the oil smoke.) Spritz or brush a tortilla on both sides with a small amount of water. Place in the pan and cook until lightly browned. The tortilla should be crisp. (If you wish, you can steam the tortilla or fry in a small amount of oil.) Spoon in the still warm filling and double over. Sprinkle each tortilla with 1 tablespoon cheese. Top with yogurt and salsa if desired.

## NUTRITIONAL VALUE FOR EACH SERVING:

### Vegetarian

| Calories | Protein | Carbs | Sodium | Total Fat | Sat. Fat | Chol. |
|----------|---------|-------|--------|-----------|----------|-------|
| 105 | 5 gms. | 12 gms. | 53 mgs. | 4.3 gms. | 2 gms. | 7.4 mgs. |

| LA | LNA | EPA | DHA | Omega-6/Omega-3 |
|----|-----|-----|-----|-----------------|
| 1 gms. | 0.5 gms. | 0 gms. | 0 gms. | 2 |

### Beef

| Calories | Protein | Carbs | Sodium | Total Fat | Sat. Fat | Chol. |
|----------|---------|-------|--------|-----------|----------|-------|
| 152 | 19 gms. | 3 gms. | 50 mgs. | 7 gms. | 3 gms. | 53 mgs. |

| LA | LNA | EPA | DHA | Omega-6/Omega-3 |
|----|-----|-----|-----|-----------------|
| 1.3 gms. | 0.7 gms. | 0 gms. | 0 gms. | 1.8 |

# BLACK BEAN SALSA

Homemade salsa is far superior to store-bought salsa, especially if you use ripe, flavorful tomatoes. It's easy to make, but it does take a fair amount of chopping.

MAKES: *3 cups*
TIME: *15–20 minutes*

2 fresh, ripe tomatoes
1/4–1/2 cup chopped cilantro (or parsley if you
   don't like cilantro)
1/3 cup finely diced white onion
1/2 to 2 serrano chili peppers, depending on your
   taste for hot
Juice of two limes (use fresh limes)
1/2 t. salt or to taste
1, 15-ounce can of black beans, drained and
   rinsed (or use home-cooked)

Dice the tomatoes and place in a medium bowl. Chop the cilantro or parsley, dice the onion, and add to the tomatoes. Cut open the chilies, remove *all* the seeds, and dice *very* finely. Add diced chilies, salt, beans, and lime juice. Cover and refrigerate for 30 minutes or more to let the vegetables marinate. If desired, pour off some of the accumulated liquid.

## NUTRITIONAL VALUE PER 2 TABLESPOONS:

| Calories | Protein | Carbs | Sodium | Total Fat | Sat. Fat | Chol. |
|----------|---------|-------|--------|-----------|----------|-------|
| 29 | 1.8 gms. | 6 gms. | 46 mgs. | .14 gms. | .03 gms. | 0 mgs. |

| LA | LNA | EPA | DHA | Omega-6/Omega-3 | |
|----|-----|-----|-----|-----------------|---|
| 0 gms. | 0 gms. | 0 gms. | 0 gms. | | |

# BRUSSELS SPROUTS
# WITH WALNUT OIL AND LEMON

MAKES: *2 servings*
TIME: *15 minutes*

2 cups brussels sprouts
1 T. walnut oil
1 t. lemon
2 T. chopped walnuts
Salt and pepper to taste

Steam the brussels sprouts for about ten minutes (be careful not to overcook). Toss them in the oil and lemon. Sprinkle with walnuts and serve.

## NUTRITIONAL VALUE PER CUP:

| Calories | Protein | Carbs | Sodium | Total Fat | Sat. Fat | Chol. |
|---|---|---|---|---|---|---|
| 168 | 6 gms. | 14.7 gms. | 34 mgs. | 12 gms. | 1.4 gms. | 0 mgs. |

| LA | LNA | EPA | DHA | Omega-6/Omega-3 |
|---|---|---|---|---|
| 6 gms. | 1.5 gms. | 0 gms. | 0 gms. | 4 |

# CHARD WITH NUTS AND RAISINS

MAKES: *4 servings*
TIME: *10–15 minutes*

12 ounces red or green Swiss chard (1 large
    bunch)
2 T. olive oil or canola oil
¼ cup walnuts, chopped
¼ cup raisins or currants
1–2 cloves garlic, minced or pressed through a
    garlic press
Juice from ½ lemon
Salt and pepper to taste

Wash the chard carefully and chop into 2-inch pieces. Steam until
almost tender. Meanwhile, heat the oil in a large frying pan and add
the raisins and walnuts. Sauté until the walnuts are lightly toasted.
Add the garlic and chard. Toss briefly. Season with salt, pepper,
lemon, and serve.

## NUTRITIONAL VALUE OF ¼ TOTAL RECIPE:

| Calories | Protein | Carbs | Sodium | Total Fat | Sat. Fat | Chol. |
|---|---|---|---|---|---|---|
| 142 | 3 gms. | 12 gms. | 182 mgs. | 11 gms. | 1 gms. | 0 mgs. |

| LA | LNA | EPA | DHA | Omega-6/Omega-3 | |
|---|---|---|---|---|---|
| 3 gms. | 0.4 gms. | 0 gms. | 0 gms. | 7.5* | |

*Use canola oil or a combination of olive oil and canola oil to lower the ratio. This
ratio is based on olive oil.

# GRILLED VEGETABLE SANDWICH

MAKES: *1 sandwich*
TIME: *10 minutes*

2 slices sourdough or whole-grain bread
2 t. olive oil
Salt and pepper to taste
$\frac{1}{4}$ red or yellow onion, sliced
$\frac{1}{2}$ red pepper, sliced
3–4 slices of fresh tomato
1 ounce cheese, such as mozzarella, jack, or
    Swiss

Coat the vegetables with the seasoned olive oil and grill (or broil or sauté) until tender. Place the cooked vegetables on the bottom slice of bread, top with cheese, and melt under the broiler. Add top slice, or for fewer calories, go topless.

Note: This sandwich is higher in calories than one would think.

**NUTRITIONAL VALUE OF ONE SANDWICH WITH TWO SLICES OF BREAD:**

| Calories | Protein | Carbs | Sodium | Total Fat | Sat. Fat | Chol. |
|---|---|---|---|---|---|---|
| 350 | 13.2 gms. | 31 gms. | 501 mgs. | 21 gms. | 7.5 gms. | 30 mgs. |

| LA | LNA | | EPA | DHA | Omega-6/Omega-3 | |
|---|---|---|---|---|---|---|
| 2.73 gms. | .246 gms. | | 0 gms. | 0 gms. | 11* | |

*Use canola oil or a combination of olive oil and canola oil to lower the ratio.

# HUMMUS

MAKES *1¹/₂ cups*
TIME: *10 minutes*

1 large can (15-ounce) garbanzo beans (chick
    peas or ceci beans)
1–3 cloves garlic, finely minced or pressed
    through a garlic press
2 T. lemon
¹/₂ cup low-fat yogurt
3 T. olive oil
¹/₄ t. salt
(1/8 t. cayenne)
(1 T. tahini) You will find tahini (ground sesame
    seeds) in the ethnic section of your supermar-
    ket, specialty store, or natural foods store. You
    can make humus without tahini if desired.

Mix all ingredients in a food processor or blender until uniform.
Serve with vegetables, fresh bread, crackers, or bread sticks.

## NUTRITIONAL VALUE OF TWO TABLESPOONS:

*Use canola oil or a combination of olive oil and canola oil to lower the ratio.

| Calories | Protein | Carbs | Sodium | Total Fat | Sat. Fat | Chol. |
|----------|---------|-------|--------|-----------|----------|-------|
| 99 | 3 gms. | 8.1 gms. | 193 mgs. | 6.4 gms. | .99 gms. | <1 mgs. |

| LA | LNA | EPA | DHA | Omega-6/Omega-3 |
|----|-----|-----|-----|-----------------|
| 1.9 gms. | 0.1 gms. | 0 gms. | 0 gms. | 19* |

# KALE WITH LEMON

MAKES: *4 servings*
TIME: *15 minutes*

½ pound kale
2 T. olive oil
½ lemon
(1 clove garlic)

Wash, dry, and chop the kale. Remove large pieces of stem. Sauté in the oil 5 minutes or more or until tender. (Add garlic if desired.) Put into serving dish and drizzle with lemon juice.

## NUTRITIONAL VALUE PER ¼ CUP COOKED:

| Calories | Protein | Carbs | Sodium | Total Fat | Sat. Fat | Chol. |
|----------|---------|-------|--------|-----------|----------|-------|
| 77 | 1 gms. | 4 gms. | 13 mgs. | 7 gms. | 1 gms. | 0 mgs. |

| LA | LNA | EPA | DHA | Omega-6/Omega-3 |
|----|-----|-----|-----|-----------------|
| .62 gms. | 0.3 gms. | 0 gms. | 0 gms. | 17* |

*To lower the omega-6 to omega-3 ratio, use canola oil or a combination of olive oil and canola oil.

# WALNUT PESTO

As you enjoy this pesto, tell yourself that it's just what the doctor ordered.

Ordinary pesto contains a number of healthy ingredients. Basil, the main ingredient, is rich in antioxidants and other phytochemicals. Garlic is also packed with phytochemicals. Olive oil, as you know, is a heart-healthy, cancer-fighting oil. This recipe is even healthier than the customary ones, however, because the traditional pine nuts have been replaced with walnuts, greatly increasing the LNA content.

MAKES: *4–6 servings, depending on appetites*
TIME: *10 minutes*

2 cups packed basil leaves (about 2 ounces),
   rinsed and stripped from the stems
⅓ cup olive oil
½ cup finely chopped walnuts
2 cloves of garlic, minced or pressed through a
   garlic press
½ t. salt
½ cup freshly grated Parmesan
(2 T. softened butter)

Place the basil, olive oil, walnuts, garlic, and salt in a blender or food processor. (Or use a mortar and pestle.) Blend until thoroughly combined. (If you don't want a "crunch" to your pesto, make sure the nuts are reduced to a meal.) Add Parmesan and softened butter and blend for 5–10 additional seconds. Just before serving, add 2 tablespoons of the hot water that you used to cook the pasta. Serve with pasta or spread on toasted bread (broil briefly).

**NUTRITIONAL VALUE PER ⅙ RECIPE:**

| Calories | Protein | Carbs | Sodium | Total Fat | Sat. Fat | Chol. |
|----------|---------|-------|--------|-----------|----------|-------|
| 305 | 9.3 gms. | 15.5 gms. | 372 mgs. | 25 gms. | 6 gms. | 16 mgs. |

| LA | LNA | EPA | DHA | Omega-6/Omega-3 | |
|----|-----|-----|-----|-----------------|--|
| 7.4 gms. | 9 gms. | 0 gms. | 0 gms. | 0.8 | |

# PROVENÇAL CASSEROLE

A recent study indicated that eating a variety of different kinds of vegetables is just as important to your health as eating a generous quantity of them. This recipe gives you both variety *and* quantity. Serve with a crusty loaf of fresh bread (and olive/butter).

MAKES: *5 cups*
TIME: *15 minutes of actual preparation, 30 or so minutes to cook*

1 medium onion, thinly sliced
1 clove garlic, finely minced or pressed through
    garlic press
2 T. canola or olive oil
1 small (10–12 ounces) eggplant, peeled and cut
    into approximately 1-inch cubes
1, 14-ounce can whole tomatoes, plus their juice
2 ounce Portobello (or other) mushrooms, wiped
    clean, stemmed, and cut into slices
1 roasted red pepper, homemade or canned
1, 15-oz. can of beans (your choice), drained and
    rinsed
1 10-oz. package frozen baby lima beans
½ t. salt
Pepper to taste
½ t. dried thyme
1 t. dried basil
1 T. vinegar

Slice the onion. Place the oil in a large casserole (range-safe) or saucepan. Sauté the onion for a few minutes. Add the garlic, eggplant, and tomatoes, and cook for several more minutes, stirring. Turn the heat to low and add the mushrooms, red pepper, canned beans, salt, thyme, and vinegar. Mix well, cover, and simmer over low heat, stirring occasionally, for about 5 minutes. Add the frozen lima beans and cook until the limas are tender.

Note: If you're looking for extra work, cook your own beans, roast your own red pepper, and use fresh tomatoes.

## NUTRITIONAL VALUE PER CUP:

| Calories | Protein | Carbs | Sodium | Total Fat | Sat. Fat | Chol. |
|----------|---------|-------|--------|-----------|----------|-------|
| 230 | 10 gms. | 36 gms. | 654 mgs. | 6.4 gms. | 0.9 gms. | 0 mgs. |

| LA | LNA | EPA | DHA | Omega-6/Omega-3 |
|----|-----|-----|-----|------------------|
| 0.9 gms. | 0.5 gms. | 0 gms. | 0 gms. | 1.8 |

# Seafood Entrées

## SALMON CILANTRO
## WITH GRILLED VEGETABLES

MAKES: *2–4 servings, depending on appetites*
TIME: *20 minutes*

1 pound salmon fillets
4 large Portobello or other mushrooms (left
    whole)
1 small eggplant, sliced in $\frac{1}{3}$-inch slices
1 red pepper, sliced

**Marinade:**
$\frac{1}{3}$ cup canola or olive oil
$\frac{1}{2}$ cup chicken broth

¼ cup lemon or lime juice (fresh)
¼ cup fresh cilantro, chopped
1–3 cloves garlic, minced or pressed through a
    garlic press
½ t. paprika
1 t. ground cumin
(¼ t. cayenne)
Salt and pepper to taste

Mix together marinade. Marinate salmon, mushrooms, eggplant, and pepper in large bowl for 1 hour or more. Barbecue, broil, or grill. (Each type of food takes a slightly different amount of time to cook, so watch closely.)

To broil, barbecue, or grill the salmon, start with skin side facing the heat source. Turn once. Total cooking time will be approximately 8–10 minutes per inch of thickness.

**NUTRITIONAL VALUE FOR 4-OUNCE PIECE OF SALMON PLUS GRILLED VEGETABLES:**

| Calories | Protein | Carbs | Sodium | Total Fat | Sat. Fat | Chol. |
|---|---|---|---|---|---|---|
| 402 | 33 gms. | 7 gms. | 169 mgs. | 27 gms. | 4.2 gms. | 56 mgs. |

| LA | LNA | EPA | DHA | Omega-6/Omega-3 | |
|---|---|---|---|---|---|
| 1.7 gms. | 0.8 gms. | 0.5 gms. | 1 gms. | 0.7 | |

# TROUT SIMMERED IN WHITE WINE SAUCE

MAKES: *2 trout*

TIME: *30 minutes*

2 trout
2 T. olive or canola oil
⅓ cup minced shallots or onions
⅔ cup minced carrots
⅔ cup chopped chanterelles (or other fresh
　　mushrooms)
1 cup vermouth or white wine
1 T. fresh thyme (½ t. dried)
3 T. fresh parsley

Cook the shallots, carrots, and mushrooms in heated oil until the shallots are soft. Add wine and seasonings. Simmer for several minutes. Add trout and cook about 6 minutes on each side. (Reduce cooking time if the trout are filleted.)

## NUTRITIONAL VALUE PER TROUT:

| Calories | Protein | Carbs | Sodium | Total Fat | Sat. Fat | Chol. |
|----------|---------|-------|--------|-----------|----------|-------|
| 413 | 25 gms. | 7 gms. | 163 mgs. | 25 gms. | 2 gms. | 0 mgs. |

| LA | LNA | EPA | DHA | Omega-6/Omega-3 | |
|----|-----|-----|-----|-----------------|--|
| 1.4 gms. | 0.3 gms. | 0.25 gms. | 1 gms. | 0.9 | |

# TROUT WITH WINE AND FINE HERBS

A friend said of this recipe: "It's the first time I've liked fish without tartar sauce."

MAKES: *2 fillet*
TIME: *20 minutes*

2 trout fillets
2 T. canola or olive oil or a butter/canola or butter/olive oil blend
4 T. dry white wine or vermouth
¼ cup fresh herbs (parsley, tarragon, chives, basil, dill, or thyme, etc.)
1 clove minced or pressed garlic
Salt and pepper

Dry fish. Coat liberally with the fresh herbs. Sauté trout briefly in the oil. Add white wine and garlic and poach until trout is just cooked. Salt and pepper to taste.

**NUTRITIONAL VALUE FOR 1 FILLET:**

| Calories | Protein | Carbs | Sodium | Total Fat | Sat. Fat | Chol. |
|---|---|---|---|---|---|---|
| 273 | 23 gms. | 1.3 gms. | 51 mgs. | 17 gms. | 2.6 gms. | 62 mgs. |

| LA | LNA | EPA | DHA | Omega-6/Omega-3 |
|---|---|---|---|---|
| 2 gms. | 0.7 gms. | 0.3 gms. | 1 gms. | 1 |

# TUNA MARINATED IN DILL

MAKES: *4, 6-ounce servings*
TIME: *20 minutes, plus 6 hours to marinate*

1½ lb. fresh tuna (not canned)

**Marinade:**
3 T. fresh dill, chopped
1 T. chopped parsley
Juice of 1 lemon
1 T. olive oil
1 t. sugar
Salt and pepper to taste

Slice the tuna into 1/2-inch-thick steaks. Marinate for 6 hours. Sauté the tuna in olive oil for 10–12 minutes or until done.

**NUTRITIONAL VALUE PER 6-OUNCE SERVING:**

| Calories | Protein | Carbs | Sodium | Total Fat | Sat. Fat | Chol. |
|----------|---------|-------|--------|-----------|----------|-------|
| 287 | 40 gms. | 4 gms. | 66 mgs. | 11 gms. | 1.8 gms. | 76 mgs. |

| LA | LNA | EPA | DHA | Omega-6/Omega-3 |
|----|-----|-----|-----|------------------|
| .7 gms. | .3 gms. | 0.45 gms. | 1.5 gms. | 0.3 |

# TUNA WITH SUN-DRIED TOMATOES

MAKES: *4, 6-ounce servings*
TIME: *20 minutes of prep, one additional hour to marinate*

1½ pounds fresh tuna (do not use canned)

**Marinade:**
Juice of 1 lime
1 clove garlic, minced or pressed through garlic
    press
1 t. prepared mustard
Ground pepper
½ cup chicken broth
2 T. olive oil

**Filling:**
½ cup sun-dried tomatoes (packed in olive oil,
    with their oil)
2 cloves garlic, minced or pressed through garlic
    press
½ cup chopped Italian parsley, spinach, or cilantro
(2 T. capers)
Salt to taste

Mix together the marinade ingredients and marinate tuna for 1 hour or more.

Make pockets in the tuna by making horizontal slits. (Do not cut all the way through.) Stuff with the filling. Broil approximately 5 minutes on each side, or until done. (Dispense with the pockets if you wish and simply spoon the filling on top of the steaks about two minutes before the fish is done.)

For variety, serve with a white sauce.

**NUTRITIONAL VALUE PER 6-OUNCE SERVING:**

| Calories | Protein | Carbs | Sodium | Total Fat | Sat. Fat | Chol. |
|----------|---------|-------|--------|-----------|----------|-------|
| 270 | 41 gms. | 5.2 gms. | 229 mgs. | 9 gms. | 1.5 gms. | 76 mgs. |

| LA | | LNA | | EPA | DHA | Omega-6/Omega-3 | |
|----|----|----|----|----|----|----|----|
| 0.45 gms. | | 0.3 gms. | | 0.45 gms. | 1.5 gms. | 0.2 | |

# THAI STIR FRY

MAKES: *5 cups*
TIME: *20 minutes*

2 T. canola oil
1 large onion, sliced into ¼-inch-wide half rings
1–3 cloves garlic, minced
1 t. minced ginger
1 red pepper, cut in half lengthwise and sliced
　　into ¼-inch-wide half rings
1 green pepper, cut in half lengthwise and sliced
　　into ¼-inch-wide half rings
1 T. sugar
Salt to taste
A sprinkle to ½ t. cayenne pepper (you be the
　　judge)
1 pound shrimp (shelled) or squid tubes, sliced
　　open and then chopped into ½-inch-wide
　　pieces

Add the oil to the wok or frying pan and heat on medium high. (Do
not let smoke.) Add the onion, garlic, ginger, and cook until onions
are soft, a few minutes. Add the peppers, sugar, salt, and cayenne
pepper and cook for another few minutes. Finally, add the shrimp or
squid and cook briefly until done. Serve over rice.

**NUTRITIONAL VALUE PER CUP (NOT INCLUDING RICE):**

| Calories | Protein | Carbs | Sodium | Total Fat | Sat. Fat | Chol. |
|---|---|---|---|---|---|---|
| 181 | 19 gms. | 9 gms. | 138 mgs. | 6 gms. | <1 gms. | 138 mgs. |

| LA | LNA | EPA | DHA | Omega-6/Omega-3 |
|---|---|---|---|---|
| 1 gms. | 0.5 gms. | 0.1 gms. | 0.1 gms. | 1.4 |

# Meat Entrées

## CHICKEN IN HELLFIRE

You may wonder—what does a sauce taste like that has two cups (that's not a misprint) of vinegar?? Delicious! As the vinegar and wine are reduced by boiling, their sharpness recedes and you are left with a bold but delightful pungency. Try it.

MAKES: *6 servings, depending on appetites*
TIME: *10 minutes of prep, 30–45 minutes to cook*

1$\frac{1}{2}$ pounds boneless skinless chicken thighs
1–2 T. canola oil or olive oil
2 cups balsamic or other red wine vinegar
$\frac{1}{2}$ cup dry white wine or vermouth
3 cloves garlic, minced or pressed through a
    garlic press
1 T. tomato paste (not sauce)
3 T. minced fresh herbs, such as tarragon, basil,
    and parsley

Sauté chicken thighs in oil. Cover and cook slowly until thoroughly cooked. Remove chicken from pan and keep warm. Skim fat off pan juices. Add vinegar, wine, garlic, and tomato paste to the pan. Reduce (boil rapidly) over high heat until the sauce has thickened. (The sauce will be reduced by about $\frac{2}{3}$.) Add herbs. Return chicken to the pan and toss in the sauce until reheated.

**NUTRITIONAL VALUE PER 4-OUNCE SERVING:**

| Calories | Protein | Carbs | Sodium | Total Fat | Sat. Fat | Chol. |
|---|---|---|---|---|---|---|
| 217 | 20 gms. | 6.6 gms. | 83 mgs. | 13 gms. | 3 gms. | 71 mgs. |
| LA | LNA | EPA | DHA | Omega-6/Omega-3 | | |
| 1.8 gms. | 0.2 gms. | 0 gms. | 0.4 gms. | 7.5 | | |

# HOISIN CHICKEN OR TOFU

MAKES: *3 servings*
TIME: *15 minutes of prep, 30–40 minutes to cook*

¾ pound boneless skinless chicken thighs or
  breasts or 10 ounces firm tofu (1% fat)
1 T. canola oil
1 T. lemon juice
¼ cup Hoisin sauce (available in Oriental section
  of most supermarkets)
½ cup chicken broth
¼ cup sliced green onions
1 t. minced fresh ginger
¼ t. cayenne or hot oil to taste
1 clove garlic, minced

Sauté chicken or tofu in oil. If using chicken, cover and cook until almost done. (Tofu will not need additional cooking.) Mix remaining ingredients in a small bowl, then pour into saucepan. Cover and cook an additional 10 minutes.

## NUTRITIONAL VALUE PER SERVING:

### Chicken

| Calories | Protein | Carbs | Sodium | Total Fat | Sat. Fat | Chol. |
|---|---|---|---|---|---|---|
| 223 | 23 gms. | 2.5 gms. | 1537 mgs. | 13 gms. | 3 gms. | 71 mgs. |

| LA | LNA | EPA | DHA | Omega-6/Omega-3 |
|---|---|---|---|---|
| 1.9 gms. | 0.4 gms. | 0 gms. | 0.3 gms. | 4.4 |

### Tofu

| Calories | Protein | Carbs | Sodium | Total Fat | Sat. Fat | Chol. |
|---|---|---|---|---|---|---|
| 90 | 9 gms. | 3 gms. | 496 mgs. | 6 gms. | <1 gms. | <1 mgs. |

| LA | LNA | EPA | DHA | Omega-6/Omega-3 |
|---|---|---|---|---|
| 0.8 gms. | 1 gms. | 0 gms. | 0.3 gms. | 0.8 |

# ORANGE CHICKEN AND RICE

MAKES: *4 servings*
TIME: *10 minutes of preparation, 60+ minutes to cook*

> 1 pound boneless, skinless chicken thighs, cut
>     into 2-inch pieces
> 1–2 T. canola or olive oil
> 1 medium onion, coarsely chopped
> 1 small can (14½ ounces) chicken broth
> 1½ cups orange juice
> 1–3 t. curry
> 2 cloves garlic, minced or pressed in a garlic
>     press
> Dash of cinnamon
> (3 T. raisins)
> ½ cup rice, white or brown
> Salt and pepper to taste

Sauté chicken and onion in the olive oil until brown. Add the broth, orange juice, and seasonings. Cover and simmer for 45 minutes. Add raisins (optional) and rice to the same pot, lower the heat, and cover. Cook until the rice is done, 25 or more additional minutes, depending on type of rice. Add water or more broth if necessary.

## NUTRITIONAL VALUE PER 4 OUNCES OF MEAT (INCLUDES RICE):

| Calories | Protein | Carbs | Sodium | Total Fat | Sat. Fat | Chol. |
|----------|---------|-------|--------|-----------|----------|-------|
| 415 | 28 gms. | 36 gms. | 432 mgs. | 18 gms. | 4 gms. | 81 mgs. |

| LA | LNA | EPA | DHA | Omega-6/Omega-3 |
|----|-----|-----|-----|-----------------|
| 1.7 gms. | 0.3 gms. | 0 gms. | 0.1 gms. | 4.2 |

# YOGURT CHICKEN

MAKES: *approximately 7 thighs*
TIME: *10 minutes prep, 1 hour to bake*

2 pounds skinless chicken thighs (weighed with
    bone in)
2 T. lemon or lime juice
1 T. olive oil or canola oil
1 cup plain low-fat yogurt
3 T. canola oil mayonnaise (low-fat, if desired)
1 T. Dijon-style mustard
1 T. Worcestershire sauce
$\frac{1}{2}$ t. dried thyme (2 t. fresh)
$\frac{1}{4}$ t. cayenne pepper (or to taste)
$\frac{1}{4}$ cup sliced green onions
($\frac{1}{4}$ cup grated Parmesan, fresh, not preshredded)

Preheat oven to 350 degrees. Blend together lemon and oil and coat chicken thighs. Place thighs in a shallow baking dish and bake for approximately 50 minutes. Remove from oven and drain off all accumulated juices. Blend remaining ingredients except Parmesan and spread over chicken. Sprinkle Parmesan on top. Return to oven and broil until the Parmesan has melted and is just beginning to brown.

## NUTRITIONAL VALUE PER 4-OUNCE SERVING (ONE LARGE THIGH WEIGHS ABOUT 4 OUNCES):

### Without Parmesan Cheese

| Calories | Protein | Carbs | Sodium | Total Fat | Sat. Fat | Chol. |
|---|---|---|---|---|---|---|
| 161 | 15 gms. | 3.5 gms. | 120 mgs. | 9 gms. | 2.2 gms. | 52 mgs. |

| LA | LNA | EPA | DHA | Omega-6/Omega-3 |
|---|---|---|---|---|
| 1.8 gms. | 0.3 gms. | 0 gms. | 0.03 gms. | 5 |

### With Parmesan Cheese

| Calories | Protein | Carbs | Sodium | Total Fat | Sat. Fat | Chol. |
|---|---|---|---|---|---|---|
| 275 | 26 gms. | 4 gms. | 585 mgs. | 17 gms. | 7 gms. | 72 mgs. |

| LA | LNA | EPA | DHA | Omega-6/Omega-3 |
|---|---|---|---|---|
| 1.9 gms. | 0.4 gms. | 0 gms. | 0.03 gms. | 4.4 |

# LAMB, PEPPER, AND APPLE CURRY

Lamb is lower in saturated fat than beef, and it also contains more omega-3 fatty acids. This Indian dish gives you the added benefit of the many phytochemicals found in the seasonings that go into curry—turmeric, cumin, garlic, and cayenne.

MAKES: *4 1/2–5 cups*
TIME: *Prep 15 minutes, cook for 2–3 hours*

1 large onion, coarsely chopped
1 1/2 pounds boneless lamb, trimmed of fat and
  cut into 1-inch cubes
1 1/2 T. canola or olive oil
1 green and 1 red pepper, cut into 1-inch pieces
2 tart apples, peeled and coarsely sliced (or 3/4 c.
  dried apples)
2 cloves garlic, minced or pressed through a
  garlic press
1–3 T. curry powder, depending on your taste
1 can (14 1/2-ounce) chicken broth
Salt and pepper to taste

Brown the lamb and onion in the oil. Add the seasonings and chicken broth, cover, and simmer on low for 2 hours or more until very tender. (Add water if needed.) Add the apples and cook for fifteen minutes. Add the peppers and cook for approximately 20–30 additional minutes, long enough for the peppers to become tender and absorb the juices, but not so long that they lose all of their bright color.

Serve with bread, rice, or bulgur.

## NUTRITIONAL VALUE PER 1 CUP:

| Calories | Protein | Carbs | Sodium | Total Fat | Sat. Fat | Chol. |
|---|---|---|---|---|---|---|
| 314 | 28 gms. | 13 gms. | 361 mgs. | 17 gms. | 5 gms. | 83 mgs. |

| LA | LNA | EPA | DHA | Omega-6/Omega-3 |
|---|---|---|---|---|
| 2.2 gms. | 0.8 gms. | 0 gms. | 0.1 gms. | 2.8 |

# PAD THAI

MAKES: *6 cups*
TIME: *40 minutes to soak noodles, 15 minutes of preparation*

> 8 ounces pad Thai (rice) noodles
> 1–2 T. canola oil
> 1 cup shrimp (shelled) or chicken
> ¼ cup catsup
> ⅓ cup white wine vinegar
> ⅓ cup fish sauce (you can substitute soy sauce
>     or oyster sauce)
> 3 T. sugar
> 2 cloves pressed or minced garlic
> ½ t. cayenne (add more if you like it *hot*)
> ⅔ cup green onions, cut into 2-inch diagonal
>     pieces
> ½ cup chopped cilantro
> ¼ pound (approximately 2 cups) fresh bean
>     sprouts
> Juice of 1–2 limes
> (3 T. chopped peanuts)

Soak noodles in warm water for 40 minutes. Drain.

Sauté shrimp or chicken in the oil until barely cooked. In a separate bowl, combine catsup, vinegar, fish sauce, sugar, garlic, and cayenne. Add sauce mixture to shrimp or chicken along with the softened noodles. Stir and cook until noodles have absorbed all the liquid. (Don't overcook or the noodles will get mushy.) Add onions, cilantro, and bean sprouts just before serving. Sprinkle with lime juice and peanuts. Serve.

**NUTRITIONAL VALUE PER 1 CUP (VALUES BELOW ARE FOR DISH MADE WITH SHRIMP):**

| Calories | Protein | Carbs | Sodium | Total Fat | Sat. Fat | Chol. |
|---|---|---|---|---|---|---|
| 365 | 15 gms. | 40 gms. | 1264 mgs. | 19 gms. | 3 gms. | 74 mgs. |

| LA | LNA | EPA | DHA | Omega-6/Omega-3 |
|---|---|---|---|---|
| 0.8 gms. | 0.4 gms. | 0.3 gms. | 0.3 gms. | 1.7 |

# PORK OR BEEF STIR FRY

MAKES: *4 servings*
TIME: *15 minutes*

8 ounces lean pork or beef, cut into thin slices or
  shreds
2 T. canola oil
4 cups mixed vegetables (frozen or fresh)
Add soy sauce or salt and pepper to taste

Sauté the pork in the canola oil. Add the vegetables and cook until tender.

**NUTRITIONAL VALUE PER 2 OUNCES PORK PLUS 1 CUP VEGETABLES:**

| Calories | Protein | Carbs | Sodium | Total Fat | Sat. Fat | Chol. |
|---|---|---|---|---|---|---|
| 366 | 19 gms. | 24 gms. | 273 mgs. | 23 gms. | 6.5 gms. | 53 mgs. |

| LA | LNA | EPA | DHA | Omega-6/Omega-3 |
|---|---|---|---|---|
| 2.3 gms. | 0.7 gms. | 0 gms. | 0 gms. | 3 |

# *Desserts*

## APPLE TORTE

MAKES: *6 servings*
TIME: *15 minutes of preparation, 35–40 minutes to bake*

1 egg or 2 egg whites
³/₄ cup sugar
¹/₂ cup white or whole-wheat pastry flour
¹/₄ t. salt
1 t. cinnamon
2 cups finely sliced apples
¹/₂ cup walnuts

Beat egg well. Slowly add sugar, beating well. Mix dry ingredients in a separate bowl and stir them into the egg mixture. Layer sliced apples and walnuts on the bottom of a lightly greased, 8-by-8-inch pan. Cover with batter. Bake at 350 degrees for 35–40 minutes.

**NUTRITIONAL VALUE FOR ¹/₆ OF THE TORTE:**

| Calories | Protein | Carbs | Sodium | Total Fat | Sat. Fat | Chol. |
|---|---|---|---|---|---|---|
| 223 | 4 gms. | 40 gms. | 129 mgs. | 6 gms. | <1 gms. | 30 mgs. |

| LA | | LNA | EPA | DHA | Omega-6/Omega-3 | |
|---|---|---|---|---|---|---|
| 3.4 gms. | | 0.6 gms. | NA | NA | 5.6 | |

# CARROT CAKE

This recipe is a delicious way to add more vegetables and omega-3 fatty acids to your diet. You get the nutritional value of the carrots plus LNA from both the canola oil and the flaxseeds.

MAKES: *8 servings*
TIME: *15–20 minutes*

3/4 cup canola oil
2 eggs, or 1 egg and 2 whites
1 cup sugar
1 1/3 cups white or whole-wheat pastry flour
    (unsifted)
1/2 t. salt
1 t. baking soda
1 T. cinnamon
1 1/2 cups grated carrots
1/2 cup ground flaxseeds (or 1/2 cup chopped
    walnuts)
1/2 cup raisins
1 t. grated orange peel or orange zest

Preheat oven to 350 degrees. Beat oil, eggs, and sugar in a mixer (or by hand) until creamy. Mix dry ingredients in a separate bowl and add to the egg mixture. Beat for an additional minute. Add remaining ingredients and stir until combined. Spoon batter into a lightly greased, 8-by-10-inch baking pan and bake for 30–40 minutes or until done. (The cake is done when you touch it lightly in the center and it springs back.)

**NUTRITIONAL VALUE PER 1/8 OF TOTAL RECIPE:**

| Calories | Protein | Carbs | Sodium | Total Fat | Sat. Fat | Chol. |
|----------|---------|-------|--------|-----------|----------|-------|
| 426 | 5 gms. | 54 gms. | 251 mgs. | 23 gms. | 2 gms. | 53 mgs. |

| LA | | LNA | | EPA | DHA | Omega-6/Omega-3 | |
|----|----|----|----|----|----|----|----|
| 4 gms. | | 3 gms. | | NA | NA | 1.3 | |

# FRUIT COMPOTE

You can make fruit compote from almost any kind of fruit. This particular recipe is convenient because it can be made with dried and frozen fruit alone—food you can have on hand at all times.

Consider making a large batch of compote and keeping leftovers in the refrigerator. Compote has a multitude of uses. For breakfast, spoon it over yogurt or cottage cheese or serve it with milk; between meals it makes an excellent snack; at dinner, compote makes a refreshing side dish for savory meat; finally, compote makes an excellent dessert. On special occasions, try serving it warm with a small scoop of vanilla ice cream. (Make sure there is more fruit than ice cream. The American tradition is to drizzle a little topping—usually very high in sugar—on a mountain of ice cream.)

MAKES: *4 servings*
TIME: *40 minutes, plus 1 hour soaking time*

> 1 cup dried prunes
> 1 cup dried figs
> 2 cups fresh or frozen raspberries or other
>   berries
> 1–3 T. sugar
> 1 t. lemon
> (2 T. brandy, triple sec, or other liqueur)

Cover dried fruit in warm water and soak for 1 hour or more. Simmer for 40 minutes or more until fruit is tender. At the last minute, add berries, sugar, and lemon and cook until heated through.

## NUTRITIONAL VALUE PER 1 CUP:

| Calories | Protein | Carbs | Sodium | Total Fat | Sat. Fat | Chol. |
|----------|---------|---------|---------|-----------|----------|--------|
| 374 | 3 gms. | 93 gms. | 7 mgs. | 0.9 gms. | <1 gms. | 0 mgs. |

| LA | LNA | EPA | DHA | Omega-6/Omega-3 |
|----|-----|-----|-----|------------------|
| 0 gms. | 0 gms. | 0 gms. | 0 gms. | |

# JO'S BROWNIES

To adapt these brownies to **The Omega Diet** guidelines, the butter was replaced with a mixture of butter and canola oil, and the sugar was reduced.

Note: Keep in mind that some people do not like nuts and others are allergic to them.

MAKES: *12 brownies*
TIME: *10 minutes to prepare, 25 minutes to bake*

2 squares (2 ounces) unsweetened baker's
   chocolate
2 T. butter
3 T. canola oil
2 eggs
³/₄ cup white sugar
¹/₂ cup white flour
¹/₄ t. salt
¹/₂ t. vanilla
(¹/₃ cup chopped walnuts)

Preheat oven to 325 degrees. Place chocolate, butter, and oil in a microwave-safe bowl. Heat in the microwave approximately 2 minutes on high or until chocolate is melted. (Or melt the chocolate in a saucepan over hot water.) Set aside.

In a separate bowl, beat the eggs with a beater as you gradually add the sugar. Stir in remaining ingredients by hand, including the melted chocolate mixture. Spoon batter into a 6-by-8-inch lightly greased pan (this is a small pan) and bake for 25 minutes or until done. (Do not overcook. The center should be slightly soft.)

Double the recipe for a large family.

## NUTRITIONAL VALUE PER $\frac{1}{12}$ OF RECIPE:

### Made with Nuts

| Calories | Protein | Carbs | Sodium | Total Fat | Sat. Fat | Chol. |
|---|---|---|---|---|---|---|
| 167 | 3 gms. | 18 gms. | 75 mgs. | 11 gms. | 3.5 gms. | 41 mgs. |

| LA | | LNA | | EPA | DHA | Omega-6/Omega-3 | |
|---|---|---|---|---|---|---|---|
| 2.6 gms. | | 3.3 gms. | | NA | NA | 0.8 | |

### Made without Nuts

| Calories | Protein | Carbs | Sodium | Total Fat | Sat. Fat | Chol. |
|---|---|---|---|---|---|---|
| 144 | 2 gms. | 18 gms. | 79 mgs. | 17 gms. | 2 gms. | 24 mgs. |

| LA | | LNA | | EPA | DHA | Omega-6/Omega-3 | |
|---|---|---|---|---|---|---|---|
| 0.7 gms. | | 0.3 gms. | | NA | NA | 2.3 | |

# LEMON APPLE TART

This lemon apple tart is adapted from a recipe that uses 100 percent butter, more sugar, and no apples. By switching from butter to a butter/canola blend, cutting back on the sugar, and adding the apples, the new recipe is lower in saturated fat and calories and has more omega-3 fatty acids. Plus, it has the added nutritional value of the apples.

But note that a small piece—2 by 3 inches—contains 253 calories. If you are following one of the weight-loss plans, you will need to hold back. Calories do count.

MAKES: *8 (2" x 3") pieces*
TIME: *10–15 minutes of preparation,*
*approximately 35–40 minutes to bake*

1 cup white or whole-wheat pastry flour
6 T. canola/butter blend (3 T. of butter and 3 T. of
    canola oil, blended together. Make in advance
    and refrigerate for 30 minutes.)
¼ cup powdered sugar (unsifted)
2 small or 1 large apple
2 eggs
1 t. grated lemon peel
2 T. lemon juice
⅔ cup granulated sugar
2 T. flour
½ t. baking powder

Preheat oven to 350 degrees. Combine the flour, canola/butter, and powdered sugar. Mix using your fingers or a fork until combined. Press into a small baking pan (approximately 10 by 7 inches) and bake for about 15 minutes or until slightly golden.

As the pastry bakes, peel the apples and then slice very thinly. Place eggs, lemon peel, lemon juice, granulated sugar, flour, and baking powder into a mixing bowl or food processor and beat until combined. (Do not overbeat.) Remove the pastry from the oven and cover with the apple slices. Pour the egg mixture over all. Reduce oven temperature to 325 and bake approximately 30 minutes more, or until done.

## NUTRITIONAL VALUE PER 2" BY 3" PIECE:

| Calories | Protein | Carbs | Sodium | Total Fat | Sat. Fat | Chol. |
|----------|---------|-------|--------|-----------|----------|-------|
| 253 | 3 gms. | 38 gms. | 70 mgs. | 10 gms. | 3 gms. | 38 mgs. |

| LA | LNA | EPA | DHA | Omega-6/Omega-3 |
|----|-----|-----|-----|------------------|
| 1 gms. | 0.5 gms. | NA | NA | 2 |

# SOUTHERN APPLE CAKE

To make this recipe more "omega-friendly," the butter was replaced with canola/butter, the sugar was reduced, and flaxmeal was substituted for some of the flour. Serve this cake for dessert, or make it the star of your Sunday brunch.

MAKES: *12 small servings*
TIME: *20 minutes of prep, 50 to 60 minutes to bake*

2/3 cup canola/butter (or 1/3 cup butter and 1/3
    cup canola oil)
1 1/2 cups white sugar
2 eggs
1/2 t. vanilla
(grated rind of one lemon or orange)
1 2/3 cup white or whole-wheat pastry flour
1/3 cup flaxmeal
2 t. baking soda (not baking powder)
1/2 t. salt
2 t. cinnamon plus 1 t. nutmeg or 1 T. pumpkin
    pie spice
3 large or 4 medium-sized apples, peeled and
    diced (5 cups)
(1/2 cup chopped walnuts)

Preheat oven to 350 degrees (325 degrees if using a glass baking pan).

Cream together the canola/butter and sugar in a large mixing bowl. Add eggs and beat again. Add all of the remaining ingredients except the diced apples and blend until combined. Stir in the diced apples (and walnuts) by hand.

Spoon into a greased 8-by-8- or 8-by-10-inch baking pan and bake 50–60 minutes or until done.

Note: To speed the preparation time, you can used dried apples instead of fresh. Simply soak them for thirty minutes or so in apple juice or orange juice.

## NUTRITIONAL VALUE PER SERVING:

### Without Walnuts

| Calories | Protein | Carbs | Sodium | Total Fat | Sat. Fat | Chol. |
|----------|---------|-------|--------|-----------|----------|-------|
| 300 | 28 gms. | 20 gms. | 381 mgs. | 13 gms. | 4 gms. | 49 mgs. |

| LA | LNA | EPA | DHA | Omega-6/Omega-3 |
|----|-----|-----|-----|-----------------|
| 1.4 gms. | 1 gms. | NA | NA | 1.4 |

### With Walnuts

| Calories | Protein | Carbs | Sodium | Total Fat | Sat. Fat | Chol. |
|----------|---------|-------|--------|-----------|----------|-------|
| 332 | 29 gms. | 20 gms. | 381 mgs. | 16 gms. | 4 gms. | 49 mgs. |

| LA | LNA | EPA | DHA | Omega-6/Omega-3 |
|----|-----|-----|-----|-----------------|
| 3 gms. | 1.5 gms. | NA | NA | 2 |

# FIFTEEN

# Shortcuts to Healthy Eating

*How to Stay on The Omega Diet
When Eating Out and on the Go*

W E AMERICANS NOW eat half of our calories away from home. We are just as likely to buy food at a restaurant, fast-food outlet, or snack vendor as we are to eat in our homes. Meanwhile, when we do eat at home, it's not unusual for dinner to be take-out food, deli pizza, or a frozen entrée heated in the microwave. Given the fact that most commercially prepared food is high in calories, salt, sugar, and bad fat, staying on **The Omega Diet** under these conditions requires knowledge and determination.

First, three general principles. (1) Virtually all the fat in commercial products is "bad" fat—it's either saturated fat, oil high in transfatty acids, or oil that is very high in omega-6 fatty acids. (2) Virtually all commercial establishments serve you far more food than you need. Since the meals are also likely to be high in salt, sugar, and fat—foods that can trigger intense food cravings—it can be difficult to hold the line. (3) Most commercially prepared food is loaded with artificial ingredients. Compare the ingredients in a recipe for homemade bread—flour, water, oil, yeast, and salt—with the ingredients found in a hamburger bun from a fast-food chain:

enriched flour (niacin, iron, thiamine mononitrate, riboflavin, and folic acid), water, sugar, vegetable shortening, salt, wheat gluten, yeast, yeast food (calcium sulfate, potassium iodate, potassium bromate, and/or ammonium sulfate), dough conditioners (polysorbate 60, calcium peroxide [oxidant], calcium salts, sulfates, phosphates, and ammonium salts), dough strengtheners (sodium and/or calcium-2 steroyllactylate or ethoxylated mono- and diglycerides), dough softeners (mono- and diglycerides, and/or protease enzyme), mold inhibitor (calcium propionate), preservative (potassium sorbate), oxidation/reduction additives (ascorbic acid, potassium/calcium phosphate).

Buyer beware.

# *What to Order*

**BREAKFAST.** If, like 25 percent of Americans, you eat breakfast away from home, you can always order juice or fresh fruit. Cooked and dry cereal are reasonable choices if you use low-fat milk. Low-fat cottage cheese or yogurt with fresh fruit is a healthy breakfast. Poached eggs and boiled eggs start your day off with protein without loading you up with calories. Watch out for omelets, however, because they tend to be mammoth affairs that cover half your plate. They're cooked in an unspecified oil and are typically top-heavy with cheese. You can request either an omelet made with egg whites, or one egg and two whites. If you want cheese, ask for a dusting of grated Parmesan, not a boatload of cheddar.

**LUNCH.** Lunch at the salad bar has become an American tradition. Choose wisely, and you can make an excellent meal. If you don't find any canola oil or olive oil dressing, order dressing on the side and use sparingly.

## HEALTHY CHOICES AT THE SALAD BAR— FROM ARUGULA TO ZUCCHINI

- Arugula (a lettucelike plant)
- Beans
- Beets
- Broccoli
- Cabbage
- Canola oil dressing
- Carrots
- Cauliflower
- Cilantro
- Feta cheese
- Hard-boiled egg
- Green, leafy lettuce
- Olive oil dressing
- Onions
- Peas
- Radishes
- Spinach
- Sunflower seeds
- Tofu
- Zucchini

Most soups are a good lunch choice, especially bean soup, borscht, bouillabaisse, cabbage soup, hot and sour soup, miso, mixed vegetable soup, onion soup, squash or pumpkin soup, and New England clam chowder. Watch out for the crackers. Unless they're fat-free, they're likely to be laced with trans-fatty acids. Bread is often the healthier choice.

Broiled or grilled fish makes an excellent lunch, especially salmon, trout, bluefish, herring, sardines, shark, swordfish, or tuna. Other kinds of fish are not as high in omega-3 fatty acids, but they are desirable nonetheless because they are low in calories and high in protein, and the little fat they *do* contain is healthy fat. Avoid deep-fat fried fish, however. Typically, the fish is pollock, cod, or flounder—fish low in omega-3s. To make matters worse, it is deep-fat fried in partially hydrogenated vegetable oil, which is rich in trans-fatty acids and omega-6 fatty acids. You get more bad fat than good fat.

If you want potatoes for lunch, skip the fries and order baked, steamed, or broiled potatoes.

**DINNER.** Much of what I've said about lunch applies to dinner as well. Order lean meat, fish, chicken, or a vegetarian entrée. Make vegetables and a salad a central part of the meal. Order the amount of food that matches your energy output, not your appetite.

Upscale American restaurants tend to offer healthier food than garden-variety ones. The portions are smaller, the vegetables are cooked with imagination and finesse, the salad is likely to be mesclun rather than anemic iceberg lettuce, olive oil salad dressings are commonplace, and a pot of olive oil may be served along with your bread. Although the portions will be smaller than those found at a restaurant chain, you can still eat far too much if you work your way through the bread and hors d'oeuvres, salad course, soup course, entrée, and dessert. Many people who sit down to an elegant, multi-course meal confess to feeling full long before the entrée arrives. Consider ordering just a soup and salad, or an entrée, or an hors d'oeuvre and salad. It's a rare experience to enjoy a great meal and not leave the restaurant feeling unpleasantly full. Some good restaurants serve "bar food," a tempting array of hors d'oeuvres, soups, salads, and à la carte entrées that are available only in the bar. If you're counting calories, consider sidestepping the main dining room.

In general, authentic ethnic restaurants offer more omega-friendly food than the Americanized versions. In an authentic Mexican restaurant, for example, you'll find healthy choices such as chicken baked in banana leaves, grilled fish, sopa marinera (seafood soup), oysters with lime juice, pescado rellano (stuffed fish), chicken with tomatillo sauce or salsa, and jicama salad. At a typical Mexican restaurant, it's burritos, enchiladas, tacos, and chimichangas, invariably accompanied by sour cream, cheese, and guacamole.

It's hard to go wrong in a Japanese restaurant because the food contains very little bad fat, and seafood dishes abound. If you don't like sushi and sashimi, you can order teriyaki or yakitori (broiled meat and seafood coated with sauce), or soup with noodles (udon).

Don't overlook vegetarian restaurants and restaurants with a natural foods orientation. Vegetables are given their due, the bread is whole-grain and freshly made, and natural ingredients are used in all the dishes. You won't have to worry about trans-fatty acids, saturated fat, MSG, BHT, BHA, or calcium-2 steroyllactylate. But be sure to ask which oils they use, because some are still using omega-6 oils rather than canola oil or olive oil.

# *Convenience Food*

Many people have such full lives that they can barely find time to eat—much less cook. For them, convenience food is a way of life. Unfortunately, it is just as "convenient" for food manufacturers to use partially hydrogenated oil in most of their products. That's the only way food can be stored for long periods of time without going bad. As you know, whenever you see the words "partially hydrogenated oil" on the label, the food will contain trans-fatty acids.

As I've mentioned earlier, you don't have to forgo convenience food in order to avoid bad fat; but you may have to do some of your shopping in a natural foods store. There you will find dozens of products made from unadulterated canola oil, including toaster waffles, cake mixes, pancake mixes, muffin mixes, pop-tarts, cereal, crackers, cookies, cakes, bread, chips, pretzels, and tortilla chips. You can also order similar products through the mail. (See page 360 for mail-order information.)

What about all the nonfat and low-fat baked goods and mixes now on the market? The good news is they do not contain any saturated fat, trans-fatty acids, or oils high in omega-6 fatty acids. The bad news is that they also don't give you any omega-3 fatty acids or monounsaturated fatty acids. Another drawback is that they are often high in sugar (or artificial sweeteners), trying to make up for the fact that they lack the flavor-enhancing properties of fat.

Buying frozen vegetables greatly cuts down on preparation time. Years ago, the only choices seemed to be corn, peas, beans, and succotash. Now ordinary supermarkets feature a dozen different "vegetable medleys." Some are quite good. Experiment until you find ones to your liking.

While you're at the freezer case, look for soy burgers. There are several varieties on the market that are quite tasty. If you keep a package in your home freezer along with a package of rolls or hamburger buns, you have the ingredients for a healthy snack, lunch, or even dinner. In some areas of the country, you will also find frozen salmon patties. Look for ones that have not been stripped of their lifesaving fat.

Bread machines are a boon to busy people. You don't have to hover over the rising dough, stay around to put the bread in the oven, or clean up a crusty mixing bowl or bread pan. It's so auto-mated, the bread can bake while you're sleeping. Having a bread machine makes it possible for even the busiest people to make their own whole-grain bread several times a week. (See the recipe for Honey Flax Bread on page 249.)

Fresh fruit is a premier "fast" food. Grab a banana, apple, pear, or a handful of grapes and you're on your way.

If you're having fish for dinner, dinner can be ready in ten min-utes. Broil or sauté the fish in a little olive oil and anoint with lemon. Tear open a package of prewashed mesclun and sprinkle with olive oil, vinegar, salt and pepper. Get out the bread and canola/butter. Dinner's ready. Dessert? Why, fresh fruit, of course.

## *Streamlining Your Shopping*

The rest of this chapter is devoted to a detailed shopping list for each of the fifty quick and easy recipes featured in the preceding chapter. (The recipes are listed in alphabetical order.) Take the lists to the store with you, and you can come home with everything you need for a fabulous meal without any preplanning.

The ingredients for each recipe are listed in two columns. The "special ingredients" column contains items you may not have on hand. As you will see, we are assuming that you will have a number of ingredients not found in all American households such as olive oil, fresh garlic, flaxseeds, flaxmeal, walnuts, canola oil mayonnaise, and canola oil. These ingredients are used frequently, so you might as well keep them stocked.

# *Shopping List*

## APPLE TORTE

TIME: *15 minutes preparation, 35–40 minutes baking*
SIZE: *6 servings*

**Special Ingredients**
2 to 4 apples
½ cup walnuts

**Pantry**
1–2 eggs
sugar
pastry flour
salt
cinnamon

## ARUGULA, WALNUT, APPLE SALAD

TIME: *20 minutes*
SIZE: *4 servings*

**Special Ingredients**
5 T. walnut oil
3 T. balsamic vinegar
2 apples
1 bunch arugula
⅓ cup chopped walnuts
2 ounces goat or other cheese
   (optional)

**Pantry**
olive oil
salt
pepper

# BANANA BREAD

TIME: *20 minutes preparation, 45 minutes baking*
SIZE: *1 loaf, 10 slices*

**Special Ingredients**
¼ cup low-fat sour cream or
 plain yogurt
1 cup mashed ripe banana
½ cup chopped walnuts

**Pantry**
canola oil
2–3 eggs
vanilla
flour
sugar
baking powder
baking soda
salt
flaxmeal

# BEAN SOUP

TIME: *20 minutes preparation, 3+ hours cooking*
SIZE: *10 cups*

**Special Ingredients**
1 pound mixed beans
6–8 cups beef or vegetable broth
2 carrots
1 large can whole tomatoes
¼ t. hot red pepper flakes
1 onion
2 garlic cloves
½ bay leaf

**Pantry**
olive oil
salt
pepper
thyme

# BEET AND BLUE CHEESE SALAD

TIME: *10 minutes*
SIZE: *2 servings*

**Special Ingredients**
1 cup canned or fresh-cooked sliced beets
1 ounce blue or Stilton cheese
2 T. chopped walnuts
bed of arugula or other lettuce, about 1 cup packed

# BEET AND CABBAGE SOUP

TIME: *15 minutes preparation, 30–45 minutes cooking*
SIZE: *8 cups*

**Special Ingredients**
$\frac{1}{2}$ red onion
1 small head cabbage
1 T. fresh dill or 1 t. dry dill
1 T. Worcestershire sauce
3 cans beef broth
2 cans diced beets and their juice
$\frac{1}{2}$ t. dry mustard
low-fat plain yogurt to garnish

**Pantry**
canola or olive oil
pepper

# BLACK BEAN SALSA

TIME: *20 minutes*
SIZE: *3 cups*

**Special Ingredients**
2 fresh tomatoes
1/4–1/2 cup cilantro or parsley
1/3 cup onion
1–2 seranno chili peppers
2 limes
1 15-oz. can black beans

**Pantry**
salt

# BLACK BEAN OR BEEF QUESADILLAS

TIME: *20 minutes*
SIZE: *4 servings*

**Special Ingredients**
1 carrot
1/2 cup chopped purple cabbage
2 cups spinach leaves
3 T. fresh cilantro or parsley
1/2 t. chili powder
4 tortillas (whole wheat or white)
4 T. cheese (such as feta, jack,
   mozzarella or Parmesan)
1 onion
1 15-oz. can black beans
1/2 t. cumin
1/2 pound of lean beef (optional)

**Pantry**
canola or olive oil
salt

# BRUSSELS SPROUTS
# WITH WALNUT OIL AND LEMON DRESSING

TIME: *15 minutes*
SIZE: *2 servings*

**Special Ingredients**
2 cups brussels sprouts, fresh or
    frozen
1 T. walnut oil
1 T. lemon juice
2 T. chopped walnuts

**Pantry**
salt
pepper

# BUTTERMILK FLAXJACKS

TIME: *10 minutes preparation, 10 minutes cooking*
SIZE: *7 5-inch pancakes*

**Special Ingredients**
1½ cups buttermilk

**Pantry**
1 egg
sugar
flour
canola oil
flaxmeal
baking soda
salt

# BUTTERMILK SALAD DRESSING

TIME: *5 minutes*
SIZE: *¾ cup*

**Special Ingredients**
½ cup canola oil mayonnaise
¼ cup buttermilk
dill
garlic

**Pantry**
salt
pepper

# CANOLA/BUTTER OR OLIVE/BUTTER

TIME: *5 minutes*
SIZE: *1 cup*

**Special Ingredients**
½ cup (1 cube) butter

**Pantry**
canola or olive oil

# CANOLA GRANOLA

TIME: *10 minutes preparation, up to 30 minutes cooking*
SIZE: *7 cups*

**Special Ingredients**
6 cups raw oats, quick-cooking or
   regular
2–4 T. honey or brown sugar
1 cup raisins or dried blueberries,
   cranberries, or papaya
1½ cups dried apples
⅓ cup chopped walnuts

**Pantry**
canola oil
flaxseed

# CANOLA OIL MAYONNAISE

TIME: *10 minutes*
SIZE: *1³/₄ cups*

**Special Ingredients**
1¹/₂ t. dried mustard
¹/₈ t. cayenne
4 T. fresh lemon juice

**Pantry**
canola oil
1 egg
sugar
salt

# CARROT CAKE

TIME: *15–20 minutes*
SIZE: *8 servings*

**Special Ingredients**
1¹/₂ cup grated carrots
1 t. orange zest
¹/₂ cup raisins

**Pantry**
canola oil
2–4 eggs
flour
cinnamon
baking soda
sugar
salt
flaxmeal

# CHARD WITH NUTS AND RAISINS

TIME: *10–15 minutes*
SIZE: *4 servings*

**Special Ingredients**
12 ounces Swiss chard
¼ cup chopped walnuts
¼ cup raisins or currants
juice of ½ lime
1–2 garlic cloves

**Pantry**
olive oil
salt
pepper

# CHICKEN IN HELLFIRE
# (POULET AU FEU D'ENFER)

TIME: *10 minutes preparation, 30–45 minutes baking*
SIZE: *6 servings*

**Special Ingredients**
1½ pounds boneless skinless
   chicken thighs
2 cups balsamic or red vinegar
½ cup dry white wine or
   vermouth
1 T. tomato paste
3 T. minced fresh herbs such as
   tarragon, basil, and parsley
3 garlic cloves

**Pantry**
canola or olive oil

# CHICKEN SALAD WITH VINAIGRETTE

TIME: *10 minutes preparation, plus cooking time for chicken*
SIZE: *2 servings*

**Special Ingredients**
6 ounces roasted skinless chicken breast, cubed or shredded (or use
   deli meat)
2 cups mixed salad greens
1 carrot
1 tomato
1/2 green or red pepper

# CITRUS VINAIGRETTE

TIME: *10 minutes*
SIZE: *4 servings*

**Special Ingredients**            **Pantry**
5 T. orange juice                  olive oil
2 T. vinegar                       salt
1 t. prepared Dijon mustard        pepper
1 t. dried tarragon or 1 T. fresh
1/2 t. paprika
1 garlic clove

# CORN BREAD

TIME: *10 minutes preparation, 20 minutes baking*
SIZE: *8 servings*

**Special Ingredients**
1 cup cornmeal

**Pantry**
1–2 eggs
canola oil
baking powder
sugar
flour
flaxmeal
nonfat milk
salt

# COTTAGE CHEESE PANCAKES

TIME: *15 minutes*
SIZE: *7–8 pancakes*

**Special Ingredients**
2/3 cup low-fat cottage cheese
1/2 cup cornmeal
1/2 t. grated orange or lemon peel
   (optional)

**Pantry**
2–3 eggs
flour
sugar
baking powder
nonfat milk
flaxmeal

# FLAXBRAN MUFFINS

TIME: *10 minutes preparation, 20 minutes cooking*
SIZE: *10 muffins*

**Special Ingredients**
1/2 cup wheat bran
2 T. molasses
orange rind, grated
2/3 cup raisins or other dried fruit

**Pantry**
canola oil
sugar
baking powder
1 egg
flaxmeal
flour
salt
low-fat milk

# FLAXMEAL

TIME: *5 minutes*
SIZE: *1³/₄ cup*

**Special Ingredients**
1 cup flaxseeds

# FRESH SAUERKRAUT SALAD

TIME: *15 minutes preparation, 12+ hours to marinate*
SIZE: *7 cups*

**Special Ingredients**
1/2 red or green cabbage
1/2 t. dry dillweed or 2 T. fresh
   dillweed
1/2 cup vinegar
1 t. prepared mustard
1 onion

**Pantry**
sugar
canola oil
salt

# FRUIT COMPOTE

TIME: *40 minutes preparation, 1 hour soaking time*
SIZE: *4 servings*

| **Special Ingredients** | **Pantry** |
|---|---|
| 1 cup dried prunes | sugar |
| 1 cup dried figs | |
| 2 cups fresh or frozen raspberries or other berries | |
| 1 t. lemon juice | |
| 2 T. brandy, triple sec, or other liqueur (optional) | |

# GRILLED VEGETABLE SANDWICH

TIME: *10 minutes*
SIZE: *1 sandwich*

| **Special Ingredients** | **Pantry** |
|---|---|
| 2 slices sourdough or whole-grain bread | olive oil |
| 1/4 red or yellow onion | salt |
| 1/2 red pepper | pepper |
| 3–4 slices tomato | |
| 1 ounce mozzarella, jack, or Swiss cheese | |

# HOISIN CHICKEN OR TOFU

TIME: *15 minutes preparation, 30–40 minutes cooking*
SIZE: *3 servings*

**Special Ingredients**
¾ pound boneless, skinless
  chicken thighs or breasts, or 10
  ounces firm tofu (1% fat)
1 T. lemon juice
¼ cup Hoisin sauce
¼ cup green onions
1 t. minced fresh ginger
½ cup chicken broth
¼ t. cayenne or hot oil
1 garlic clove

**Pantry**
canola oil

# HONEY FLAX BREAD

TIME: *5 minutes preparation with bread machine*
SIZE: *1 loaf, 14 slices*

**Special Ingredients**
3 cups whole-wheat bread flour
3 T. honey or sugar
1 T. plus 1 t. yeast

**Pantry**
canola oil
white flour
flaxmeal
salt

# HOT AND SOUR SOUP

TIME: *40 minutes*
SIZE: *8 cups*

## Special Ingredients
3 cans beef stock (or 6 cups homemade stock)
10 fresh or dried shiitake mushrooms
$\frac{1}{2}$ cup bamboo shoots
$\frac{1}{2}$ cup water chestnuts
1 t. minced fresh ginger
4 ounces firm tofu
1 T. soy sauce
2 T. rice wine vinegar
$\frac{1}{2}$ t. chili oil
1 t. sesame oil
2 ounces bean thread noodles
$\frac{1}{2}$ pound chopped spinach or mustard greens

# HUMMUS

TIME: *10 minutes*
SIZE: *1$\frac{1}{2}$ cups*

## Special Ingredients
1 15-ounce can garbanzo beans
2 T. lemon juice
$\frac{1}{2}$ cup low-fat yogurt
1 T. tahini (ground sesame seeds)
1–3 garlic cloves
$\frac{1}{8}$ t. cayenne (optional)

## Pantry
olive oil
salt

# JO'S BROWNIES

TIME: *10 minutes preparation, 25 minutes baking*
SIZE: *12 servings*

**Special Ingredients**
2 squares unsweetened bakers
  chocolate
2 T. butter
1/3 cup chopped walnuts
  (optional)

**Pantry**
canola oil
flour
sugar
vanilla
2 eggs
salt

# KALE WITH LEMON

TIME: *15 minutes*

SIZE: *4 servings*

**Pantry**
olive oil

**Special Ingredients**
1/2 pound kale
1 lemon
1 garlic clove (optional)

# LAMB, PEPPER, AND APPLE CURRY

TIME: *15 minutes preparation, 2–3 hours cooking*
SIZE: *4¹/₂–5 cups*

**Special Ingredients**
1 green pepper
1 red pepper
2 tart apples (or ³/₄ cups dried
   apples)
1–3 T. curry powder
1 can chicken broth
1 onion
1¹/₂ pounds boneless lamb,
   trimmed of fat
2 garlic cloves

**Pantry**
canola or olive oil
salt
pepper

# LEMON APPLE TART

TIME: *10 minutes preparation, 35–40 minutes baking*
SIZE: *8 pieces*

**Special Ingredients**
2 apples
1 t. lemon peel plus 2 T. juice (use
   fresh, not bottled, lemon juice)

**Pantry**
pastry flour
6 T. canola/butter blend
2 eggs
powdered sugar
granulated sugar
baking powder

# ORANGE CHICKEN AND RICE

TIME: *10 minutes preparation, 40 minutes baking*
SIZE: *4 servings*

**Special Ingredients**
1 pound skinless boneless
   chicken thighs
1 can chicken broth
1$\frac{1}{2}$ cups orange juice
1–3 t. curry powder
1 onion
2 garlic cloves
$\frac{1}{2}$ cup rice
3 T. raisins (optional)

**Pantry**
canola or olive oil
cinnamon
salt
pepper

# ORANGE WALNUT SALAD

TIME: *15 minutes*
SIZE: *6 servings*

**Special Ingredients**
6 cups mixed salad greens
2 oranges or 1 small can mandarin oranges
$\frac{1}{3}$ cup walnuts
1 cup celery
5 green onions
2 ounces blue cheese (optional)

# PAD THAI

TIME: *40 minutes to soak noodles, 15 minutes preparation*
SIZE: *6 cups*

**Special Ingredients**
8 ounces pad Thai (rice) noodles
1 cup shrimp (shelled) or chicken
1/3 cup fish sauce, soy sauce, or
   oyster sauce
2/3 cup green onion
1/2 cup cilantro
2 cups fresh bean sprouts
1/3 cup white wine vinegar
2 garlic cloves
1/2 t. cayenne
Juice of 2 limes
3 T. chopped peanuts (optional)

**Pantry**
canola oil
1/4 cup catsup
sugar

# PORK OR BEEF STIR FRY

TIME: *15 minutes*
SIZE: *4 servings*

**Special Ingredients**
8 ounces pork or beef
4 cups mixed vegetables (frozen
   or fresh)
soy sauce

**Pantry**
canola oil
salt
pepper

# PROVENÇAL CASSEROLE

TIME: *15 minutes preparation, 30 minutes baking*
SIZE: *5 cups*

**Special Ingredients**
1 small eggplant
1 14-oz. can whole tomatoes
2 ounces Portobello (or other)
   mushrooms
1 fresh or canned roasted red
   pepper
1 15-oz. can beans (your choice)
1 10-oz. package frozen baby
   lima beans
1 garlic clove
1 onion

**Pantry**
canola or olive oil
vinegar
basil
thyme
salt
pepper

# SALMON CILANTRO
# WITH GRILLED VEGETABLES

TIME: *20 minutes*
SIZE: *2–4 servings*

**Special Ingredients**
1 pound salmon filets
4 large Portobello or other
   mushrooms (left whole)
1 small eggplant
1 red pepper
$\frac{1}{2}$ cup chicken broth
$\frac{1}{4}$ cup lemon or lime juice
$\frac{1}{4}$ cup fresh cilantro
$\frac{1}{2}$ t. paprika
1 t. ground cumin
1–3 garlic cloves
cayenne (optional)

**Pantry**
olive or canola oil
salt
pepper

# SOUTHERN APPLE CAKE

TIME: *20 minutes preparation, 50–60 minutes baking*
SIZE: *12 servings*

**Special Ingredients**
grated rind of lemon or orange
3–4 apples
½ cup walnuts (optional)

**Pantry**
2 eggs
canola/butter
sugar
vanilla
flour
flaxmeal
baking soda
salt
cinnamon
nutmeg

# SPLIT PEA SOUP

TIME: *Soak overnight, 15 minutes preparation, 2+ hours cooking*
SIZE: *5½ cups*

**Special Ingredients**
2 cups split peas
2 carrots
1 quart chicken broth
1 onion
1 T. Worcestershire sauce
2 garlic cloves
⅔ cup evaporated skim milk
   (optional)
1 cup smoked salmon (optional)

**Pantry**
canola or olive oil
thyme
salt
pepper

# THAI STIR FRY

TIME: *20 minutes*
SIZE: *5 cups*

**Special Ingredients**
1 t. minced ginger
1 red pepper
1 green pepper
cayenne pepper
1 pound (shelled) shrimp or squid
   tubes
1 large onion
1–3 garlic cloves

**Pantry**
canola oil
sugar
salt

# TROUT WITH WINE AND FINE HERBS

TIME: *20 minutes*
SIZE: *2 servings*

**Special Ingredients**
2 trout fillets
4 T. dry white wine or vermouth
fresh herbs (parsley, tarragon,
   chives, basil, dill, thyme, etc.)
1 garlic clove

**Pantry**
canola or olive oil
salt
pepper

# TROUT SIMMERED IN WHITE WINE SAUCE

TIME: *30 minutes*
SIZE: *2 servings*

**Special Ingredients**
2 trout
⅓ cup minced shallots or onions
⅔ cup carrots
⅔ cup chopped chanterelles (or
   other fresh mushrooms)
1 cup vermouth or white wine
1 T. fresh thyme (½ t. dried)
3 T. fresh parsley

**Pantry**
olive or canola oil

# TUNA MARINATED IN DILL

TIME: *20 minutes preparation, 6 hours to marinate*
SIZE: *4 servings*

**Special Ingredients**
1½ pounds fresh tuna
3 T. fresh dill
1 T. chopped parsley
juice of 1 lemon

**Pantry**
olive oil
sugar
salt
pepper

# TUNA PASTA SALAD

TIME: *30 minutes*
SIZE: *4¹/₂ cups*

## Special Ingredients
2 cups colorful pasta shells
1 can tuna or 1 cup fresh cooked tuna
1 red pepper
3 T. canola oil mayonnaise
1 T. lime juice
¹/₂ cup chopped green onion

# TUNA WITH SUN-DRIED TOMATOES

TIME: *20 minutes preparation, 1 hour to marinate*
SIZE: *4 servings*

## Special Ingredients
1¹/₂ pounds fresh tuna
juice of 1 lime
1 t. prepared mustard
¹/₂ cup sun-dried tomatoes
   (packed in olive oil, with their
   oil)
¹/₂ cup fresh Italian parsley,
   spinach, or cilantro
3 garlic cloves
¹/₂ cup chicken broth
2 T. capers (optional)

## Pantry
olive oil
salt
pepper

# WALNUT OIL DRESSING

TIME: *5 minutes*
SIZE: *½ cup*

**Special Ingredients**
⅓ cup walnut oil
2 T. rice wine or other vinegar
½ t. dried tarragon or 1 T. fresh
½ t. prepared mustard

**Pantry**
salt
pepper

# WALNUT PESTO

TIME: *10 minutes*
SIZE: *4–6 servings*

**Special Ingredients**
2 cups basil leaves, packed
½ cup walnuts, chopped
2 garlic cloves
½ cup Parmesan, freshly grated
2 T. butter (optional)

**Pantry**
olive oil
salt

# YOGURT CHICKEN

TIME: *10 minutes preparation, 1 hour baking*
SIZE: *7 servings*

**Special Ingredients**
2 pounds boneless skinless
   chicken thighs
2 T. lemon or lime juice
1 cup plain nonfat yogurt
3 T. canola oil mayonnaise
1 T. Dijon mustard
1 T. Worcestershire sauce
¼ t. cayenne
¼ cup sliced green onions
¼ cup grated fresh Parmesan
   (optional)

**Pantry**
olive or canola oil
thyme

# Comments and Endnotes

*Chapter 1: Found: The Missing Ingredients for Optimal Health*

1. Simopoulos, A. P. "Omega-3 fatty acids in health and disease and in growth and development." *Am J Clin Nutr,* 1991; 54:438–63.

2. Simopoulos, A. P., R. R. Kifer, R. E. Martin, eds. *Health effects of polyunsaturated fatty acids in seafoods.* Orlando, FL: Academic Press, 1986.

3. Galli, C., A. P. Simopoulos. *Dietary w3 and w6 fatty acids. Biological effects and nutritional essentiality.* New York: Plenum Press, 1989.

4. Simopoulos, A. P., R. R. Kifer, R. E. Martin, S. M. Barlow, eds. "Health effects of w3 polyunsaturated fatty acids in seafoods." *World Rev Nutr Diet,* 1991; 66:1–592.

5. Galli, C., A. P. Simopoulos, E. Tremoli, eds. "Fatty acids and lipids: biological aspects." *World Rev Nutr Diet,* 1994; 75:1–196.

6. Galli, C., A. P. Simopoulos, E. Tremoli, eds. "Effects of fatty acids and lipids in health and disease." *World Rev Nutr Diet,* 1994; 76:1–152.

7. Salem, N., Jr., A. P. Simopoulos, C. Galli, M. Lagarde, H. R. Knapp, eds. "Fatty acids and lipids from cell biology to human disease." *Lipids,* 1996; 31 (suppl):S-1–S-326.

8. Keys, A., A. Menotti, and H. Toshima. "The diet and 15-year death rate in the seven countries study." *Amer J Epidemiology,* 1986; 124(6):903–15.

9. Simopoulos A. P., Salem, N., Jr. "Purslane: a terrestrial source of omega-3 fatty acids." *N Engl J Med,* 1986; 315:83

10. de Lorgeril, M., S. Renaud, and J. Delaye. Mediterranean alpha-linolenic acid-rich diet in secondary prevention of coronary heart disease. *The Lancet,* 1994; 343:1454–145.

11. Renaud, S., T. Paul. "Cretan Mediterranean diet for prevention of coronary heart disease." *Am J Clin Nutr,* 1995; 61 (suppl):1360S–7S.

12. de Lorgeril, M., P. Salen, and J. Delaye. "Effect of a Mediterranean type of diet on the rate of cardiovascular complications in patients with coronary artery disease." *J Amer Coll Cardiology,* 1996; 28(5):1103–8.

13. The chart has been adapted from a chart that appeared in reference 10 above. It compares the number of patients who were free from cardiac death and nonfatal heart attacks.

*Chapter 2: The Skinny on Fat*

1. Dorgan, J., et al. "Effects of dietary fat and fiber on plasma and urine androgens and estrogens in men: a controlled feeding study." *Am J Clin Nutr,* 1996; 64(6):850–855.

2. Gartner, C., W. Stahl, and H. Sies. Lycopene is more bioavailable from tomato paste than from fresh tomatoes. *Am J Clin Nutr,* 1997; 66:116–22.

3. Katahn, M. *The T-Factor Diet.* 1989, New York: Norton.

4. Golay, A. et al. Weight loss with a low or high carbohydrate diet? *Int J Obesity,* 1996; 20:1062–72.

5. A study conducted at Vanderbilt University came up with an even stronger indictment against the "faster metabolism" weight-loss theory. In this more stringent study, volunteers were placed on an ultralean, 17 percent-fat diet for four months. After this long period of self-denial, the dieters had an even *lower* metabolic rate than they had had at the beginning. A weight-loss diet that was low in fat and high in carbohydrates had actually dampened their metabolic furnaces. Schlundt, D. Randomized evaluation of a lowfat diet for weight reduction. *Int J Obesity,* 1993; 17:623–629.

6. Rouse, L. R., K. D. Hammel, and M. D. Jensen. Effects of isoenergetic, lowfat diets on energy metabolism in lean and obese women. *Amer J Clin Nutr,* 1994; 60:470–5.

7. Hudgins, L. C., M. Hellerstein, C. Seidman, and J. Hirsch. Human fatty acid synthesis is stimulated by a eucaloric low fat, high carbohydrate diet. *J Clin Invest,* 1996; 97:2081–2091.

8. Cotton, J., J. Weststrate, and J. Blundell. Replacement of dietary fat with sucrose polyester: effects on energy intake and appetite control in nonobese males. *Am J Clin Nutr,* 1996; 63(6):891.

9. Allred, J. B. Too much of a good thing? An overemphasis on eating low-fat foods may be contributing to the alarming increase in overweight among US adults. *J Amer Dietetic Assoc,* 1995; 95(4)417–18.

10. The illustration is from the above journal article. The data came from the National Health and Nutrition Examination Surveys, 1960–1991; and the third National Health and Nutrition Examination Survey, Phase 1, 1988–91.

11. Simopoulos, A. P. Characteristics of obesity: An overview. *Ann NY Acad Sci,* 1987; 499:4–13.

*Chapter 3: Why We Eat the Wrong Fats*

1. Eaton, S. B., S. B. I. Eaton, and M. Shostak. An evolutionary perspective enhances understanding of human nutritional requirements. *J. Nutrition,* 1996; 126:1732–40.

2. Simopoulos, A. P. The role of fatty acids in gene expression: Health implications. *Ann Nutr Metab,* 1996; 40:303–11.

3. Singh, J., R. Hamid, and B. S. Reddy. Dietary fat and colon cancer: modulating effect of types and amount of dietary fat on ras-p21 function during promotion

and progression stages of colon cancer. *Cancer Research,* 1997; 57:253–258.

4. Simopoulos, A. P. Omega-3 fatty acids in health and disease and in growth and development. *Am J Clin Nutr,* 1991; 54:438–63. Both omega-6 and omega-3 fatty acids instruct your genes to produce less fat, but omega-3 fatty acids are more effective.

5. Eaton, S. B. An evolutionary perspective enhances understanding of human nutritional requirements. *J. Nutr,* 1996; 126:1732–40.

6. Simopoulos, A. P., H. A. Norman, and J. E. Gillaspy. Purslane in Human Nutrition and Its Potential for World Agriculture. *World Rev Nutr: Diet, Plants in Human Nutrition,* ed. A. P. Simopoulos. Vol. 77. 1995, Basel: Karger. 47–74.

7. Simopoulos, A. P., Terrestrial Sources of Omega-3 Fatty Acids: Purslane. *Horticulture and Human Health: Contributions of Fruits and Vegetables,* ed. Quebedeaux, B., and Bliss, F. Englewood Cliffs, NJ: Prentice-Hall, 1988: 93–107.

8. Simopoulos, A. P. and N. J. Salem. Purslane: a terrestrial source of w-3 fatty acids. *N Engl J Med,* 1986; 315: 833.

9. Simopoulos, A. P., H. A. Norman, and J. A. Duke. Common Purslane: A Source of Omega-3 Fatty Acids and Antioxidants. *J Amer Coll of Nutr,* 1992; 11(4):374–82.

10. Simopoulos, A. P. and N. Salem Jr. n-3 Fatty acids in eggs from range-fed Greek chickens. *N Engl J Med,* 1989:1412.

11. Crawford, M. A. Fatty-acid ratios in free-living and domestic animals. *The Lancet,* 1968; 1:1329–33.

12. The illustration is adapted from reference 11.

13. Dolecek, T. A. and G. Grandits. Dietary polyunsaturated fatty acids and mortality in the multiple risk factor intervention trial (MRFIT). *World Rev Nutr Diet,* 1991; 66:205–16.

14. From our modern perspective, we know that having high cholesterol levels is just one of many risk factors linked with cardiovascular disease. Others are just as important, including blood levels of antioxidants, omega-3 fatty acids, and homocysteine. The fixation on lowering cholesterol obscured the importance of these and other factors for decades.

15. Rose, G. A., W. B. Thomson, and R. T. Williams. Corn oil in treatment of ischaemic heart disease. *Brit Med J,* 1965. 1:1531–33.

16. Pearce, M. L. and S. Dayton. Incidence of cancer in men on a diet high in polyunsaturated fat. *The Lancet,* 1971:464–467.

17. Pinckney, E. R. The potential toxicity of excessive polyunsaturates. *Amer Heart J,* 1973; 85(6):723–6.

18. Chow, C. K. *Fatty Acids in Foods and Their Health Implications.* 1992, New York: Marcek Dekker, Inc. 889.

19. Litin, L. and F. Sacks. Trans-fatty-acid content of common foods. *N Engl J Med,* 1996; 329(26).

20. The data are from the Economic Research Service and Human Nutrition Information Service of the U.S. Department of Agriculture and the Institute of Shortening and Edible Oils.

21. Simopoulos, A. P. The Mediterranean food guide. Greek column rather than an Egyptian pyramid. *Nutrition Today,* 1995; 30(2):54–61.

22. Given the strength of the new research about fats, there are signs that the tide is already beginning to turn. For example, a conference that I organized, held in Bethesda, Maryland, in September 1997, titled "The Return of w-3 Fatty Acids into the Food Supply: I. Land-Based Animal Food Products and Their Health Effects," brought together medical researchers and food producers from around the world to explore the feasibility of restoring omega-3 fatty acids to the food chain. One of the conclusions of the conference is that the technology is available to accomplish this goal. All that is needed to take advantage of the technology is consumer demand or enlightened government policy.

*Chapter 4: A Fatty Acid Primer*

1. Other diseases and conditions associated with a preponderance of eicosanoids coming from omega-6 fatty acids include cardiovascular disease, hypertension, diabetes, obesity, and aging.

2. Harel, Z., F. M. Biro, and S. L. Rosenthal. Supplementation with omega-3 polyunsaturated fatty acids in the management of dysmenorrhea in adolescents. *Am J Obstet Gynecol,* 1996; 174(4):1335–8.

*Chapter 5: The Genesis of a Heart Attack*

1. Browner, W. S., J. Westenhouse, and J. A. Tice. What if Americans ate less fat? *J Amer Med Assoc,* 1991; 265(24):3285–91.

2. "Research Group Hails Folic Acid as a Preventer of Heart Disease," in *New York Times*. 1995, p. A11.

3. Olszewski, A. J. Fish oil decreases homocysteine in hyperlipemic men. *Coron Artery Dis,* 1993; 4:53–60.

4. We learned this fact in the 1950s, when army physicians performed autopsies on 300 young servicemen who had been killed during the Korean War. Even though the men had been fit, healthy, and in their late teens or early twenties, most of their arteries had shown significant amounts of abrasion. The researchers believed that normal wear and tear was partly to blame because they had located the most extensive damage just above the branch in an artery, a place where blood can swirl and eddy. Enos, M. W. F., L. C. R. H. Holmes, and C. J. Beyer. Coronary disease among United States soldiers killed in action in Korea. *J Amer Med Assoc,* 1953; 152(12):1090–3.

5. Howe, P. R. C. Fish oil supplements and hypertension. *ISSFAL Newsletter,* 1996; 3(4):2–5.

6. Berry, M. E., and J. Hirsch. Does dietary linolenic acid influence blood pressure? *Amer J Clin Nutr,* 1986; 44:336–340.

7. Ruiz-Gutierrez, V., F. J. G. Muriana, A. Guerrero, and J. Villar. Plasma lipids, erythrocyte membrane lipids and blood pressure of hypertensive women after ingestion of dietary oleic acid from two different sources. *J Hypertension,* 1996; 14:1483–1490.

8. Harris, W. S., G. S. Rambjor, S. L. Windsor, and D. Diederich. n–3 Fatty acids and urinary excretion of nitric oxide metabolites in humans. *Amer J of Clin Nutr,* 1997; 65:459–64.

9. Ridker, P. M., et al. Inflammation, aspirin, and the risk of cardiovascular disease in apparently healthy men. *N Engl J Med,* 1997; 336(14):973–9.

10. Fisher, M., K. S. Upchurch, and J. J. Hoogasian. Effects of dietary fish oil supplementation on polymorphonuclear leukocyte inflammatory potential. *Inflammation,* 1986; 10(4):387–92.

11. Daviglus, M. L. Fish consumption and the 30-year risk of myocardial infarction. *N Engl J Med,* 1977; 336:1046–53.

12. Reaven, P., S. Parthasarathy, and J. L. Witztum. Effects of oleate-rich and linoleate-rich diets on the susceptibility of low density lipoprotein to oxidative modification in mildly hypercholesterolemic subjects. *J Clin Invest,* 1993; 91:668–76.

13. Kushi, L. H., A. R. Folsom, R. J. Prineas, and R. M. Bostick. Dietary antioxidant vitamins and death from coronary heart disease in postmenopausal women. *N Engl J Med,* 1996; 334:1156–62.

14. Miller, M. and R. A. Vogel. *The Practice of Coronary Disease Prevention.* 1996, Baltimore: Williams & Wilkins. 293.

15. Chan, P., B. Tomlinson, and Y.-S. Lee. Effectiveness and safety of low-dose pravastatin and squalene, alone and in combination, in elderly patients with hypercholesterolemia. *J Clin Pharacology,* 1996; 36:422–7.

16. Grundy, S. M. Monounsaturated fatty acids and cholesterol metabolism: Implications for dietary recommendations. *Amer Inst Nutr,* 1989:529–532.

17. Ascherio, A., C. H. Hennekens, and W. C. Willett. Trans-fatty acid intake and risk of myocardial infarction. *Circulation,* 1994; 89(1):94–101.

18. Schaefer, E. J., A. H. Lichtenstein, and J. M. Ordovas. Body weight and low-density lipoprotein cholesterol changes after consumption of a low-fat ad libitum diet. *J Amer Med Assoc,* 1995; 274(18):1450–5.

19. Dyerberg, J., H. O. Bang, and O. Aagaard. "Small is beautiful": alpha linolenic acid and eicosapentaenoic acid in man. *The Lancet,* May 21, 1983; 1169.

20. Radack, K., C. Deck, and G. Huster. Dietary supplementation with low-dose fish oils lowers fibrinogen levels: a randomized, double-blind controlled study. *Ann Int Med,* 1989; 11(9):757–58.

21. Leaf, A., G. E. Billman, and H. Hallaq. Prevention of ischemia-induced ventricular fibrillation by omega–3 fatty acids. *Proc National Acad Sci,* 1994; 91:4427–30.

22. Burr, M. L., J. F. Gilbert, and N. M. Deadman. Effects of changes in fat, fish, and fibre intakes on death and myocardial reinfarction: Diet and Reinfarction Trial (DART). *The Lancet,* 1989. September 30, 1989:757–761.

*Chapter 6: Taming the Savage Cell*

1. "Cancer-War Skeptic Confirms Drop in Death Rate," in *New York Times*. 1997: New York, p. A13.

2. Willett, W. C. Diet and health: What should we eat? *Science,* 1994; 264:532–7.

3. Schloss, I., M. S. G. Kidd, and S. J. D. O'Keefe. Dietary factors associated with a low risk of colon cancer in coloured West Coast fisherman. *South African Med J,* 1997; 82(2):152–8.

4. Cave, W. T. J. *W-3 Fatty Acid Diet Effects on Tumorigenesis in Experimental Animals.* In *Health Effects of W-3 Polyunsaturated Fatty Acids in Seafoods.* A. P. Simopoulos, et al., eds. 1991, Karger: Basel, 462–476.

5. Karmali, R. A. n-3 fatty acids and cancer. *J of Internal Med,* 1989. 225(1):197–200.

6. Sauer, L. A. and R. T. Dauchy. Stimulation of tumor growth in adult rats in vivo during an acute fast. *Cancer Research,* 1986; 46:3469–75.7.

7. Noguchi, M., D. P. Rose, and I. Miyazaki. The role of fatty acids and eicosanoid synthesis inhibitors in breast carcinoma. *Oncology,* 1995; 52:265–271.

8. Galli, Claudio, and D. Butrum. *Dietary W-3 Fatty Acids and Cancer: An Overview.* In *Health Effects of W-3 Polyunsaturated Fatty Acids in Seafoods.* A. P. Simopoulos, et al., eds. 1991, Karger: Basel, 462–76.

9. The following chart summarizes the fourteen studies and their results.

| DESCRIPTION AND SOURCE OF STUDY | RESULTS |
| --- | --- |
| **Study:** Researchers determined the ratio of linoleic to alpha-linolenic acid in the diets of 12,866 American men.<br><br>Source: Dolecek, Theres A., Greg Grandits. *Dietary Polyunsaturated Fatty Acids and Mortality in the Multiple Risk Factor Intervention Trial (MRFIT)* in Health Effects of W-3 Polyunsaturated Fatty Acids in Seafoods, World Rev Nutr Diet. Basel, Karger, 1991, vol. 66, pp. 205–216. | **Results:** Those who had the lowest ratio (in other words they were eating relatively low amounts of the omega-6 fatty acid linoleic acid and high amounts of the omega-3 fatty acid alpha-linolenic acid) had a 33 percent lower risk of dying from cancer. |
| **Study:** Tissues taken from 100 melanoma (skin cancer) patients and 100 healthy individuals was analyzed for its fatty acid content.<br><br>Source: Mackie, B. S., L. E. Mackie, and D. J. Bourne, *Melanoma and Dietary Lipids.* Nutrition and Cancer, 1987; 9(4): pp. 219–26. | **Results:** The more omega-6 fatty acids (linoleic and arachidonic acid) in a person's tissues, the higher the risk of melanoma. People with the lowest levels of linoleic acid had the lowest risk of the deadly disease. |
| **Study:** The dietary intake of 88,751 women was compared with the incidence of colon cancer.<br><br>Source: Willett, W. C., M. J. Stampfer, and F. E. Speizer, *Relation of Meat, Fat, and Fiber Intake to the Risk of Colon Cancer in a Prospective Study Among Women.* N Eng J Med, 1990. Dec. | **Results:** Women whose diets were relatively high in fish (and therefore, in omega-3 fatty acids) and low in red meat were less likely to have colon cancer. |

| DESCRIPTION AND SOURCE OF STUDY | RESULTS |
|---|---|
| **Study:** The fatty acid content of human brain tumors was compared with that of normal brain tissue.<br><br>Source: Martin, D.D., Robbins, M.E.C., Hussey, D.H., *The Fatty Acid Composition of Human Gliomas Differs from That Found in Nonmalignant Brain Tissue.* Lipids, 1996. 31(12): pp. 1283–1288. | **Results:** Compared to normal brain tissue, tissue from brain tumors (malignant gliomas) contained more than four times as much LA and half as much DHA. |
| **Study:** A comparison was made between cancer mortality in Israeli Jews whose diet is very high in linoleic acid and Israeli Arabs whose diet is based on olive oil .<br><br>Source: Yam, D., Eliraz, Abraham, Eliraz, Berry, Elliot, M., *Diet and Disease—The Israeli Paradox: Possible dangers of a high omega-6 polyunsaturated fatty acid diet.* Isr J Med Sci, 1996. 32: pp. 1134–1143. | **Results:** People with diets high in linoleic acid were more than three times as likely to die from cancer as those whose diets were rich in olive oil. |
| **Study:** A comparison was made between the fatty acid content of breast tissue from women with breast cancer and women with benign breast disease.<br><br>Source: Zhu, Z. R., J. Agren, and M. Uusitupa, *Fatty Acid Composition of Breast Adipose Tissue in Breast Cancer Patients and in Patients with Benign Breast Disease.* Nutrition and Cancer, 1995. 24: pp. 151–160. | **Results:** Tissue from postmenopausal women with breast cancer had lower levels of DHA, an omega-3 fatty acid, than tissue from women without cancer. |
| **Study:** Tissues from 91 human breast tumors were analyzed for their prostaglandin content.<br><br>Source: Rolland, P. H., P. M. Martin, and M. Toga, *Prostaglandin in Human Breast Cancer: Evidence Suggesting that Elevated Prostaglandin Production Is a Marker of High Metastatic Potential for Neoplastic Cells.* JNCI, 1980. 64(5): pp. 1061–1070. | **Results:** Tissue from women with metastatic breast cancer had higher levels of prostaglandin ($PGE_2$), a prostaglandin derived from linoleic acid, than tissue from people whose tumors had not spread. |
| **Study:** Researchers compared the fat intake of Japanese and Caucasian breast cancer patients with their mortality<br><br>Source: Nomura, A.M.Y., L. Le Marchand, and J.H. Hankin, *The effect of dietary fat on breast cancer survival among Caucasian and Japenese women in Hawaii.* Breast Cancer Research and Treatment, 1991. 18: pp. S135–S141. | **Results:** Women whose diets contained relatively high amounts of omega-6 fatty acids had a greater risk (RR 1.72) of dying from breast cancer. |

## DESCRIPTION AND SOURCE OF STUDY

## RESULTS

**Study:** Food intake in 32 countries was compared with the incidence of breast cancer.

Source: Kaizer, L., N. Boyd, and D. Tritchler, *Fish Consumption and Breast Cancer Risk: An Ecological Study.* 1989. 12(1): pp. 61–68.

**Results:** Of all the dietary factors considered, fish intake had the strongest protective effect.

**Study:** A food questionnaire was administered to 820 women with breast cancer and 1548 women free of the disease.

Source: Trichopoulou, A., K. Katsouyanni, and D. Trichopoulos, *Consumption of Olive Oil and Specific Food Groups in Relation to Breast Cancer Risk in Greece.* Journal of the National Cancer Institute, 1995. 87(2): pp. 110–6.

**Results:** A high intake of vegetables, fruits, and olive oil (three of the main components of **The Omega Diet**) was linked with a lower risk of cancer. The more olive oil consumed, the lower the risk. Margarine was associated with a possible *increased* risk. (Olive oil has been shown to increase blood levels of omega-3 fatty acids.)

**Study:** Women at high risk for breast cancer were placed on a diet rich in omega-3 fatty acids.

Source: Karmali, R. A., *n-3 fatty acids and cancer.* Journal of Internal Medicine, 1989. 225(1): pp. 197–200.

**Results:** There was a reduction in a process (16 alpha-hydroxylation of estrogen) that is strongly linked with breast cancer. The researcher commented, ". . . the use of omega-3 fatty acids in high-risk women is attractive and requires further exploration."

**Study:** The incidence of breast cancer in women in Greenland and Iceland was compared with changes in the traditional diet.

Source: Bjarnason, O., *The effect of year of birth on the breast cancer age-incidence curve of Iceland.* Int. J. Cancer, 1974. 13(689–96): pp. 689–96.

**Results:** A declining consumption of fish and marine animals was linked with an increased risk of breast cancer.

**Study:** In an eight-year study, 846 men were assigned to a conventional diet relatively high in saturated fat or to one in which omega-6 oils were substituted for saturated fat.

Source: Pearce, M.L. and S. Dayton, *Incidence of Cancer in Men on a Diet High in Polyunsaturated Fat.* The Lancet, 1971: pp. 464–467.

**Results:** Men assigned to the diet high in omega-6 oils and linoleic acid had almost twice the rate of cancer mortality as those eating the standard diet.

**Study:** The rising U.S. death rate from cancer in the period between 1909 to 1972 was compared with changes in fat consumption.

Source: Enig, M. G., Munn, R. J., Keeney, M., *Dietary fat and cancer trends—a critique.* Federation Proc., 1978. 37: pp. 2215–2220.

**Results:** During this time period, Americans ate *less* saturated fat and more linoleic acid, linking linoleic acid but not saturated fat with a greater risk of cancer.

10. Anti, M., G. Marra, and G. Miggiano. Effect of omega-3 fatty acids on rectal mucosal cell proliferation in subjects at risk for colon cancer. *Gastroenterology,* 1992;103:883–91.

11. Huang, Y.-C., J. M. Jessup, and G. L. Blackburn. n-3 fatty acids decrease colonic epithelial cell proliferation in high-risk bowel mucosa. *Lipids,* 1996. 31(Supplement):S-313–316.

12. Sauer, L. A. and R. T. Dauchy. The effect of omega-6 and omega-3 fatty acids on 3H-thymidine incorporation in hepatoma 7288CTC perfused in situ. *Br J Cancer,* 1992; 66:297–303.

13. Das, U. N. and D. F. Horrobin. Polyunsaturated fatty acids augment free radical generation in tumor cells in vitro. *Biochemical and Biophysical Research Communications,* 1987; 145(1):15–24.

14. This study has yet to be published.

15. Bougnoux, P., V. Chajes, and O. Le Floch. *Role of 18:3n-3 content of breast adipose tissue: Br J Cancer,* 1994; 70: 330–4.

16. In her animal studies, Thompson has found that flaxseeds contain not only LNA but a second cancer-fighting ingredient as well: an estrogen-blocking substance called "lignan." These two elements appear to have different actions: lignan is more effective at blocking the formation of new tumors, while LNA is better at slowing established tumors. Together, she has found that they can shrink breast tumors in rats by more than 50 percent. (Thompson, L. U., S. E. Rickard, and M.M. Seidl. Flaxseed and its lignan and oil components reduce mammary tumor growth at a late stage of carcinogenesis. *Carcinogenesis,* 1996; 17(6):1373–1376.)

17. In a personal communication, Thompson added another word of caution: "Breast cancer patients who are being treated with estrogen-blocking drugs such as taxol might be wise to refrain from eating flaxseeds. Flaxseeds and taxol are both anti-estrogens, and we don't know how the two will interact." (Note: This restriction does not apply to flaxseed oil, which is rich in LNA but does *not* contain lignan.)

18. Johanning, G. L. Modulation of breast cancer cell adhesion by unsaturated fatty acids. *Nutrition,* 1996; 12(11/12):810–816.

19. Reich, R. and G. R. Martin. Identification of arachidonic acid pathways required for the invasive and metastatic activity of malignant tumor cells. *Prostaglandins,* 1996; 51:01–17.

20. Personal communication.

21. Jonas, W. B. Researching alternative medicine. *Nature Medicine,* 1997; 3(8)824–827.

22. Rose, D. P., J. M. Connolly, and M. Coleman. Effect of omega-3 fatty acids on the progression of metastases after the surgical excision of human breast cancer cell solid tumors growing in nude mice. *Clinical Cancer Research,* 1996; 2:1751–6.

23. Kenler, A. S., W. S. Swails, and B. R. Bistrian. Early enteral feeding in postsurgical cancer patients: Fish oil structured lipid-based polymeric formula versus a standard polymeric formula. *Ann of Surgery* 1996; 223(3):316–333.

24. Shao, Y., L. Pardini, and R. Pardini. Dietary menhaden oil enhances mito-

mycin C antitumor activity toward human mammary carcinoma MX-1. *Lipids,* 1995; 30(11):1035–1045.

25. Chart created from data published in reference 24.

26. In press.

27. Personal communication.

28. Personal communication.

29. Vartak, S., M. E. C. Robins, and A. A. Spector. Polyunsaturated fatty acids increase the sensitivity of 36B10 rat astrocytoma cells to radiation-induced cell kill. *Lipids,* 1997; 32(3):283–292.

30. Grady, D. "Unusual Molecule Could Be Key to Cancer Patients' Weight Loss," in *New York Times.* 1996, p. B10.

31. Wigmore, The effect of polyunsaturated fatty acids on the progress of cachexia in patients with pancreatic cancer. *Nutrition,* 1996; 12:527–530.

*Chapter 7: Defeating Syndrome-X, Obesity, and Diabetes*

1. Haffner, S. M., R. A. Valdez, and M. P. Stern. Prospective analysis of the insulin-resistance syndrome (syndrome X). *Diabetes,* 1992; 41:715–22.

2. Simopoulos, A. Is insulin resistance influenced by dietary linoleic acid and trans-fatty acids? *Free Radical Biology and Medicine,* 1994; 17(4):367–372.

3. Simopoulos, A. P. Fatty acid composition of skeletal-muscle membrane phospholipids, insulin resistance, and obesity. *Nutrition Today,* 1994; 29(1):12–16.

4. Salmeron, J., J. E. Manson, and W. C. Wilett. Dietary fiber, glycemic load, and risk of non-insulin-dependent diabetes mellitus in women. *JAMA,* 1997; 277(6):472–477.

5. Hainault, I., M. Carlotti, and M. Lavau. Fish oil in a high lard diet prevents obesity, hyperlipemia, and adipocyte insulin resistance in rats. *Annals of New York Academy of Sciences,* :98–101.

6. Ikemoto, S., O. Ezaki, and M. Takahashi. High-fat diet-induced hyperglycemia and obesity in mice: Differential effects of dietary oils. *Metabolism,* 1996; 45(12):1539–46.

7. The graph was created from data from reference 6, above.

8. Storlien, L. H. Skeletal muscle membrane lipids and insulin resistance. *Lipids,* 1996; 31(Supplement):S-261–265.

9. Yam, D., Abraham Eliraz, Berry Eliraz, and M. Elliot. Diet and disease—The Israeli paradox: Possible dangers of a high omega–6 polyunsaturated fatty acid diet. *Isr J Med Sci,* 1996; 32:1134–1143.

10. Kuller, L. H. (letter). *The Lancet,* 1993; 341:1093–4.

11. Ostlund-Lindqvist, A., L. Albanus, and L. Croon. Effect of dietary trans-fatty acids on microsomal enzymes and membranes. *Lipids,* 1985; 20(9):620–624.

12. Torjesen, P. A., et al. Lifestyle changes may reverse development of the insulin resistance syndrome. *Diabetes Care,* 1997; 30:26–31.

13. Fanaian, M., J. Szilasi, L. Storlien, and G. D. Calvert. The effect of modified fat diet on insulin resistance and metabolic parameters in type II diabetes. *Diabetologia,* 1996; 39(1):A7.

## Chapter 8: Food for Thought

1. Salem, N., Omega-3 fatty acids: Molecular and biochemical aspects. In *New Protective Roles for Selected Nutrients*, J. Spiller, ed. 1989, Alan R. Liss: New York, 109–228.

2. Lamptey, M. S. and B. L. Walker. A possible essential role for dietary linolenic acid in the development of the young rat. *J of Nutrition,* 1976; 106:86–92.

3. Nakashima, Y., S. Yuasa, Y. Hukamizu, and T. Nabeshima. Effect of a high linoleate and a high apha-linolenate diet on general behavior and drug sensitivity in mice. *J of Lipid Research,* 1993; 34:239–247.

4. Gibson, R. A., M. A. Neumann, and M. Makrides. Effect of dietary docosahexaenoic acid on brain composition and neural function in term infants. *Lipids,* 1996; 31(Supplement):S-177–181.

5. Simopoulos, A. P. Omega-3 fatty acids part I: Metabolic effects of omega-3 fatty acids and essentiality. In Handbook of Lipids in Human Nutrition. 1996, CRC Press Inc.: Boca Raton, p. 51–73.

6. Uauy, R., et al. Role of essential fatty acids in the function of the developing nervous system. *Lipids,* 1996; 31 (Suppl):S-167–176.

7. Carlson, S. and S. Werkman. A randomized trial of visual attention of preterm infants fed docosahexaenoic acid until two months. *Lipids,* 1996. 31(1):85–90.

8. See reference 4.

9. Stevens, L. J., et al. Omega-3 fatty acids in boys with behavior, learning, and health problems. *Physiology & Behavior,* 1996; 59(4/5):915–20.

10. Myanaga, K., K. Yonemura, and K. Yazawa. DHA shortens P300 latency in healthy persons. In *International Conference on Highly Unsaturated Fatty Acids in Nutrition and Disease Prevention.* 1996. Barcelona, Spain.

11. Yoshida, S., A. Yasuda, and H. Okuyama. Synaptic vesicle ultrastructural changes in the rat hippocampus induced by a combination of alpha-linolenic deficiency and a learning task. *J of Neurochemistry,* 1997; 68:1261–1268.

12. Schaefer, E. J. Decreased plasma phosphatidylcholine docosahexaenoic acid content in dementia. Unpublished abstract.

13. Kalmijn, S., E. J. M. Feskens, and D. Kromhout. Polyunsaturated fatty acids, antioxidants, and cognitive function in very old men. *Amer J of Epidemiology,* 1997; 145(1):33–41.

14. Yazawa, K. Clinical experience with docosahexaenoic acid in demented patients. In *International Conference on Highly Unsaturated Fatty Acids in Nutrition and Disease Prevention.* 1996. Barcelona, Spain.

15. Hibbeln, J. R., J. C. Umhau, and N. J. Salem. Do plasma polyunsaturates predict hostility and depression? *World Rev Nutr Diet,* 1997; 82:175–86.

16. Smith, R. S. The macrophage theory of depression. *MedHypotheses,* 1991. 35:298–306.

17. Hibbeln, J. R. and N. Salem. Dietary polyunsaturated fatty acids and depression: when cholesterol does not satisfy. *Amer J of Clin Nutr,* 1995; 62:1–9.

18. Adams, P. B., et al. Arachidonic acid to eicosapentaenoic acid ratio in blood correlates positively with clinical symptoms of depression. *Lipids,* 1996; 31:S157–S161.

19. Klerman, G. L. and M. M. Weissman. Increasing rates of depression. *JAMA*, 1989; 261(15):2229–35.

20. Zigler, E. F. and M. Finn-Stevenson. *Children: Development and Social Issues*. 1987, Washington, D.C.: Heath and Co.

21. Hibbeln unearthed this information when he came across Burden's treatise, *The Anatomy of Melancholy*, published in 1652. In his book, Burden acknowledges he learned about the antidepressant properties of cow brains while reading early Arabic medical texts. People may have been using omega-3 fatty acids to treat depression for thousands of years.

22. Maggioni, M., G. B. Picotti, and F. Brambilla. Effects of phosphatidylserine therapy in geriatric patients with depressive disorders. *Acta Psychiatr Scand*, 1990; 81:265–70.

23. Rudin, D. O. and C. Felix. *Omega-3 Oils*. 1996, Honesdale, PA: Paragon Press. 216.

24. Rudin, D. O. The major psychoses and neuroses as omega-3 essential fatty acid deficiency syndrome: Substrate pellagra. *Biological Psychiatry*, 1981; 16(9):827–50.

25. Gitlin, M. J. and R. O. Pasnau. Psychiatric syndromes linked to reproductive function in women: A review of current knowledge. *Am J Psychiatry*, 1989; 146(11):1413–1422.

26. Holman, R. T., S. B. Johnson, and P. L. Ogburn. Deficiency of essential fatty acids and membrane fluidity during pregnancy and lactation. *Proc Natl Acad Sci*, USA, 1991; 88:4835–9.

27. Al, M. D. M. *Essential fatty acids, pregnancy, and pregnancy outcome. Relationship between mother and child*. CIP-Gegevens Koninklijke Bibliotheek, Den Haag, The Netherlands, 1994.

28. Stevens, L. J., S. S. Zentall, and J. R. Burgess. Essential fatty acid metabolism in boys with attention-deficit hyperactivity disorder. *Amer J of Clinical Nutrition*, 1995; 62:761–8.

29. Stevens, L. J., et al. Omega-3 fatty acids in boys with behavior, learning, and health problems. *Physiology & Behavior*, 1996; 59(4/5):915–20.

30. The violent offenders also had unusually high levels of long-chain omega-6 fatty acids. Virkkunen, M. E., D. F. Horrobin, and M. S. Manku. Plasma phospholipid essential fatty acids and prostaglandins in alcoholic, habitually violent, and impulsive offenders. *Biological Psychiatry*, 1987; 22:1087–96.

31. Kaplan, J. R., S. B. Manuck, and C. Shively. The effects of fat and cholesterol on social behavior in monkeys. *Psychosomatic Medicine*, 1991; 53:634–642.

32. Hamazaki, T., S. Sawazaki, and M. Kobayashi. The effect of docosahexaenoic acid on aggression in young adults. *J of Clinical Investigation*, 1996. 97(4):1129–34.

33. Singer, P. Effects of dietary oleic, linoleic and alpha-linolenic acids on blood pressure, serum lipids, lipoproteins and the formation of eicosanoid precursors in patients with mild essential hypertension. *J of Human Hypertension*, 1990; 4:227–33.

34. Williams, R. B. Neurobiology, cellular and molecular biology, and psychosomatic medicine. *Psychosomatic Medicine*, 1994; 56:308–15.

35. Laugharne, J. D. E., J. E. Mellor, and M. Peet. Fatty acids and schizophrenia. *Lipids,* 1996; 31 Supplement:S-163–165.

*Chapter 9: How The Omega Diet Fine-tunes Your Immune System*

1. Two of the main offenders are leukotriene $B_4$ ($LTB_4$) and prostaglandin $E_2$ ($PGE_2$).

2. Fisher, M., K. S. Upchurch, and J. J. Hoogasian. Effects of dietary fish oil supplementation on polymorphonuclear leukocyte inflammatory potential. *Inflammation,* 1986; 10(4):387–92.

3. Endres, S., T. Eisenhut, and B. Sinha. Lipids in immune function and inflammatory disorders. 1995; 23:277–281.

4. Fernandes, G. Modulation of antioxidant enzymes and programmed cell death by n-3 fatty acids. *Lipids,* 1996; 31(Supplement):S-91–96.

5. Kremer, J. M., W. Jubiz, and L. Lininger. Fish-oil fatty acid supplementation in active rheumatoid arthritis. *Annals of Internal Medicine,* 1987; 106(4):497–502.

6. Kremer, J. M. and S. Malcolm. Dietary fish oil and olive oil supplementation in patients with rheumatoid arthritis. *Arthritis and Rheumatism,* 1990; 33(6):810–820.

7. Kremer, J.M.L., and A. David. Effects of high-dose fish oil on rheumatoid arthritis after stopping nonsteroidal antiinflammatory drugs. *Arthritis & Rheumatism,* 1995; 36(8):1107–1114.

8. Cleary, E. G. and M. W. Whitehouse. Linseed (flax) oil: anti-inflammatory activity when applied transcutaneously to treat experimental and clinical arthritis. In *Third International Congress on Essential Fatty Acids and Eicosanoids.* 1992. Adelaide, Austrailia.

9. Hodge, L., C. M. Salome, J. K. Peat, and A. J. Woolcock. Consumption of oily fish and childhood asthma risk. *MJA,* 1996. 164:137–140.

10. Schwartz, J. and S. T. Weiss. The relationship of dietary fish intake to level of pulmonary function in the first National Health and Nutrition Survey (NHANES 1). *European Respiratory J,* 1994; 7:1821–4.

11. Dry, J. and D. Vincent. Effect of a fish oil diet on asthma: Results of a 1-year double-blind study. *Int Arch Allergy Appl Immunoll,* 1991; 95:156–157.

12. Broughton, K. S., C. S. Johnson, and K. M. Kleppinger. Reduced asthma symptoms with n-3 fatty acid ingestion are related to 5-series leukotriene production. *Am J Clin Nutr,* 1997; 65(1011–7):1011–7.

13. Cacabelos, R., X. A. Alvarez, and T. Nishimura. Brain interleukin-1B in Alzheimer's disease and vascular dementia. *Meth Find Exp Clin Pharmacol,* 1994. 16(2):141–151.

14. Kalmijn, S., E. J. M. Feskens, and D. Kromhout. Polyunsaturated fatty acids, antioxidants, and cognitive function in very old men. *Amer J of Epidemiology,* 1997; 145(1):33–41.

15. Shahar, E., A. R. Folsom, and M. Szklo. Dietary n-3 polyunsaturated fatty acids and smoking-related chronic obstructive pulmonary disease. *N Engl J of Med,* 1994; 331(4):S- 228–33.

16. McCarty, M. F. Fish oil may be an antidote for the cardiovascular risk of smoking. *MedHypotheses,* 1995; 46:343.

17. Belluzzi, A., C. Brignola, M. Campieri, and M. Miglioli. Effect of an enteric-coated fish-oil preparation on relapses in Crohn's desease. *N Engl J of Med,* 1996; 24:1557–60.

18. Stenson, W. F., D. Cort, and W. Beeken. Dietary supplementation with fish oil in ulcerative colitis. *Ann Int Med,* 1992; 116:609–14.

19. Campan, P., P. O. Planchand, and D. Duran. Polyunsaturated omega-3 fatty acids in the treatment of experimental human gingivitis. *Bull Group Int Rech Sci Stomatol Odontol,* 1996; 29(1–2):25–31.

20. Donadio, J. V., E. J. Bergstralh, K. P. Offord, and K. E. Holley. A controlled trial of fish oil in IgA nephropathy. *N Engl J Med,* 1994; 331:1194–9.

21. Thorner, A., G. Walldius, E. Nilsson, and R. Gullberg. Beneficial effects of reduced intake of polyunsaturated fatty acids in the diet for one year in patients with systemic lupus erythematosus. *Annals of the Rheumatic Diseases,* 1990; 49:134.

22. Walton, A. J. E., M. L. Snaith, M. Locniskar, and D. A. Isenberg. Dietary fish oil and the severity of symptoms in patients with systemic lupus erythematosus. *Annals of the Rheumatic Diseases,* 1991; 50:463–466.

23. Das, U. Beneficial effects of eicosapentaenoic and docosahexaenoice acids in the management of systemic lupus erythematosus and its relationship to the cytokine network. *Prostaglandins, Leukotrienes, and Essential Fatty Acids,* 1994. 51:207–13.

24. Deutch, Menstrual pain in Danish women correlated with low n-3 polyunsaturated fatty acid intake. *European J of Clinical Nutrition,* 1995; 49:508–516.

25. Harel, Z., F. M. Biro, and S. L. Rosenthal. Supplementation with omega-3 polyunsaturated fatty acids in the management of dysmenorrhea in adolescents. *Am J Obstet Gynecol,* 1996; 174(4):1335–8.

26. Press, A. "Skin-Cancer Risk Is Found in Psoriasis Therapy," in *New York Times.* 1997, p. A22.

27. Bittiner, S. B., I. Cartwright, W. F. G. Tucker, and S. S. Bleehen. A double-blind, randomised, placebo-controlled trial of fish oil in psoriasis. *The Lancet,* 1988; 1:378–380.

28. Simopoulos, A. P., R. R. Kifer, and S. M. Barlow, eds. Health effects of omega-3 polyunsaturated fatty acids in seafoods. *World Review of Nutrition and Dietetics,* ed. A. P. Simopoulos. Vol. 66. 1991, Karger: Basel, p. 591.

29. Watkins B. A., M. F. Seifert, and K. G. Allen. Importance of dietary fat in modulating $PGE_2$ responses and influence of vitamin E on bone morphometry. *World Rev Nutr Diet,* 1997; 82:250-9.

*Chapter 10: Your Health Is in the Balance*

1. People familiar with my work will note that the illustration of The Omega Diet Food Guide is an adaptation of the Greek column that I have written about in a number of publications. (Simopoulos, A. P. The Mediterranean food guide. *Nutri-*

*tion Today,* 1995; 30(2):54–60.) In creating The Omega Diet, the traditional diet of Crete has been modified in a number of ways, including adding canola oil with its high LNA content to compensate for the fact that Americans eat fewer green leafy vegetables, legumes, and walnuts than the Greeks, and rarely eat wild plants—all good sources of LNA, vitamins, minerals, fiber, and phytochemicals.

2. De Oliveira e Silva, E. R., C. E. Seidman, and J. L. Breslow. Effects of shrimp consumption on plasma lipoproteins. *Amer J of Clinical Nutrition,* 1996; 64:712–7.

3. Sauer, L. A. and R. T. Dauchy. The effect of omega-6 and omega-3 fatty acids on 3H-thymidine incorporation in hepatoma 7288CTC perfused in situ. *Br J Cancer,* 1992; 66:297–303.

4. Rose, D. P., J. M. Connolly, and M. Coleman. Influence of diets containing eicosapentaenoic or docosahexaenoic acid on growth and metastasis of breast cancer cells in nude mice. *J of the National Cancer Institute,* 1995; 87(8):587–92.

5. Saynor, R. and T. Gillott. Changes in blood lipids and fibrinogen with a note on safety in a long-term study on the effects of n-3 fatty acids in subjects receiving fish oil supplements and followed for seven years. *Lipids,* 1992; 27(7):533–8.

6. Dehmer, G. J., J. J. Popma, and J. M. Schmitz. Reduction in the rate of early restenoisis after coronary angioplasty by a diet supplemented with n-3 fatty acids. *N Engl J of Med,* 1988; 319(12):733–40.

7. Broughton, K. S., C. S. Johnson, and K. M. Kleppinger. Reduced asthma symptoms with n-3 fatty acid ingestion are related to 5-series leukotriene production. *Am J Clin Nutr,* 1997; 65:1011–7.

8. Heimendinger, J., and M. A. S. Van Duyn. Dietary behavior change: the challenge of recasting the role of fruit and vegetables in the Amer diet. *Amer J Clin Nutr,* 1995; 61(suppl):1397S–401S.

9. Sabate, J., G. E. Fraser, and K. D. Lindsted. Effects of walnuts on serum lipid levels and blood pressure in normal men. *N Engl J of Med,* 1993; 328(9):603–7.

10. *Clinical Pearls News,* July 1997, 7 (7)75.

11. Data from: Chow, C. K., *Fatty Acids in Foods and Their Health Implications.* 1992, New York: Marcel Dekker, Inc. 889. All nuts also contain monounsaturated fatty acids, which are not shown in this table.

12. Renaud, S., M. Ciavatti, and J. P. Ripoll. Protective effects of dietary calcium and magnesium on platelet function and atherosclerosis in rabbits fed saturated fat. *Atherosclerosis,* 1983; 47:189–198.

13. Pelletier, X., Thouvenot, and G. Debry. Effect of egg consumption in healthy volunteers: Influence of yolk, white or whole-egg on gastric emptying and on glycemic and hormonal responses. *Annals of Nutrition and Metabolism,* 1996; 40:109–15.

*Chapter 11: The Omega Shopper*

1. Vaisey-Genser, M. *Flaxseed.* 1994, Winnipeg: The Flax Council of Canada.

2. Hamlin, S. "Canned Tuna: In Search of Flavor and Texture," in *New York Times.* 1997, pp. B1, B8.

*Chapter 12: The 3-Week Omega Diet*

1. Salem, N. J., H.-Y. Kim, and J. A. Yergey. Docosahexaenoic acid: Membrane function and metabolism. In *Health Effects of Polyunsaturated Fatty Acids in Seafoods*, A. P. Simopoulos, ed. 1986, Academic Press, Inc. 263–317.

*Chapter 13: The Omega Weight-Loss Diet*

1. Stunkard, A. J. Conservative treatments for obesity. *Am J Clin Nutr,* 1987; 45:1142–54.

2. Ravussin, E. and C. Bogardus. Relationship of genetics, age, and physical fitness to daily energy expenditure and fuel utilization. *Am J Clin Nutr*, 1989; 49:968–75.

3. Pavlov, K., et al. Exercise as an adjunct to weight loss and maintenance in moderately obese subjects. *Am J. Clin Nutr.* 1989; 49: 1115–23.

4. Himaya, A., et al. Satiety power of dietary fat: a new appraisal. *Am J Clin Nutr,* 1997; 65:1410–8.

5. Sakata, F. K., K. Kurata, et al. Charting of daily weight pattern reinforces maintenance of weight reduction in moderately obese patients. *Am J Med Sci,* 1992; 303(3):145–50.

6. This list is adapted from the article "Conservative Treatments for Obesity," by Albert J. Stunkard, which appeared in the *Amer J Clin Nutr,* 1987, 45:1142–54.

*Chapter 14: In the Omega Kitchen*

1. For example, ordinary eggs in the market have a 20:1 ratio of omega-6 to omega-3. Omega-3 enriched eggs have a ratio that ranges from 2–6:1; whereas the egg under completely natural conditions has a ratio of 1:1. Recipes that use eggs from chickens fed fish meal or fish oil will have DHA and EPA. But eggs from chickens fed on flaxmeal or flax oil will contain LNA.

# Appendix

Date _____ Weight _____

Today's Goal: _____

_____

| Time of Day | Food | Calories | Mood or situation |
|---|---|---|---|
|  |  |  |  |
|  |  |  |  |
|  |  |  |  |
|  |  |  |  |
|  |  |  |  |

|  | Total Calories | Overall Comments |  |
|---|---|---|---|
| Type of Exercise | Amount | Comments |  |
|  |  |  |  |

Date _____ Weight _____

Today's Goal: _____

_____

| Time of Day | Food | Calories | Mood or situation |
|---|---|---|---|
|  |  |  |  |
|  |  |  |  |
|  |  |  |  |
|  |  |  |  |
|  |  |  |  |

| | Total Calories | Overall Comments |
|---|---|---|

| Type of Exercise | Amount | Comments |
|---|---|---|
|  |  |  |

Date _____ Weight_____

Today's Goal:_____

_____

| Time of Day | Food | Calories | Mood or situation |
|---|---|---|---|
|  |  |  |  |
|  |  |  |  |
|  |  |  |  |
|  |  |  |  |
|  |  |  |  |

|  | Total Calories | Overall Comments |  |
|---|---|---|---|
| Type of Exercise | Amount | Comments |  |
|  |  |  |  |

APPENDIX

## Weight Chart

Date

+3
+2
+1
0
-1
-2
-3
-4
-5
-6
-7
-8
-9
-10
-11
-12
-13

Linoleic Acid                          Alpha-Linolenic Acid

```
 HO  O                                    HO  O
   \ //   ← carboxyl group (C–O– O–H)       \ //   carboxyl group (C–O– O–H)
    C                                         C
    |                                         |
 H – C– H                                   H – C– H
    |                                         |
 H – C– H                                   H – C– H
    |                                         |
 H – C– H                                   H – C– H
    |                                         |
 H – C– H                                   H – C– H
    |                                         |
 H – C– H                                   H – C– H
    |                                         |
 H – C– H                                   H – C– H
    |                                         |
 H – C– H                                   H – C– H
    |                                         |
 H – C·                                     H – C·
   ||   ← double bond in the 9th position     ||   ← double bond in the 9th position
 H – C                                      H – C
    |                                         |
 H – C– H                                   H – C– H
    |                                         |
 H – C                                      H – C
   ||   ← double bond in the 6th position     ||   ← double bond in the 6th position
 H – C                                      H – C
    |                                         |
 H – C– H                                   H – C– H
    |                                         |
 H – C– H                                   H – C– H
    |                                         ||   ← double bond in the 3rd position
 H – C– H                                   H – C– H
    |                                         |
 H – C– H                                   H – C– H
    |                                         |
 H – C– H   ← methyl group                  H – C– H   ← methyl group
    |                                         |
    H                                         H
```

As you can see, the only difference between linoleic and alpha-linolenic acid is that alpha-linolenic has an additional double bond at the 3rd position, which gives it the designation of an "omega-3" fatty acid. Linoleic acid, which has its first double bond 6 carbon atoms from the end (methyl group) is referred to as an "omega-6" fatty acid.

# GRAMS OF FATTY ACIDS PER 100 GRAMS

| Type of Food | Omega-6 Fatty Acid | Omega-3 Fatty Acids | | |
|---|---|---|---|---|
| | | Alpha-Linolenic Acid | EPA | DHA |
| **FISH** | | | | |
| Anchovy | 0.2 | — | 0.5 | 0.9 |
| Bass, freshwater | 0.4 | Tr | 0.1 | 0.2 |
| Bass, striped | — | Tr | 0.2 | 0.6 |
| Bluefish | 0.4 | — | 0.4 | 0.8 |
| Burbot | 0.1 | — | 0.1 | 0.1 |
| Capelin | 0.3 | 0.1 | 0.6 | 0.5 |
| Carp | 0.8 | 0.3 | 0.2 | 0.1 |
| Catfish, brown bullhead | 0.3 | 0.1 | 0.2 | 0.2 |
| Catfish, channel | 0.7 | Tr | 0.1 | 0.2 |
| Cisco | 0.1 | 0.1 | 0.1 | 0.3 |
| Cod, Atlantic | Tr | Tr | 0.1 | 0.2 |
| Cod, Pacific | Tr | Tr | 0.1 | 0.1 |
| Croaker, Atlantic | 0.3 | Tr | 0.1 | 0.1 |
| Dogfish, spiny | 0.7 | 0.1 | 0.7 | 1.2 |
| Dolphin fish | 0.1 | Tr | Tr | 0.1 |
| Drum, black | 0.3 | Tr | 0.1 | 0.1 |
| Drum, freshwater | 0.6 | 0.1 | 0.2 | 0.3 |
| Eel, European | 0.5 | 0.7 | 0.1 | 0.1 |
| Flounder, unspecified | 0.1 | Tr | 0.1 | 0.1 |
| Flounder, yellowtail | 0.1 | Tr | 0.1 | 0.1 |
| Grouper, jewfish | 0.1 | Tr | Tr | 0.3 |
| Grouper, red | Tr | — | Tr | 0.2 |
| Haddock | — | Tr | 0.1 | 0.1 |
| Hake, Atlantic | 0.1 | Tr | Tr | Tr |
| Hake, Pacific | 0.2 | Tr | 0.2 | 0.2 |
| Hake, red | 0.1 | — | 0.1 | 0.1 |

Notes: 100 grams is approximately ½ cup. Tr = trace amounts
— = lack of reliable data for nutrient known to be present. The best sources of omega-3 fatty acids are highlighted. This is a composite table, with the bulk of the data coming from *Health Effects of Polyunsaturated Fatty Acids in Seafoods,* edited by Artemis P. Simopoulos, Robert R. Kifer, Roy E. Martin, published by Academic Press in 1986.

| Type of Food | Omega-6 | Alpha-Linolenic Acid | EPA | DHA |
|---|---|---|---|---|
| Hake, silver | 0.3 | 0.1 | 0.2 | 0.3 |
| Hake, unspecified | — | — | 0.1 | 0.4 |
| Halibut, Greenland | 0.5 | Tr | 0.5 | 0.4 |
| Halibut, Pacific | 0.2 | 0.1 | 0.1 | 0.3 |
| Herring, Atlantic | 0.4 | 0.1 | 0.7 | 0.9 |
| Herring, Pacific | 0.6 | 0.1 | 1.0 | 0.7 |
| Herring, round | 0.2 | 0.1 | 0.4 | 0.8 |
| Mackerel, Atlantic | 1.1 | 0.1 | 0.9 | 1.6 |
| Mackerel, chub | 0.8 | 0.3 | 0.9 | 1.0 |
| Mackerel, horse | 0.3 | Tr | 0.3 | 0.3 |
| Mackerel, Japanese horse | 0.4 | 0.1 | 0.5 | 1.3 |
| Mackerel, king | 1.0 | — | 1.0 | 1.2 |
| Mullet, striped | 0.5 | 0.1 | 0.3 | 0.2 |
| Mullet, unspecified | 0.4 | Tr | 0.5 | 0.6 |
| Ocean perch | 0.3 | Tr | 0.1 | 0.1 |
| Perch, white | 0.3 | 0.1 | 0.2 | 0.1 |
| Perch, yellow | 0.1 | Tr | 0.1 | 0.2 |
| Pike, northern | 0.1 | Tr | Tr | 0.1 |
| Pike, walleye | 0.1 | Tr | 0.1 | 0.2 |
| Plaice, European | 0.2 | Tr | 0.1 | 0.1 |
| Pollock | — | — | 0.1 | 0.4 |
| Pompano, Florida | 0.5 | — | 0.2 | 0.4 |
| Ratfish | — | Tr | Tr | 0.1 |
| Rockfish, brown | 0.3 | Tr | 0.3 | 0.4 |
| Rockfish, canary | 0.1 | Tr | 0.2 | 0.3 |
| Rockfish, unspecified | 0.1 | Tr | 0.2 | 0.3 |
| Sablefish | 0.5 | 0.1 | 0.7 | 0.7 |
| Salmon, Atlantic | 0.7 | 0.2 | 0.3 | 0.9 |
| Salmon, Atlantic, farmed | ? | 0.1 | 0.6 | 1.2 |
| Salmon, chinook | 0.6 | 0.1 | 0.8 | 0.6 |
| Salmon, chum | 0.4 | 0.1 | 0.4 | 0.6 |
| Salmon, coho | 0.7 | 0.2 | 0.3 | 0.5 |
| Salmon, coho, farmed | ? | 0.1 | 0.4 | 0.8 |
| Salmon, pink | 0.4 | Tr | 0.4 | 0.6 |
| Salmon, sockeye | 0.6 | 0.1 | 0.5 | 0.7 |
| Sardines, canned, drained | ? | 0.5 | 0.4 | 0.6 |
| Saury | 0.4 | 0.1 | 0.5 | 0.8 |
| Scad, Muroaji | 0.5 | 0.1 | 0.5 | 1.5 |
| Scad, other | 0.1 | — | Tr | Tr |

| Type of Food | Omega-6 | Alpha-Linolenic Acid | EPA | DHA |
|---|---|---|---|---|
| Sea bass, Japanese | 0.1 | Tr | 0.1 | 0.3 |
| Seatrout, sand | 0.1 | Tr | 0.1 | 0.2 |
| Seatrout, spotted | 0.2 | Tr | 0.1 | 0.1 |
| Shark, unspecified | 0.3 | – | Tr | 0.5 |
| Sheepshead | 0.3 | Tr | 0.1 | 0.1 |
| Smelt, pond | – | – | 0.1 | 0.2 |
| Smelt, rainbow | 0.1 | 0.1 | 0.3 | 0.4 |
| Smelt, sweet | 0.4 | 0.3 | 0.2 | 0.1 |
| Snapper, red | 0.2 | Tr | Tr | 0.2 |
| Sole, European | 0.1 | Tr | Tr | 0.1 |
| Sprat | 0.2 | – | 0.5 | 0.8 |
| Sturgeon, Atlantic | 0.6 | Tr | 1.0 | 0.5 |
| Sturgeon, common | 0.1 | 0.1 | 0.2 | 0.1 |
| Sunfish, pumpkinseed | 0.1 | Tr | Tr | 0.1 |
| Swordfish | – | – | 0.1 | 0.1 |
| Trout, arctic char | 0.3 | Tr | 0.1 | 0.5 |
| Trout, brook | 0.3 | 0.2 | 0.2 | 0.2 |
| Trout, lake | 1.4 | 0.4 | 0.5 | 1.1 |
| Trout, rainbow | 0.6 | 0.1 | 0.1 | 0.4 |
| Tuna, albacore | 0.3 | 0.2 | 0.3 | 1.0 |
| Tuna, bluefin | 0.4 | – | 0.4 | 1.2 |
| Tuna, skipjack | 0.2 | – | 0.1 | 0.3 |
| Tuna, unspecified | – | – | 0.1 | 0.4 |
| Whitefish, lake | 0.7 | 0.2 | 0.3 | 1.0 |
| Whiting, European | – | Tr | Tr | 0.1 |
| Wolffish, Atlantic | 0.2 | Tr | 0.3 | 0.3 |

**CRUSTACEANS**

| | | | | |
|---|---|---|---|---|
| Crab, Alaska king | – | Tr | 0.2 | 0.1 |
| Crab, blue | 0.1 | Tr | 0.2 | 0.2 |
| Crab, Dungeness | – | – | 0.2 | 0.1 |
| Crab, queen | 0.1 | Tr | 0.2 | 0.1 |
| Crayfish, unspecified | 0.2 | Tr | 0.1 | Tr |
| Lobster, European | – | – | 0.1 | 0.1 |
| Lobster, northern | – | – | 0.1 | 0.1 |
| Shrimp, Atlantic brown | 0.2 | Tr | 0.2 | 0.1 |
| Shrimp, Atlantic white | 0.2 | Tr | 0.2 | 0.2 |
| Shrimp, Japanese (kuruma) prawn | 0.5 | Tr | 0.3 | 0.2 |

| Type of Food | Omega-6 | Alpha-Linolenic Acid | EPA | DHA |
|---|---|---|---|---|
| Shrimp, northern | 0.1 | Tr | 0.3 | 0.2 |
| Shrimp, other | 0.1 | Tr | 0.1 | 0.1 |
| Shrimp, unspecified | 0.1 | Tr | 0.2 | 0.1 |
| Spiny lobster, Caribbean | 0.3 | Tr | 0.2 | 0.1 |
| Spiny lobster, southern rock | — | Tr | 0.2 | 0.1 |

**MOLLUSKS**

| Type of Food | Omega-6 | Alpha-Linolenic Acid | EPA | DHA |
|---|---|---|---|---|
| Abalone, New Zealand | 0.2 | Tr | Tr | — |
| Abalone, South African | 0.2 | Tr | Tr | Tr |
| Clam, hardshell | 0.1 | Tr | Tr | Tr |
| Clam, hen | 0.1 | — | Tr | Tr |
| Clam, littleneck | 0.1 | Tr | Tr | Tr |
| Clam, Japanese hardshell | — | — | 0.1 | 0.1 |
| Clam, softshell | 0.2 | Tr | 0.2 | 0.2 |
| Clam, surf | — | Tr | 0.1 | 0.1 |
| Conch, unspecified | 0.1 | Tr | 0.6 | 0.4 |
| Cuttlefish, unspecified | 0.1 | Tr | Tr | Tr |
| Mussel, blue | 0.1 | Tr | 0.2 | 0.3 |
| Mussel, Mediterranean | 0.1 | — | 0.1 | 0.1 |
| Octopus, common | 0.1 | — | 0.1 | 0.1 |
| Oyster, eastern | 0.3 | Tr | 0.2 | 0.2 |
| Oyster, European | 0.1 | 0.1 | 0.3 | 0.2 |
| Oyster, Pacific | 0.3 | Tr | 0.4 | 0.2 |
| Periwinkle, common | 0.4 | 0.2 | 0.5 | Tr |
| Scallop, Atlantic deepsea | 0.1 | Tr | 0.1 | 0.1 |
| Scallop, calico | — | Tr | 0.1 | 0.1 |
| Scallop, unspecified | 0.1 | Tr | 0.1 | 0.1 |
| Squid, Atlantic | 0.1 | Tr | 0.1 | 0.3 |
| Squid, short-finned | 0.1 | Tr | 0.2 | 0.4 |
| Squid, unspecified | 0.1 | Tr | 0.1 | 0.2 |

**FISH OILS**

| Type of Food | Omega-6 | Alpha-Linolenic Acid | EPA | DHA |
|---|---|---|---|---|
| Cod liver oil | 6.6 | 0.7 | 9.0 | 9.5 |
| Herring oil | 4.1 | 0.6 | 7.1 | 4.3 |
| Menhaden oil | 7.8 | 1.1 | 12.7 | 7.9 |
| MaxEPA, concentrated fish body oils | 11.7 | 0 | 17.8 | 11.6 |
| Salmon oil | 9.0 | 1.0 | 8.8 | 11.1 |

| Type of Food | Omega-6 | Alpha-Linolenic Acid | EPA | DHA |
|---|---|---|---|---|
| **BEEF** | | | | |
| Chuck, blade roast, all grades, separable lean & fat, raw | 0.6 | 0.3 | – | – |
| Ground, regular, raw | 0.8 | 0.2 | – | – |
| Round, full cut, choice grade, separable lean & fat, raw | 0.5 | 0.2 | – | – |
| Separable from retail cuts, raw | 1.6 | 1.0 | – | – |
| T-Bone steak, choice grade, lean only, raw | 0.3 | Tr | – | – |
| T-Bone steak, choice grade, separable lean & fat, raw | 0.7 | 0.3 | – | – |
| **CEREAL GRAINS** | | | | |
| Barley, bran | 2.4 | 0.3 | – | – |
| Corn, germ | 17.7 | 0.3 | – | – |
| Oats, germ | 11.0 | 1.4 | – | – |
| Rice, bran | 6.4 | 0.2 | – | – |
| Wheat, bran | 2.2 | 0.2 | – | – |
| Wheat, germ | 5.9 | 0.7 | – | – |
| Wheat, hard red winter | 1.1 | 0.1 | – | – |
| **DAIRY AND EGG PRODUCTS** | | | | |
| Cheese, Cheddar | 0.5 | 0.4 | – | – |
| Cheese, Roquefort | 0.6 | 0.7 | – | – |
| Cream, heavy whipping | 0.9 | 0.5 | – | – |
| Milk, whole | – | 0.1 | – | – |
| Egg yolk, chicken, raw | 4.2 | 0.1 | | |
| **FATS AND OILS** | | | | |
| Beef fat | ? | 0.6 | – | – |
| Butter | 1.8 | 1.2 | – | – |
| Butter oil | 2.2 | 1.5 | – | – |
| Canola oil (Rapeseed) | 22.2 | 11.1 | – | – |
| Chicken fat | 19.9 | 1.0 | – | – |

| Type of Food | Omega-6 | Alpha-Linolenic Acid | EPA | DHA |
|---|---|---|---|---|
| Duck fat | 11.9 | 1.0 | — | — |
| Flaxseed oil (Linseed) | 12.7 | 53.5 | — | — |
| Lard | 10.2 | 1.0 | — | — |
| Margarine, hard, soybean | 19.4 | 1.5 | — | — |
| Margarine, hard, soybean and soybean (hydrog.) | 24.3 | 1.9 | — | — |
| Margarine, hard, soybean (hydrog.) & palm | 25.9 | 2.3 | — | — |
| Margarine, hard, soybean (hydrog.) & cottonseed | 22.5 | 2.8 | — | — |
| Margarine, hard, soybean (hydrog.) & palm (hydrog.) | 26.8 | 3.0 | — | — |
| Margarine, liquid, soybean (hydrog.), soybean, & cottonseed | 33.4 | 2.4 | — | — |
| Margarine, soft, soybean (hydrog.) & cottonseed | 27.5 | 1.6 | — | — |
| Margarine, soft, soybean (hydrog.) & palm | 32.7 | 1.9 | — | — |
| Margarine, soft, soybean, soybean (hydrog.) & cottonseed (hydrog.) | 27.3 | 2.8 | — | — |
| Mustard oil | NA | 1.8 | — | — |
| Mutton tallow | 5.5 | 2.3 | — | — |
| Rice bran oil | 33.4 | 1.6 | — | — |
| Safflower oil | 77 | <1 | — | — |
| Salad dressing, comm., blue chesse, reg. | 24.1 | 3.7 | — | — |
| Salad dressing, comm., Italian, reg. | 24.7 | 3.3 | — | — |
| Salad dressing, comm., mayonnaise, imitation, soybean, w/o cholesterol | 23.0 | 4.6 | — | — |
| Salad dressing, comm., mayonnaise, safflower & soybean | 52.0 | 3.0 | — | — |

| Type of Food | Omega-6 | Alpha-Linolenic Acid | EPA | DHA |
|---|---|---|---|---|
| Salad dressing, comm., mayonnaise, soybean | 37.1 | 4.2 | – | – |
| Salad dressing, comm., mayonnaise-type | 16.0 | 2.0 | – | – |
| Salad dressing, comm., Thousand Island, reg. | 17.3 | 2.5 | – | – |
| Salad dressing, home recipe, French | 31.8 | 1.9 | – | – |
| Salad dressing, home recipe, vinegar & soybean oil | 22.7 | 1.4 | – | – |
| Shortening, household, lard & veg. oil | 9.8 | 1.1 | – | – |
| Shortening, household, soybean (hydrog.) & cottonseed (hydrog.) | 24.5 | 1.6 | – | – |
| Shortening, special-purpose, for bread, soy (hydrog.) & cottonseed | 36.6 | 4.0 | – | – |
| Shortening, special-purpose, for cake mixes, soybean (hydrog.) | 13.0 | 1.1 | – | – |
| Shortening, special-purpose, heavy-duty, frying, soybean (hydrog.) | 31.1 | 2.4 | – | – |
| Soybean lecithin | 40.0 | 5.1 | – | – |
| Soybean oil | 51.1 | 6.8 | – | – |
| Soybean oil (hydrog.) & cottonseed oil | 34.8 | 2.8 | – | – |
| Spread, margarine-like, about 60% fat, soybean (hydrog.) & palm (hydrog.) | 16.5 | 1.6 | – | – |
| Spread, margarine-like, about 60% fat, soybean (hydrog.), palm (hydrog.) & palm | 18.8 | 1.6 | – | – |
| Tomato seed oil | 50.8 | 2.3 | – | – |

| Type of Food | Omega-6 | Alpha-Linolenic Acid | EPA | DHA |
|---|---|---|---|---|
| Walnut oil | 52.9 | 10.4 | – | – |
| Wheat germ oil | 54.8 | 6.9 | – | – |
| | | | | |
| **FRUITS** | | | | |
| Avocados, California, raw | 1.9 | 0.1 | – | – |
| Raspberries, raw | 0.2 | 0.1 | – | – |
| Strawberries, raw | 0.1 | 0.1 | – | – |
| | | | | |
| **LAMB AND VEAL** | | | | |
| Lamb, leg, raw (83% lean, 17% fat) | 0.7 | 0.3 | – | – |
| Lamb, loin, raw (72% lean, 28% fat) | 1.1 | 0.5 | – | – |
| Veal, leg round with rump, raw (87% lean, 13% fat) | 0.5 | 0.1 | | |
| | | | | |
| **LEGUMES** | | | | |
| Beans, common, dry | 0.3 | 0.6 | – | – |
| Black gram | – | 0.7 | – | – |
| Chickpeas, dry | 2.2 | 0.1 | – | – |
| Cowpeas, dry | 0.5 | 0.5 | – | – |
| Green gram | – | 0.2 | – | – |
| Lentils, dry | 0.4 | 0.16 | – | – |
| Lima beans, dry | 0.5 | 0.2 | – | – |
| Peas, garden, dry | 0.2 | 0.2 | – | – |
| Red gram | – | 0.1 | – | – |
| Soybeans, dry | 10.7 | 1.6 | – | – |
| | | | | |
| **NUTS AND SEEDS** | | | | |
| Beechnuts, dried | 18.4 | 1.7 | – | – |
| Butternuts, dried | 34.0 | 8.7 | – | – |
| Chia seeds, dried | 3.4 | 3.9 | – | – |
| Hickory nuts, dried | 20.9 | 1.0 | – | – |
| Soybean kernels, roasted & toasted | 11.2 | 1.5 | – | – |
| Walnuts, black | 34.2 | 3.3 | – | – |
| Walnuts, English/Persian | 32.3 | 6.8 | – | – |

| Type of Food | Omega-6 | Alpha-Linolenic Acid | EPA | DHA |
|---|---|---|---|---|
| **PORK** | | | | |
| Pork, cured, bacon, raw | 6.0 | 0.8 | – | – |
| Pork, cured, breakfast strips, raw | 4.7 | 0.9 | – | – |
| Pork, cured salt pork, raw | 8.7 | 0.7 | – | – |
| Pork, fresh, ham, raw | 2.0 | 0.2 | – | – |
| Pork, fresh, jowl, raw | 7.5 | 0.6 | – | – |
| Pork, fresh, leaf fat, raw | 6.4 | 0.9 | – | – |
| Pork, fresh, separable fat, raw | 7.5 | 0.7 | – | – |
| | | | | |
| **POULTRY** | | | | |
| Chicken, dark meat, w/o skin, raw* | 1.0 | Tr | 0.01 | 0.04 |
| Chicken, light meat, w/o skin, raw* | 0.4 | Tr | Tr. | 0.02 |
| Turkey, dark meat, w/o skin, raw | 1.06 | 0.04 | Tr | 0.03 |
| Turkey, light meat, w/o skin, raw | 0.27 | 0.01 | Tr. | 0.02 |
| | | | | |
| **VEGETABLES** | | | | |
| Beans, cluster, fresh | NA | 0.03 | – | – |
| Beans, French, fresh | NA | 0.03 | – | – |
| Beans, Navy, sprouted, cooked | 0.2 | 0.3 | – | – |
| Beans, pinto, sprouted, cooked | 0.2 | 0.3 | – | – |
| Broccoli, raw | 0.03 | 0.1 | – | – |
| Cauliflower, raw | – | 0.1 | – | – |
| Kale, raw | 0.1 | 0.2 | – | – |
| Lettuce, buttercrunch | – | 0.03 | – | – |
| Lettuce, butterhead, raw | – | 0.1 | – | – |
| Lettuce, red leaf | – | 0.03 | – | – |
| Mint | – | 0.01 | – | – |
| Mustard | – | 0.04 | – | – |
| Purslane | 0.09 | 0.4 | – | – |
| Seaweed, Spirulina, dried | 1.2 | 0.8 | – | – |

| Type of Food | Omega-6 | Alpha-Linolenic Acid | EPA | DHA |
|---|---|---|---|---|
| Soybeans, green, raw | 0.6 | 3.2 | – | – |
| Soybeans, mature seeds, sprouted, cooked | 0.4 | 2.1 | – | – |
| Spinach, raw | 0.1 | 0.9 | – | – |

*Contains trace amounts of 20:5, 22:5, and 22.6.

# Resource Section

## Recommended Products

*Barlean's Organic Oils*
Flaxseed oil can have a strong and, some would say, unpleasant taste. Barlean's Flax Oil tastes better than most. Look for it in the refrigerator case of your natural foods store. For more information, call (800) 445 FLAX (3529) or write to: Barlean's Organic Oils, 4936 Lake Terrell Road, Ferndale, Washington 98248. To receive a 1-ounce free sample, send a self-addressed stamped envelope ($.55 postage, business size #10 envelope).

*Bob's Red Mill*
Bob's Red Mill Natural Foods, Inc., mills, manufactures, and distributes a wide variety of whole-grain food products, including flaxmeal (flaxseed meal), flaxseeds, cereals, and bread, cake, and muffin mixes made from whole grains and without additives or preservatives. (Most of the mixes require you to add your own oil, making it easy to use canola oil or olive oil.) If you don't find Red Mill products where you shop, you can call or write for a free, 33-page mail-order catalogue. Phone: (503) 654-3215. Fax: (503) 653-1339. Monday through Friday from 8:30–4:30, West Coast time. Bob's Red Mill Natural Foods, Inc., 5209 S.E. International Way, Milwaukie, Oregon 97222.

*Born 3 Marketing Company*
A Canadian source for omega-3 fortified eggs. Born 3 Marketing Corporation, 141 Ross Road, Abbotsford, B.C. Canada V4X 2M6. (604) 856-1243. Fax: (604) 607-7333.

*The Country Hen*
Country Hen omega-3 fortified eggs are currently available in the northeastern section of the United States. The Country Hen, P.O.

Box 333, Hubbardston, MA 01452. (508) 928-5333. Fax: (508) 928-5414. The Country Hen eggs, introduced ten years ago, were the first omega-3 enriched eggs on the market. They are now sold throughout the northeast section of the United States. Each egg contains 170 mg. of omega-3 fatty acids. The hens are free walking and the feed is certified as organic.

### Denver Buffalo Company
Buffalo meat has more omega-3 fatty acids and less saturated fat than standard beef. You can order buffalo meat airmail by calling (800) BUY-BUFF (289–2833). (The meat is shipped frozen and packed in dry ice to preserve its quality.)

### King Oscar Sardines
For more information on the health benefit of sardines and for a free sardine cookbook, send a postcard with your address to King Oscar USA, 120 Montgomery Street #1960, San Francisco, CA 94104.

### The Missing Link® Master Nutrient Formula™
The Missing Link® Master Nutrient Formula™ is a dietary supplement produced in both powdered and food bar form. The formulas are rich in flaxseed, lignans, fiber, and naturally occuring phytochemicals. Only the finest whole food ingredients are used—no fillers, wheat, gluten, or synthetics are added. Each tablespoon of the powder (and each food bar) contains a full gram of omega-3 essential fatty acids. The powdered form can be taken with juice or sprinkled on salads or cereals. The product is produced using proprietary cold processing and packaging that ensures long-lasting freshness without preservatives. The company also offers a line of products for dogs, cats, horses, and birds. Available through retail outlets worldwide or directly by calling (800) 774-7387. Visit the website at www.designinghealth.com. Manufactured by Designing Health, 28310 Avenue Crocker, Unit G, Valencia, CA 91311.

### Natural Ovens
Wisconsin baker and food researcher Paul Stitt has been specializing in making bread and muffins fortified with flax for ten years. His company also sells its own brand of fortified flaxmeal. Place your

mail order by calling (800) 772-0730 or writing to Natural Ovens, 4300 County Trunk CR, P.O. Box 730, Manitowoc, WI 54221-0730, e-mail: flax@lakefield.net.

## Omega Nutrition USA Inc.
The original company to produce organic flax oil. Beside the good tasting original flax oil, they produce a special blend, Essential Balance (1:1 ratio of omega-3/omega-6) with or without butterscotch flavor for children. For a free sample of flax or organic olive oil or flax powder call (800) 661-FLAX or write to Omega Nutrition, 6515 Aldrich Road., Bellingham, WA 98226, or email omega@istar.ca.

## OmegaTech, Inc. (Gold Circle Farms)
OmegaTech, Inc. is a leader in producing the highest quality DHA-rich foods and food ingredients to help improve and maintain human health. DHA, an important omega-3 fatty acid, is vital for the health of our cardiovascular, nervous, and immune systems. OmegaTech's DHA comes from nature's original source—a marine microalgae. Unlike other sources, such as fish oil, this source is vegetarian, renewable, stable, and highly bioavailable. In the United States, OmegaTech markets Gold Circle Farms eggs. Just two Gold Circle Farms eggs provide 350 mg. of DHA and six times more vitamin E than ordinary eggs. OmegaTech looks forward to bringing you more DHA-enriched products such as chicken, pasta, mayonnaise, dairy products, baby foods, and much more to help you live a happy, healthy life. OmegaTech, 4904 Nautilus Court. N., Suite 208, Boulder, CO 80301. Call (888) 599-4DHA or (303) 527-3000 or find them on the web at www.omegadha.com or www.goldcirclefarms.com.

## Polarica
If your taste in meat runs to the exotic, Polarica is for you. Among other products, they offer free-range chickens and turkeys, partridge, pheasant, elk, moose, eland, buffalo, boar, rabbit, lamb, rattlesnake, turtle, alligator, ostrich, emu, kangaroo, escargot, goose, and duck. As a general rule, these types of meat have less overall fat, less saturated fat, and more omega-3 fatty acids than the products you find in stores. Polarica has West Coast and East Coast offices. On the West Coast, call (800) GAME USA. On the East Coast call (800) GAME 4US.

*Whole Foods*

This nationwide chain of natural food stores carries flaxbread and other wholesome products They are located in eighteen states plus Washington, D.C. To find the store closest to you, visit their website: www.wholefoods.com.

*Pilgrim's Pride EggsPlus*

Pilgrim's Pride, the fifth largest poultry company in the United States, has introduced omega-3-fortified eggs into the national market. Each egg contains 200 mg. of omega-3 fatty acids. Look for EggsPlus in the refrigerator case of your local store. For more product or distribution information, call Pilgrim's Pride in Texas at (800) 824-1159. Pilgrim's Pride, 2777 Stemmons Freeway, Suite 850, Dallas, TX 75207-2268.

*Zingerman's*

If you want to learn more about fine olive oil, send away for a free catalogue from Zingerman's, a delicatessen with a large mail-order business that has been called "a global culinary shrine." Among other catalogue offers are Zingerman's *Guide to Good Olive Oil* (a 64-page booklet, price $10), a wide array of premium (expensive) olive oils, or a high-priced olive oil taster, which is a collection of three or five different olive oils. Call (313) 769-1625 from 9–5 EST. Send e-mail to zing@chamber.ann-arbor.mi.us or write to Zingerman's, 422 Detroit Street., Ann Arbor, MI 48104.

# On the Web

*http://www.teleport.com/~jor*   This is our own website. We will be posting new research findings and information about **The Omega Diet** on a regular basis.

   *http://www.nlm.nih.gov*   Recently, the federal government has granted free public access to Medline, the most comprehensive compendium of medical journal articles. If you want to read original research articles on any medical topic, this is the place to go.

   *http://www.healthfinder.gov/*   The U.S. government provides this free service to guide the general public to reliable health information. You will be directed to selected websites, self-help groups, and government agencies.

*http://www.olen.com/food/* This website gives you a nutritional analysis of food from popular fast-food restaurants. You can search by restaurant chain, type of food, or even look for food that stays within a specific calorie or fat gram limit. Unfortunately, it offers no insight into the fatty acid content.

*http://www.flax.com* If you want to know more about flax, visit this home page for the Essential Nutrient Research Company, or ENRECO. You'll find information about the history and nutritional benefits of flax plus hundreds of scientific abstracts on omega-3 fatty acids.

## Miscellaneous

Purslane seeds can be hard to find. You can order a package of seeds, plus a delightful, 75-page book full of purslane lore and recipes from: Columbia Media, 2401 N. Cedar, Tacoma, WA, 98406. The cost is $13.00 (includes shipping and handling).

You can also order purslane seeds from Seeds of Change, P.O. Box 15700, Santa Fe, NM 87506-5700 or from Territorial Seed Company, P.O. Box 157, Cottage Grove, OR 97424.

For information about euterically coated fish oil pills, write to Allergy Research/Nutricology, P.O. Box 489, San Leandro, CA 94577, or call 800-545-9960.

## Newsletters

*The ISSFAL Newsletter* is the quarterly scientific report on fatty acid research issued by the International Society for the Study of Fatty Acids and Lipids. The cost is $50 a year ($15 for students and predoctoral fellows) and is payable in British pounds by check or by Visa or Mastercard. For more information, contact Dr. Ray Rice, Secretary/Treasurer, ISSFAL, P.O. Box 24, Tiverton, Devon EX16 4QQ, United Kingdom. Fax: 44-1884-242757. Email: rayrice@eclipse.co.uk.

*The Felix Letter*, 1329 Talbot Avenue, Berkeley, CA 94702. (510) 526-6268.

*The Nutrition Reporter*, published ten times a year, summarizes recent medical journal articles on vitamins, minerals, and other micronutrients. The emphasis is on the therapeutic use of these substances. Free sample copy available by sending a self-addressed, stamped envelope to The Nutrition Reporter, P.O. Box 5505, Aloha, OR 97006-5505. Subscription rate (no charge cards) US, $25 a year, Canada, $43 CND or $32 US. All other countries, $38 US payable through a U.S. bank. (503) 642-1372.

*OmegaTech Research Communique*, published quarterly, features abstracts of the most recent studies and literature reports on the subjects of omega-3 fatty acids in general and DHA in particular. For information contact OmegaTech, 4909 Nautilus Court. N., Suite 208, Boulder, CO 80301. Fax: (303) 381-8181. Website: www.omegadha.com.

# Recommended Reading

*The Healing Diet: How to Reduce Your Risks and Live a Longer and Healthier Life If You Have a Family History of Cancer, Heart Disease, Diabetes, Alcoholism, Obesity, or Food Allergies.* Simopoulos, Artemis P., M.D., Victor Herbert, M.D., J.D., and Beverly Jacobson. Macmillan, 1995. This book helps you tailor your diet to help compensate for a family history of a number of common diseases. A good companion to *The Omega Diet*.

*Leafy Greens,* Bittman, Mark. Macmillan, 1995. If you want to expand your familiarity with omega-3 and antioxidant-packed greens, this book will get you started.

*The Mediterranean Diet Cookbook,* Jenkins, Nancy. Bantam, 1994. A highly regarded cookbook featuring healthy Mediterranean cooking.

*Mediterranean Grains and Greens: A Book of Savory, Sun-Drenched Recipes*, Wolfert, Paula. HarperCollins, 1998.

*The Paleolithic Prescription: A Program of Diet & Exercise and a Design for Living*, Eaton, S. Boyd, Shostak, Marjorie, and Konner, Melvin. Harper & Row, 1988.

*The Woman's Guide to Good Health,* Gray, Mary Jane, Haseltine, Florence, Love, Susan, Mayzel, Kathleen, Simopoulos, Artemis P. Consumer Reports Books, 1991.

## Suggested Reading for Medical Professionals

Simopoulos, A. P., R. E. Kifer, and R. R. Martin, eds. *Health Effects of Polyunsaturated Fatty Acids in Seafoods, Proceedings from the Conference,* June 1985. Academic Press, Orlando, FL 1986.

Simopoulos, A. P., and V. Herbert, consultants. *The Eat Well, Be Well Cookbook.* Simon & Schuster, New York, 1986.

Simopoulos, A. P. "Terrestrial sources of omega-3 fatty acids: Purslane." In: *Horticulture and Human Health, Contributions of*

*Fruits and Vegetables.* Quebedeaux, B., and F. Bliss, eds. Prentice-Hall, Englewood Cliffs, NJ, 1988, pp. 93–107.

Simopoulos, A. P. "Opening address: Nutrition and fitness from the first Olympiad in 776 BC to 393 AD and the concept of positive health." *Am J Clin Nutr,* 1989; 49 (suppl):921-926.

Galli, C., and A. P. Simopoulos, eds. *Dietary w-3 and w-6 Fatty Acids: Biological Effects and Nutritional Essentiality.* Plenum Publishing Corporation, New York, 1989.

Simopoulos, A. P., and B. Childs, eds. "Genetic Variation and Nutrition: Volume 63." *World Review of Nutrition and Dietetics.* Proceedings of the International Conference on Genetic Variation and Nutrition, June 22–23, 1989, Washington, D.C. Karger Publishing Press, Basel, Switzerland, 1990.

Simopoulos, A. P., R. R. Kifer, R. E. Martin, and S. N. Barlow, eds. "Health Effects of w-3 Polyunsaturated Fatty Acids in Seafoods," *World Rev Nutr Diet.* Basel, Karger, 1991, vol. 66.

Simopoulos, A. P. "Omega-3 fatty acids in health and disease and in growth and development." *Am J Clin Nutr,* 1991; 54:438–463.

Simopoulos, A. P., and N. Salem, Jr. "Egg yolk as a source of long-chain polyunsaturated fatty acids in infant feeding." *Am J Clin Nutr,* 1992; 55:411–414.

Simopoulos, A. P., and C. Galli, eds. "Osteoporosis: Nutritional Aspects." *World Rev Nutr Diet.* Basel, Karger, vol. 73, 1993.

Galli, C., A. P. Simopoulos, and E. Tremoli, eds. "Fatty Acids and Lipids: Biological Aspects." *World Rev Nutr Diet.* Basel, Karger, vol. 75, 1994.

Galli, C., A. P. Simopoulos, and E. Tremoli, eds. "Effects of Fatty Acids and Lipids in Health and Disease." *World Rev Nutr Diet.* Basel, Karger, vol. 76, 1994.

Simopoulos, A. P. "Evolutionary Aspects of Diet: Fatty Acids, Insulin Resistance and Obesity." In: Vanltallie T. B., and A. P. Simopoulos, sr. eds. *Obesity: New Directions in Assessment and Management.* Charles Press, Philadelphia, 1995, pp. 241-261.

Simopoulos, A. P., ed. "Behavioral and Metabolic Aspects of Breastfeeding: International Trends." *World Rev Nutr Diet.* Basel, Karger, vol. 78, 1995.

Salem, N., Jr., A. P. Simopoulos, C. Galli, M. Lagarde, and H. Knapp, eds. "Proceedings of the 2nd Congress of ISSFAL on

Fatty Acids and Lipids from Cell Biology to Human Disease."
  *Lipids*, 1996; 31 (suppl.): S1–S326.

Simopoulos, A. P., ed. "Metabolic Consequences of Changing
  Dietary Patterns." *World Rev Nutr Diet*, vol. 79, 1996.

Simopoulos, A.P. "Trans Fatty Acids." In: Spiller, G. A. *Handbook of
  Lipids in Human Nutrition*. CRC Press, Boca Raton, Florida,
  1996.

Simopoulos, A. P., ed. Volume I. "Nutrition and Fitness: Evolutionary Aspects. Children's Health, Programs and Policies." Proceedings of the Third International Conference on Nutrition and
  Fitness. *World Rev Nutr Diet*, vol. 81, 1997.

Simopoulos, A. P., ed. Volume II. "Nutrition and Fitness: Metabolic
  and Behavioral Aspects in Health and Disease." Proceedings of
  the Third International Conference on Nutrition and Fitness.
  *World Rev Nutr Diet*, vol. 82, 1997.

Simopoulos, A. P. "W-3 fatty acids in the prevention-management of
  cardiovascular disease." *Can J Physio Pharmacol*,1997;
  75:234–239.

Simopoulos, A. P. "The Return of W-3 Fatty Acids Into the Food
  Supply. I. Land-Based Animal Food Products and Their Health
  and Effects." *World Rev Nutr Diet*. Basel, Karger, 1998, vol. 83.

Yehuda, S. and D. I. Mostofsky, eds. *Essential Fatty Acid Biology:
  Biochemistry, Physiology, and Behavioral Neurobiology*. Human
  Press, Totowa, New Jersey, 1997.

# Index

Adult-onset diabetes, 77. *See also* Diabetes

African Americans, and inflammatory disease, 101–102

Aggression, 95–96

Agriculture Department, 120

Alcoholism, 93

Allergies, 99

Alpha-linolenic acid (LNA), 28, 40, 127, 349
  adding to your diet, 129–131
  blood pressure reduction and, 51
  brain functioning and, 87
  cancer and, 68
  in common fats and oils, 41
  dietary sources of, 129–130, 138
  insulin resistance and, 83
  in recipe nutritional breakdown, 236

Alzheimer's disease, 6, 90, 99, 106–107

American Heart Association (AHA) diet, 8–9

Animal fat, 38. *See also* Fat, dietary

Antioxidants, 28, 62–63, 113

Antipsychotic drugs, 97

Apples
  arugula, walnut, and apple salad, 151, 304
  lamb, pepper, and apple curry, 286, 319
  lemon apple tart, 294–295, 319
  southern apple cake, 296–297, 323

Apple torte
  recipe for, 289
  shopping list for, 304

Arachidonic acid (AA), 40, 42

Arrhythmia, in heart attacks, 57–59

Arthritis, 6

Arugula, 156

Arugula, walnut, and apple salad
  recipe for, 251
  shopping list for, 304

Aspirin, 53, 100

Asthma, 6, 99, 100, 105–106

Atherosclerosis, 99

Attention deficit disorder (ADD), 95

Attention-deficit hyperactivity disorder (ADHD), 6, 95

Autoimmune diseases, 103–104

Avocado oil, 38

Baked goods
  commercially prepared foods, 298–299
  convenience foods, 302

Baking, with flaxmeal and flaxseeds, 237–238

Banana bread
  recipe for, 244–245
  shopping list for, 305

Bang, H. O., 56

Beans. *See also specific beans*
  in the Seven Dietary Guidelines, 136–138

Bean soup
  recipe for, 260
  shopping list for, 305

Beef
  fatty acid content of, 41, 354
  shopping for, 140

Beef quesadillas
  recipe for, 264–265
  shopping list for, 307

369

bottom line on, 74
boost for therapies in, 69–72
clinical studies on, 66–67
commonly seen cancers, 61–62
fat consumption and, 63–64
fatty acids and, 64–66
fruits and vegetables and, 62–63
metastatic spread of, 67–68
omega-3 fatty acids and prevention
of, 65–66, 67
wasting syndrome in, 72–73
Canned fish, shopping for, 154–155
Canola/butter
recipe for, 238–240
shopping list for, 309
Canola granola
recipe for, 245–246
shopping list for, 309
Canola oil, 10, 38, 39, 42
blood pressure reduction and, 51
in canned fish, 154
compared with olive oil, 132
fatty acid content of, 41
margarine with, 143–144
mayonnaise with, 130, 148–149,
240–241
popularity of, 5
in the Seven Dietary Guidelines,
131–132
shopping for, 145
as a source of LNA (alpha-linolenic
acid), 130
spread with, 139, 238–240, 310
Canola oil mayonnaise, 130
recipe for, 240–241
shopping list for, 310
Carbohydrates
insulin resistance and, 78–79
metabolism and, 17–18
weight gain and consumption of, 18–19
Cardiovascular disease, 49. *See also*
Heart attack
cholesterol levels and, 55
Omega Diet and, 12–13, 59

Carrot cake
recipe for, 290
shopping list for, 310
Cereals and bread
in diet of early man, 26
recipes for, 242–250
Cereal grains, fatty acids in, 354
Cervical cancer, 62, 63. *See also* Cancer
Chard with nuts and raisins
recipe for, 268
shopping list for, 311
Chart, for weight, 348
Cheese, 139–140
Chemotherapy, 70–72
Chicken, Hoisin
recipe for, 282
shopping list for, 316
Chicken in hellfire
recipe for, 281
shopping list for, 311
Chicken, orange, and rice
recipe for, 283
shopping list for, 320
Chicken, Yogurt
recipe for, 284–285
shopping list for, 328
Chicken salad with vinaigrette
recipe for, 253
shopping list for, 312
Chickpeas (garbanzo beans), 136
Chicory, 156
Children
asthma in, 105–106
attention-deficit hyperactivity
disorder (ADHD) in, 95
breast-feeding and intelligence of, 88
essential fatty-acid levels in, 88–89
ways to get kids to eat vegetables,
134–35
Cholesterol
arterial inflammation and, 52
coronary artery disease and, 31, 55
heart attack and stroke and, 52, 53,
54, 56

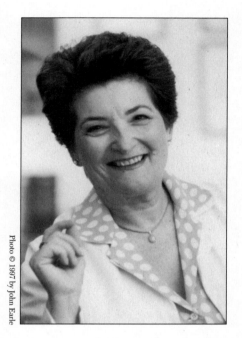

ARTEMIS P. SIMOPOULOS, M.D., is the president of the Center for Genetics, Nutrition, and Health in Washington, D.C. She chaired the Nutrition Coordinating Committee of the National Institutes of Health for nine consecutive years and served as a nutritional advisor to the Office of Consumer Affairs at the White House. She is also the author of *The Healing Diet* and the editor-in-chief of *World Review of Nutrition and Dietetics*.

Bestselling author JO ROBINSON has coauthored nine books in the fields of psychology and health. More than 1.5 million copies of her books have been sold.